Diabetes Cookbook For Dummies®

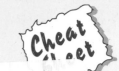

D1152338

Determining Your Body Mass Index Kilocalorie Intake

The following is a general rule for calculating your ideal weight:

- A man should weigh roughly 51 kilograms at a height of 1.5 metres and 3.5–4 kilograms more for every 5 centimetres he is taller than 1.5 metres.

- A woman should weigh 48 kilograms at a height of 1.5 metres and 3–3.5kg more for every 5 centimetres she is taller than 1.5 metres.

Body mass index is a formula to determine a person's body weight relative to height. This number is a good indicator of the amount of fat in your body. To obtain your body mass index (BMI):

1. **Work out your height in metres and multiply the figure by itself.**
2. **Measure your weight in kilograms.**
3. **Divide the weight by the height squared (the answer to step 1).**

For example, you might be 1.6 metres tall and weigh 65 kilograms. The height calculation would then be:

$1.6 \times 1.6 = 2.56$.

Your BMI would be 65 divided by 2.56 = 25.39.

A body mass index under 20 is slim, 20 to 25 is normal, 25 to 30 is overweight, and greater than 30 is obese.

To work out your daily kilocalorie needs:

1. **Multiply your ideal weight in kilograms by 22.**
2. **If you get no exercise, multiply the result of Step 1 by 10 per cent or 0.1. If you exercise moderately, multiply the result of Step 1 by 20 per cent or 0.2. If you get heavy exercise, multiply this number by 40 per cent or 0.4.**
3. **Add the result of Step 2 to the result of Step 1.**

   This number is the amount of kilocalories you need to consume every day in order to maintain your ideal weight.

Food Standards Agency Definitions for Fat Content

- Fat-free is less than 0.15 grams of fat per 100 gram serving.

- Low-fat is less than 3 grams of fat per 100 gram serving.

For Dummies: Bestselling Book Series for Beginners

Diabetes Cookbook For Dummies®

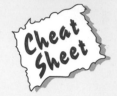

Cheat Sheet

Cooking Terms That Indicate Low or High Fat Content in a Food

If you're overweight, you must be able to evaluate recipes for their fat content.

These terms indicate a low fat content:

- Baked
- Grilled
- Cooked in its own juice
- Poached

These terms indicate a high fat content:

- Buttered or in butter sauce
- Creamed or in cream sauce
- Deep fried
- Fried
- In cheese sauce
- In plum sauce
- Sautéed
- Sweet and sour

Ten (Or So) Simple Steps to Improve Your Eating Habits

Here are ten (or so) steps that aren't very difficult to do but that can make a difference in your health. See Chapter 19 for more information.

- Keep a food diary.
- Work out why you eat the way that you do.
- Avoid missing a meal; eat at regular times.
- Sit down for meals.
- Use water in place of sugary drinks.
- Include vegetables in all meals.
- Cook with half the fat you usually use.
- Remove all visible fat.
- Don't add salt.
- Flavour food with condiments, herbs, and spices.
- Try to cook in three low-fat ways: Braise, grill, or boil.

Eyeballing Portion Size

To determine the size of a portion, compare it to something you see regularly. For example:

- 100g of meat is the size of a deck of cards.
- A medium fruit is the size of a tennis ball.
- A medium potato is the size of a computer mouse.
- 30g of cheese is the size of a domino.
- A portion of fruit is the size of a cricket ball.
- A portion of broccoli is the size of a light bulb.

For Dummies: Bestselling Book Series for Beginners

Diabetes Cookbook

FOR

DUMMIES®

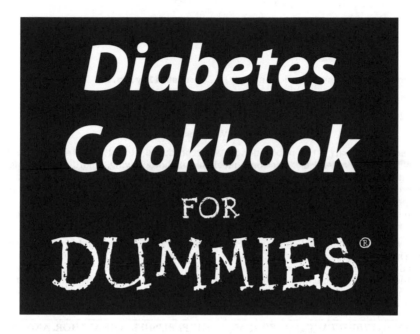

Diabetes Cookbook FOR DUMMIES®

by Dr Alan L Rubin and Dr Sarah Brewer, GP,
with Alison G Acerra and Denise Scharf

John Wiley & Sons, Ltd

Diabetes Cookbook For Dummies®

Published by
John Wiley & Sons, Ltd
The Atrium
Southern Gate
Chichester
West Sussex
PO19 8SQ
England

E-mail (for orders and customer service enquires): `cs-boo`

Visit our Home Page on `www.wiley.com`

For general information on our other products and services, please contact our Customer Care Department within the U.S. at 800-762-2974, outside the U.S. at 317-572-3993, or fax 317-572-4002.

For technical support, please visit `www.wiley.com/techsupport`.

Wiley also publishes its books in a variety of electronic formats. Some content that appears in print may not be available in electronic books.

British Library Cataloguing in Publication Data: A catalogue record for this book is available from the British Library

ISBN: 978-0-470-51219-7

Printed and bound in Great Britain by Bell & Bain Ltd., Glasgow

10 9 8 7 6 5 4 3 2 1

WILEY

About the Authors

Dr Alan L Rubin is one of America's foremost experts on diabetes. He is a professional member of the American Diabetes Association and the Endocrine Society and has been in private practice specialising in diabetes and thyroid disease for over 25 years. Dr. Rubin was assistant clinical professor of medicine at the University of California Medical Center in San Francisco for 20 years. He has spoken about diabetes to professional medical audiences and nonmedical audiences around the world. He has been a consultant to many pharmaceutical companies and companies that make diabetes products.

Dr Sarah Brewer, GP, qualified as a doctor in 1983 from Cambridge University. She was a full-time GP for five years and now works in nutritional medicine and sexual health. Sarah is currently completing an MSc in Nutritional Medicine at the University of Surrey, Guildford.

Although her first love is medicine, her major passion is writing. Sarah writes widely on all aspects of health and has written over 40 popular self-help books. She is a regular contributor to a number of newspapers and women's magazines, and appears regularly on TV and radio. She was voted Health Journalist of the Year 2002.

Alison G Acerra is a registered dietitian/nutrition consultant. She received her undergraduate degree in applied nutrition at Pennsylvania State University and continued her graduate studies at New York University, where she earned her Master of Science degree in clinical nutrition. Alison is currently working as an outpatient dietitian in San Francisco, where she conducts individual and group nutrition counseling sessions. She also consults privately with clients, specialising in weight management, diabetes prevention and management, cardiovascular health, sports nutrition, and gastric bypass surgery. A lover of good food and wine, Alison cooks often but enjoys dining out more! She stays active exploring San Francisco and is currently considering the location of her second marathon.

Denise Sharf, who created many of the breakfast, lunch, and appetizer recipes in this book, has received accreditation by the American Culinary Federation as a Certified Chef de Cuisine. She is a retired personal chef and has held positions as an executive chef and *chef de garde manger* for several major hotel chains and restaurants. Chef Sharf has achieved recognition as a culinary competitor, judge, and presenter of seminars.

Authors' Acknowledgements

Acquisitions editors Mikal Belicove – who shepherded the original edition through all the committees that had to approve it – and Samantha Clapp of the UK *For Dummies* team, deserve special commendation. Our project editors, Traci Cumbay,Georgette Beatty, and Simon Bell along with copy editors Tina Sims and Andy Finch, made certain that the book is understandable and readable in the great *For Dummies* tradition.

Denise Sharf produced most of the recipes for breakfast, lunch, and appetisers. Her help has been invaluable, and she has set an example for really nutritious food.

Heather Dismore is responsible for most of the discussions of food and the organisation of the recipes in the book, and she also contributed a number of excellent recipes.

Recipe tester Emily Nolan has not only checked every recipe to verify that it can be successfully prepared and tastes very good but has also offered numerous suggestions for replacing or reducing ingredients so that the finished product is a perfect fit for a person with diabetes.

Reviewers Dawn M. Ayers, MD, and Patty Santelli did a fantastic job of ensuring that the information in the book is accurate.

Dr Rubin's wife, Enid, has shown great patience, perseverance, and love in providing the time and the environment in which he could write this book.

Publisher's Acknowledgements

We're proud of this book; please send us your comments through our Dummies online registration form located at www.dummies.com/register/.

Some of the people who helped bring this book to market include the following:

Acquisitions, Editorial, and Media Development

Commissioning Editor: Samantha Clapp

Project Editor: Simon Bell

Content Editor: Steve Edwards

Copy Editor: Andy Finch

Technical Reviewers: Marc Owen, Emily Nolan

Executive Editor: Jason Dunne

Executive Project Editor: Martin Tribe

Cover Photo: GettyImages/Jan Mammey

Cartoons: Ed McLachlan

Composition Services

Project Coordinators: Kristie Rees, Erin Smith

Layout and Graphics: Carl Byers, Stephanie D. Jumper, Barbara Moore

Proofreader: Dwight Ramsey

Indexer: Claudia Bourbeau

Brand Reviewer: Jennifer Bingham

Publishing and Editorial for Consumer Dummies

Diane Graves Steele, Vice President and Publisher, Consumer Dummies

Joyce Pepple, Acquisitions Director, Consumer Dummies

Kristin A. Cocks, Product Development Director, Consumer Dummies

Michael Spring, Vice President and Publisher, Travel

Kelly Regan, Editorial Director, Travel

Publishing for Technology Dummies

Andy Cummings, Vice President and Publisher, Dummies Technology/General User

Composition Services

Gerry Fahey, Vice President of Production Services

Debbie Stailey, Director of Composition Services

Contents at a Glance

Recipes at a Glance

Table of Contents

Introduction

*P*eople with diabetes *can* eat great food! We don't have to prove that statement any more. The recipes in *Diabetes For Dummies*, by Alan L. Rubin and Sarah Jarvis (published by Wiley), and in this book show that people with diabetes can follow a delicious and healthy diet at home or anywhere they travel – and still enjoy a five-star meal. You just have to know how to cook it or where to go to get it.

More and more eating is taking place away from home or, if at home, from food in the form of a takeaway from a local supermarket or restaurant, and people with diabetes want to know what they can and can't eat. This book is both a cookbook that shows you how to prepare great foods in your own home, and a guide to eating out in restaurants, on picnics, and when preparing a packed lunch.

Is diet important for a person with diabetes? Do salmon swim upstream? Various clinical trials show that a good diet can improve long-term glucose control enough to lower the level of haemoglobin A1c (a test of overall blood glucose control) by over 1 per cent. That much improvement reduces your risk of developing the complications of diabetes such as eye disease, nerve disease, and kidney disease by 25 per cent or more. The progression of complications that have already started to occur is also significantly slowed.

Of course, there's much more to managing diabetes than diet alone. In this book, you can discover the place of diet in a complete programme of diabetes care.

About This Book

You wouldn't read a cookbook from cover to cover, and this book is no exception to that rule. There's no reason to read about setting up your kitchen if you simply want advice about selecting healthy food when eating out. You may want to read the first few chapters to get an overview of the place of diet in your overall diabetes management, but if you just need a great dish for tonight's supper, or a great soup for lunch, go right to that chapter. The book is designed so you can dip in and out for the information you need, at will.

Conventions Used in This Book

The recipes in this book are produced in a standard form that tells you what you're cooking, how much you're cooking, and how to cook it. The preparation time, cooking time (which is in addition to the prep time), and the number of people the recipe serves are all presented at the beginning of the recipe, followed by a list of ingredients. We suggest that you always read through a recipe completely before you start preparing it so that you can make sure that you have all the ingredients and equipment you need.

Chefs sometimes use exotic ingredients that are not easily available to you. These recipes mostly contain common ingredients. On the other hand, walking into a shop that sells special ingredients for a Chinese meal or an Indian meal, for example, is a fascinating experience. We always define ingredients that are unfamiliar to English-speaking eaters in the introduction to the recipe.

You can find nutrition information and diabetic exchanges at the end of most recipes so you can incorporate the recipe into your nutrition plan. The nutrition information is always given in the following order:

- Kilocalories (see Chapter 1)
- Grams of fat
- Grams of saturated fat
- Milligrams of cholesterol
- Milligrams of sodium
- Grams of carbohydrate
- Grams of fibre
- Grams of protein

Wherever possible, salt is not listed as an ingredient, as it's wise to retrain your taste buds to do without it. Very soon, prepared food that is pre-salted during cooking will start to taste too salty for you, as a result. The sodium that's listed in a recipe that does not contain salt comes from the natural ingredients used such as the vegetables. Serving sizes are always calculated as the total recipe divided by the number of servings listed at the beginning of the recipe.

You can find more information about the exchange lists in Chapter 2 and a comprehensive list of food exchanges in Appendix B.

Here are a few other guidelines to keep in mind about the recipes:

- ✔ All butter is unsalted. Margarine is not a suitable substitute for butter, because of the difference in flavour and nutritional value. Butter is a natural product, whereas margarine is man-made and may contain trans fatty acids.
- ✔ All eggs are large.
- ✔ All flour is plain unless otherwise specified.
- ✔ All milk is semi-skimmed unless otherwise specified.
- ✔ All onions are white unless specified as red.
- ✔ All pepper is freshly ground black pepper unless otherwise specified.
- ✔ All salt is table salt unless otherwise specified.
- ✔ All mentions of Splenda refer to the sugar substitute, sucralose.
- ✔ All dry ingredient measurements are level – use a dry teaspoon or tablespoon, fill it to a heap, then scrape it even with a straight object, such as the flat side of a knife.
- ✔ All temperatures are given in Celsius and Fahrenheit, and recipes also give the standard Gas Mark. (See Appendix D for information about converting temperatures.)
- ℧ If you need or want vegetarian recipes, scan the list of 'Recipes in This Chapter' on the first page of each chapter in Part II. A little tomato, rather than a triangle, in front of the name of a recipe marks that recipe as vegetarian. (See the tomato to the left of this paragraph.)

This isn't a complete book about diagnosing and treating diabetes and its complications. Check out *Diabetes For Dummies* if you need diagnosis and treatment information.

What You're Not to Read

All *For Dummies* books have shaded areas called *sidebars*. They contain interesting but non-essential information. If you aren't interested in the nitty-gritty, you can skip these sidebars. We promise not to include that information on the test.

Foolish Assumptions

The book assumes that you've done some cooking, you're familiar with the right knife to use to slice an onion without cutting your finger, and you can tell one pan from another. Beyond that, you can find many cooking terms in Appendix C at the end of the book.

How This Book Is Organised

The book is divided into five parts to help you incorporate the benefits of a good diet into your diabetes management programme, while showing you that the food can taste great.

Part 1: Thriving with Diabetes

This part takes you on the road to long life and great health as you incorporate the needs of having diabetes into the rest of your life. It begins by showing you all aspects of a healthy lifestyle and continues with the focus on food and its importance to you. When you cook for a person with diabetes (either yourself or a loved one), you need to keep some special considerations in mind, but this part shows you that a diet for diabetes is an excellent diet for anyone. In fact, there is really no such thing as a 'diabetic diet'. We guide you around the kitchen and take you to the supermarket to find out about meal-enhancing ingredients, as well as the ones to bypass as you navigate the aisles.

Part 11: Healthy Recipes That Taste Great

This part presents recipes from A to Z – that's apples to zebra steaks (not really, though they're probably quite tasty and lean) plus everything in between. The chapters take you through your eating day, starting with breakfast, providing snacks for mid-morning and mid-afternoon, and offering larger meals at lunch and dinner. They end, naturally, with wonderful desserts, which show that you're not doomed to give up what you may consider the best part of the meal. You just need to take care about calories and fat content.

Part III: Eating Away from Home

Part III tells you how to eat well and stay healthy wherever you are. You can always visit a fast-food franchise, but a lot of that food isn't good for you. If you pick and choose well, however, you'll select a healthy meal, plan a picnic, or prepare a packed lunch for work or school.

Part IV: The Part of Tens

We love to help you solve your problems in groups of ten. If you have 13 problems, you'll just have to wait for the next book to solve the last 3 (or check out the Internet). In this part, we provide ten (or so) steps to improve your eating habits and ten food substitutions you can easily make within a recipe. You can explore ten strategies to normalise your blood glucose and ten ways to promote healthy eating in children.

Part V: Appendixes

Appendix A has info about food supplements – the vitamins, minerals, and essential fatty acids that can boost the nutritional value of your diet. Appendix B contains exchange lists for the person with diabetes. In Appendix C, you find a glossary of key cooking terms. Appendix D offers guidelines if you want to substitute other sweeteners for sugar, as well as cooking equivalents, such as how many tablespoons of sucralose are equivalent to 100 grams of sugar. In Appendix E, you find other resources in books and on the Web for recipes and nutritional information for people with diabetes.

Icons Used in This Book

The icons in this book are like bookmarks, pointing out information that we think is especially important. You may want to pick out one particular icon that appeals to you. For example, if you like hints, pick out the Tip icons for shortcuts and useful information. If your interests lie in the direction of very mild fear, look for the Warning icon. Here are the icons used in this book:

Whenever we want to emphasise the importance of the current information to your nutritional plan, we use this icon.

When you see the Remember icon, pay special attention because the information is essential.

This helpful icon marks important information that can save you time and energy.

Watch for this icon; it warns about potential problems (for example, the possible results if you don't treat a condition).

Where to Go from Here

Where you go from here depends on your immediate needs. If you want an introduction to the place of nutrition in diabetes management, start with Chapter 1. If you are hungry and want some lunch, go to Chapter 8 or 9. If you are about to travel or eat out, head for Part III. At any time, the Part of Tens can provide useful tips for healthy eating. Finally, the Appendixes help you cook for yourself or choose a food supplement. Feel free to jump around, but take the time to go through Part II so that you realise that diabetes and great food are not mutually exclusive.

Part I
Thriving with Diabetes

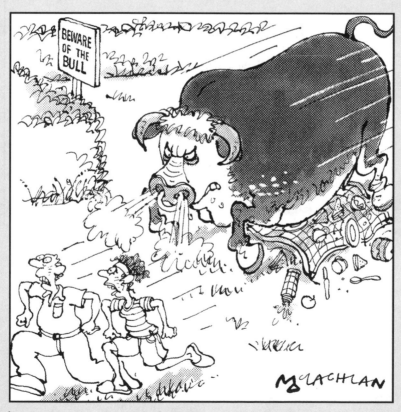

'You and your healthy picnic in the countryside with plenty of exercise.'

In this part . . .

Diabetes is a disease with which you can live. In this part, we show you not only how to live with diabetes but also how to thrive with diabetes. Diabetes requires that you think about every aspect of your lifestyle, and we cover all the issues. But the part starts with the way you eat, because diet is central to a healthy lifestyle. We show you what to eat, how much to eat, and, especially, how to prepare your food so that the fact that you have diabetes doesn't prevent you from enjoying a variety of delicious cuisine.

Chapter 1

Living to Eat with Diabetes

Many people with diabetes are surprised to find that, after receiving their diagnosis, they start to feel better than ever. You are likely to notice the same after you start eating a healthy diet; losing excess weight and becoming more active helps to improve your physical and mental wellbeing.

This chapter gives you the latest information about what diabetes means, how doctors diagnose it, and all the other things you need to know in order to thrive following a diagnosis of diabetes. Don't waste another minute. Get stuck in right away so that you can feel as healthy as possible, as soon as possible.

Recognising Diabetes

With so much diabetes around these days, you may think that recognising it is easy. The truth is, however, that spotting diabetes is actually quite difficult, because its diagnosis depends on blood tests. You can't just look at someone and know the level of glucose in his or her blood. In addition, symptoms are often quite general, and so the diagnosis of diabetes doesn't just jump out and grab you (or your doctor).

Glucose is the name of the type of sugar found in your body that provides most of the energy that your cells and organs need to carry on all the chemical reactions that let you live, think, breathe, and move around.

Diabetes by the numbers

The level of glucose that means you have diabetes is as follows:

- A *random* blood glucose test result (one not taken first thing in the morning after fasting) that is greater than, or equal to, 11.1 millimoles per litre (mmol/l), along with symptoms such as fatigue, frequent urination and thirst, slow healing of skin, urinary infections, and vaginal itching in women. A normal random blood glucose level is between 4 and 8 mmol/l.

- A *fasting* blood glucose level (taken after consuming nothing but water for at least eight hours) that is greater than, or equal to, 7 mmol/l. A normal fasting blood glucose level is less than 5.6 mmol/l.

- A blood glucose level that is greater than, or equal to, 11.1 mmol/l two hours after consuming 75 grams of glucose during an *oral glucose tolerance test.*

Although an oral glucose tolerance test is the gold standard for diabetes, this test isn't always practical, and is expensive. Diabetes UK, the leading charity for people with diabetes, recommends using a fasting glucose level, which is more convenient. Taking a random blood glucose test isn't as sensitive for diagnosing diabetes.

The United Kingdom and most of the rest of the world uses the International System (SI) of units – millimole per litre (mmol/l) – to measure the concentration of something in a liquid, such as glucose in blood. For some reason, the United States is different and uses milligrams/decilitre (mg/dl) as the unit of measurement. You may come across mg/dl values on some Web sites or in American books. To convert mg/dl to mmol/l, simply divide the value of mg/dl by 18. For example, 126 mg/dl becomes 7 mmol/l.

Some people have blood glucose levels that are not (yet) high enough to diagnose diabetes, but aren't as low as normal. Such people have *impaired glucose tolerance,* or *pre-diabetes.* Pre-diabetes is diagnosed when a fasting blood glucose level is between 5.6 and 7 mmol/l and a blood level taken two hours after drinking a sugar solution in an oral glucose tolerance test is between 7.8 and 11 mmol/l. Without changing their diet and lifestyle, between 29 and 55 per cent of people with pre-diabetes develop type 2 diabetes over the course of three years, and most people with pre-diabetes go on to develop diabetes within ten years. Although people with pre-diabetes don't usually develop small blood vessel complications of diabetes like blindness, kidney failure, and nerve damage, they're more prone to large vessel disease like heart attacks and strokes. Therefore, you want to get that glucose level down. An estimated 388 million people are currently living with pre-diabetes worldwide, although most are unaware that they are affected.

Types of diabetes

Three main types of diabetes exist:

✔ **Type 1 diabetes:** Previously known as *juvenile diabetes* or *insulin-dependent diabetes,* this type mostly begins in childhood and results from the body's self-destruction of its own pancreas cells. The pancreas is an organ of the body that sits behind the stomach and makes *insulin,* the chemical or *hormone* that is needed to get glucose into cells for use as a fuel. You can't live without insulin, and so people with type 1 diabetes take insulin shots (injected or, most recently, inhaled). Of the known 2.2 million people in the United Kingdom with diabetes, about 10 per cent have type 1.

✔ **Type 2 diabetes:** Once called *adult-onset diabetes,* type 2 tends to come on around the age of 40, but is now occurring younger and younger – even in children – due to rising levels of obesity and lack of exercise. The problem in type 2 diabetes is not a total lack of insulin, as occurs in type 1, but a resistance to insulin, so that cells no longer respond to it properly; as a result, glucose isn't let into cells and builds up in the blood so levels rise.

✔ **Gestational diabetes:** This type of diabetes is like type 2 but occurs in women during pregnancy, when a lot of chemicals in the mother's blood oppose the action of insulin. About 4 per cent of all pregnant women develop gestational diabetes. If the mother isn't treated to lower her blood glucose, the glucose gets into the baby's bloodstream. The baby doesn't have diabetes, and so produces plenty of insulin. As a result, the baby begins to store the excess glucose as fat and becomes much larger than usual, so that delivery is often difficult. When born, the baby is cut off from the large sugar supply but is still making lots of insulin, and so the blood glucose can drop severely after birth. The mother is at risk of gestational diabetes in later pregnancies and is likely to develop type 2 diabetes as she gets older, especially if she puts on weight and doesn't exercise.

Consequences of diabetes

If your blood glucose isn't well controlled, it can damage your body cells temporarily or even permanently, depending on how high your blood glucose becomes, and for how long it stays that high. The damage is divided into three categories: irritations, short-term complications, and long-term complications.

Irritations

Irritations are mild and reversible, but still unpleasant, results of high blood glucose levels. The levels aren't so high that the person is in immediate life-threatening danger. The most important of these irritations are the following:

- Blurred vision
- Fatigue
- Frequent urination and thirst
- Genital itching, especially in females
- Gum and urinary tract infections
- Obesity
- Slow healing of the skin

Short-term complications

These complications are potentially very serious and can even lead to death if not treated. They're associated with very high levels of blood glucose – in the 20 mmol/l range and above. The three main short-term complications are:

- **Ketoacidosis:** This complication is found mostly in type 1 diabetes. Without insulin, glucose levels rise very high, and the body starts to use fat for energy. As fat breaks down, it produces chemicals called *ketones* that make the blood very acid. The acid condition makes the patient nauseated and unable to eat or drink. He or she becomes very dehydrated but continues to lose fluids due to excessive urination or vomiting. The increased urine takes important body constituents with it, such as potassium. The patient becomes very sick and dies if not treated with large volumes of fluids and large amounts of insulin. After the situation is reversed, however, the patient is fine.

- **Hyperosmolar syndrome:** This condition is often seen in neglected older people. Their blood glucose rises due to severe dehydration and the fact that the kidneys of older people often can't get rid of glucose as well as younger kidneys. The blood becomes like thick syrup. The person can die if large amounts of fluids aren't restored, but replenishing fluids is tricky in older people, who often have heart failure as well. When heart failure is present, the heart can't handle too much fluid at one time. The excess fluid can get into the lungs and also cause swelling of the legs. People with hyperosmolar syndrome don't need that much insulin to recover. After the condition is treated, the person returns to a normal state.

  ✔ **Hypoglycaemia or low blood glucose:** This complication happens when someone is on a drug like insulin, or a pill that drives down glucose levels, at a time when they aren't getting enough food or are getting too much exercise. If glucose levels fall much below 3 mmol/l, the patient starts to feel bad because not enough glucose reaches the brain. Typical symptoms include sweating, rapid heartbeat, hunger, nervousness, confusion, and even coma if the low glucose level is prolonged. The usual treatment is to take glucose by mouth or, if the person is unconscious, to inject a glucose solution directly into a vein. This complication usually causes no permanent damage.

Long-term complications

The long-term complications of diabetes have a substantial impact on quality of life and are divided into two groups: *microvascular,* which are due at least in part to small blood vessel damage, and *macrovascular,* associated with damage to large blood vessels.

These problems occur after ten or more years of poorly controlled diabetes or, in the case of macrovascular complications, after years of pre-diabetes or diabetes. After these complications are established, reversing them is hard, but treatment is available early in their course, and so your doctor screens you for them on a regular basis after your initial diagnosis of diabetes. See *Diabetes For Dummies,* 2nd Edition, by Dr Sarah Jarvis and Dr Alan Rubin (Wiley) for information on screening for these complications.

Microvascular complications include the following:

  ✔ **Diabetic retinopathy:** Eye damage that leads to blindness if untreated.

  ✔ **Diabetic nephropathy:** Kidney damage that can lead to kidney failure.

  ✔ **Diabetic neuropathy:** Nerve damage that results in many clinical symptoms, the most common of which are tingling and numbness in the feet. Lack of sensation in the feet can result in severe injury without awareness unless you carefully check your feet regularly. Such injury can result in infection and may even lead to amputation.

Macrovascular complications also occur in pre-diabetes and consist of the following:

  ✔ **Coronary heart disease:** Furring up of the arteries supplying the heart. Blockage of the coronary arteries can lead to a heart attack, which is the most common cause of death in people with diabetes.

  ✔ **Cerebrovascular disease:** Furring up and blockage of arteries supplying the brain, resulting in a stroke.

✔ **Peripheral vascular disease involving the blood vessels of the legs:** These vessels can become clogged and lack of blood can lead to ulceration and gangrene, which may eventually require amputation of the feet or legs.

If you control your blood glucose well, none of these complications need ever occur. Controlling your blood pressure and your cholesterol also helps prevent these complications.

Treating diabetes

Treatment of diabetes involves three essential elements:

✔ **Diet:** If you follow the recommendations in this book, you can significantly lower your average blood glucose level, and reduce your risk of developing diabetes-related complications.

✔ **Exercise:** Exercise lowers blood glucose levels, because it improves insulin resistance and allows more glucose into muscle cells for use as a fuel. This chapter and Chapter 3 touch on exercise, and *Diabetes For Dummies,* 2nd Edition (Wiley) discusses it more fully.

✔ **Medication:** Diabetes medications abound – far too many are available to discuss here, in a recipe book, but you can find out about them in *Diabetes For Dummies,* 2nd Edition (Wiley).

Controlling Kilocalories

Just as the three most important factors in the value of a house are location, location, location, the three most important factors in diet for people with diabetes are moderation, moderation, moderation. If you're overweight or obese, which is true of most people with type 2 diabetes and a lot of people with type 1 diabetes who are on intensive insulin treatment (four shots of insulin daily), weight loss makes a huge difference to your blood glucose levels. If you maintain the weight loss, you can avoid the complications of diabetes and may even find that your blood glucose levels return to normal.

Successful weight loss means controlling the amount of kilocalories you consume (see the 'Kilocalories versus calories' sidebar for an explanation of kilocalories), and increasing the amount of exercise you take. If you don't burn the same amount of kilocalories as you eat, you gain weight. Conversely, losing weight involves burning up more kilocalories than you eat. Sounds simple, eh!

Kilocalories versus calories

A kilocalorie is 1,000 times greater than a calorie. This book uses the term *kilocalories* (or *kcals*) because it's more accurate – experts in health and medicine always use kilocalories as the unit of measurement when working out the energy provided in a diet plan or in different foods. Unfortunately, however, the term *calories* is in common use on food labels and in diet books, and health officials don't want to confuse the public by attempting to correct this error.

Calorie counts in the text of this book and in the nutritional analyses of the recipes are given in kilocalories.

As you reduce your portions of food, also make sure that you reduce your intake of added sugars, fats, and alcohol. These items contain few nutrients such as vitamins and minerals and are simply sources of empty kilocalories.

If you are predisposed to develop diabetes because, for example, both your parents have diabetes, you can help to prevent it by maintaining a healthy weight. If you already have diabetes, you can minimise its impact by losing weight and keeping it off.

Do you need a highly complicated formula to figure out how to moderate your food intake? No! The process is as simple as looking at the portions you currently eat and cutting them in half. This approach is relatively easy in your own home, but in restaurants that serve super-sized portions, the rule of eating half isn't always strong enough. In these fast-food emporiums, the advice is often to eat only a third of their usual portions! You may also need to apply the same portion control when you eat at someone else's home. And NEVER go back for seconds! Figure 1-1 shows you the difference between reasonably sized portions and ones that are too big.

Figure 1-1: Eating in moderation means choosing the portion sizes on the left, rather than those on the right.

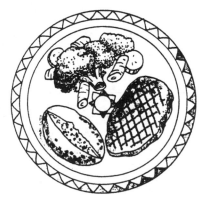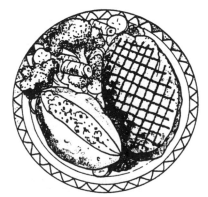

Controlling kilocalories isn't easy when TV commercials often imply that eating certain foods helps make you sexier and more beautiful. Another challenge is eating in a restaurant where the menu makes everything sound perfectly delectable. And when the portions arrive at your table, they're twice the size that you normally eat. Use these tips to help you visualise portion sizes:

- ✔ A serving of meat is around the size of a deck of cards.
- ✔ A medium fruit is the size of a tennis ball.
- ✔ A medium potato is the size of a computer mouse.
- ✔ A serving of cheese is the size of a domino.
- ✔ A serving of vegetables such as broccoli is the size of a light bulb.

An average woman needs around 2,000 kilocalories per day to maintain her weight, and an average man needs around 2,500 kilocalories per day. You don't need to take in many more kilocalories than you need, over time, to gain weight. Just 100 extra kilocalories on a daily basis results in a weight gain of 5.5 kilograms (12 pounds) in a year. An extra glass of wine is that many kilocalories. On the other hand, if you reduce your daily intake by 100 kilocalories, you can lose those 5.5 kilograms (12 pounds) over a year. Just cut out that glass of wine!

Look at a few examples of today's typical portion sizes and compare them to a serving offered 20 years ago. Table 1-1 shows the kilocalories in the portions of 20 years ago and today and how much exercise you need to burn up the extra kilocalories in order not to gain weight.

Table 1-1	Consequences of Today's Larger Portions		
Food	*Kilocalories 20 Years Ago*	*Kilocalories Today*	*Exercise to Burn Up the Difference*
Bagel	140	350	50 minutes raking leaves
Cheeseburger	333	590	90 minutes lifting weights
Chicken Caesar salad	390	790	80 minutes walking
Chips	210	610	80 minutes walking
Chocolate chip cookie	55	275	75 minutes washing the car
Coffee	45	350	60 minutes walking
Popcorn	270	630	75 minutes of water aerobics
Turkey sandwich	320	820	85 minutes cycling

Including Exercise (and Rest)

Exercise is just as important as diet in controlling your blood glucose. When people at risk of developing diabetes (because both their parents have diabetes) walk for just 30 minutes a day, 80 per cent of them don't develop the disease. These people don't necessarily lose weight, but they do exercise.

Exercise isn't only for someone with diabetes. Anyone who wants a healthy lifestyle needs to exercise, but for people with diabetes, exercise is especially important as it protects against both the microvascular and the macrovascular complications of diabetes.

And you don't have to spend hours exercising. About 30 minutes a day of moderate exercise, such as walking, gives you all that you need. If walking doesn't interest you, you can cycle, swim, jog, play a sport, or do just about anything that gets your heart pumping faster and your muscles moving.

Too many people complain that they just can't find time to exercise. This excuse isn't really acceptable, is it? Especially when you realise how much difference exercise makes in your life and to your diabetes control. Here are some ways that different amounts of exercise can help you:

- ✔ Thirty minutes of exercise a day gets you in excellent physical shape and reduces your blood glucose substantially.

- ✔ Sixty minutes of exercise a day helps you maintain a weight loss and gets you in even better physical shape; it can even help you to discontinue medications for diabetes, unless you have type 1 diabetes.

- ✔ Ninety minutes of exercise a day helps you lose weight.

If you say that you can't find 90 extra minutes in your day, that's probably not an unreasonable assessment of your schedule, but do consider the benefits before ruling out the possibility! How about walking the kids to school, or walking to the shops rather than taking the car?

An exercise partner helps ensure that you get out and do your thing. Having someone waiting for you so that you can exercise together is extremely helpful.

Here are some more facts about exercise to keep in mind:

- ✔ You don't have to get all your minutes of exercise in one session. Two 30-minute workouts are just as good as, and possibly better than, one 60-minute workout.

- ✔ Although walking is excellent exercise, especially for older people, the benefits of more vigorous exercise for a longer time are greater still.

Keeping up to speed on treatment developments

Every month, researchers are making important discoveries about diabetes and related medical areas that you may need to know about. For example, inhaled insulin is now available – although it doesn't suit everyone. How can you keep up to date with all the latest and greatest treatments?

✔ Attend any meetings designed for people with diabetes that are organised through your local hospital or diabetes self-help groups. You can discover how to manage your diabetes right now and find out about what's coming up.

✔ Do a Web search for diabetes. If you want to ensure that the sites you come up with are both accurate and helpful, go to Appendix B, which has a list of useful Web sites.

✔ When you visit your doctor, ask questions. If you don't get satisfactory answers, ask if you can see a specialist.

✔ After several years, attend another set of meetings or a course. You're sure to be amazed at the changes in the understanding and treatment of diabetes.

✔ Everything counts when it comes to exercise. Your decision to take the stairs instead of the lift may not seem like much, but if you do so day after day, it makes a profound difference. Another suggestion that helps over time is to park your car farther from your office or the shops.

✔ A pedometer (a small gadget worn on your belt that counts your steps) may help you achieve your exercise goals. The objective is to increase your step count every week and get up to 10,000 steps a day.

You also need to strengthen your muscles. Stronger (larger) muscles take in more glucose, providing another way of keeping your diabetes under control. A programme of light weight training is often all you need. You may want to book a personal trainer to show you a routine at the start, and then take over on your own (or keep up with weekly trainer sessions to maintain your motivation). You can buy hand-held weights inexpensively from most sport shops. You don't need to weight train every day, as is advisable for walking – three or four times a week is enough. You may be surprised at how much your stamina increases and how much your blood glucose falls when you keep this routine up.

Place a daily limit on activities that are completely sedentary, such as watching television or surfing the Web. Use the time you may have once spent on these activities to exercise. This advice is especially helpful for overweight children.

You want to keep active, but don't do it at the cost of getting plenty of rest each day. People who sleep eight hours a night tend to get less hungry and are leaner than people who sleep less. Strange but true!

Controlling Your Blood Pressure

Keeping your blood pressure in check is particularly important in preventing the macrovascular (large blood vessel) complications of diabetes. But elevated blood pressure also plays a role in bringing on eye disease, kidney disease, and neuropathy. Have your blood pressure checked every time you see your doctor. The goal is to keep your blood pressure under 130/80 mmHg – even lower if you have kidney problems. You may want to get your own blood pressure monitor so that you can check your blood pressure at home yourself.

The statistics about diabetes and high blood pressure are daunting. Over 70 per cent of people with diabetes have high blood pressure, but almost a third are unaware of it. And almost half of them aren't receiving proper treatment for high blood pressure. Among those treated, more than half still have a blood pressure greater than 130/80.

You can do plenty of things to lower your blood pressure, including losing weight, avoiding salt, eating more fruit and vegetables, and, of course, exercising. But if all else fails, your doctor prescribes medication. Many blood pressure medicines are available, and one or two are exactly right for you. See *High Blood Pressure For Dummies,* 2nd edition, by Alan L. Rubin (Wiley) for an extensive discussion of the large number of blood pressure medications at your doctor's fingertips.

One class of drugs in particular is very useful for people with diabetes who have high blood pressure: *angiotensin converting enzyme inhibitors* (ACE inhibitors), which protect your kidneys. If kidney damage is detected early, ACE inhibitors can reverse the damage. Some experts believe that all people with diabetes benefit from taking ACE inhibitors, but as long as no evidence exists of kidney damage and the diabetes is well controlled, most doctors prefer to keep these drugs in reserve.

Considering the Rest of Your Lifestyle

Diabetes is just one part of your life. It can affect the rest of your lifestyle, however, and your lifestyle certainly affects your diabetes. This section explores the other parts of your lifestyle that you can alter to benefit both your overall health and your diabetes.

Try making changes one at a time, and when you think that you have one aspect under control, move on to the next. If you try to tackle too much at once, you soon give up as we're all creatures of habit and changing more than one aspect of our behaviour at the same time isn't easy.

Drinking alcohol safely

A glass of wine is a pleasant addition to dinner, and studies show that alcohol in moderation can lower the risk of a heart attack (see the sidebar 'How alcohol helps prevent heart disease', later in this chapter). For someone with diabetes, however, ensuring that food accompanies the wine is especially important because alcohol reduces blood glucose levels; a complication called hypoglycaemia may occur if you drink too much alcohol and eat too little food (see the section 'Short-term complications', earlier in this chapter).

Never drink alcohol without food, especially when you're taking glucose-lowering medication.

The following people shouldn't drink alcohol at all:

- ✔ Children and adolescents
- ✔ People with medical conditions that are worsened by alcohol, such as liver disease and certain diseases of the pancreas
- ✔ People who take medications that interact with alcohol
- ✔ Pregnant women
- ✔ Women who are breastfeeding

Don't drink more than two 100-millilitre glasses (two small glasses) of medium-strength, dry wine daily if you're a man, or one 100-millilitre glass if you're a woman. Men metabolise alcohol more rapidly than women, which means that they're able to drink more. But don't drink more than a maximum of five days out of every seven overall, so you have two alcohol-free days per week. In terms of alcohol content, 100 millilitres of wine (a small glass) is equivalent to 300 millilitres (½ pint) of beer or 25 millilitres (a single measure) of spirits.

Alcohol adds kilocalories without providing any nutrition. Alcohol contains no vitamins or minerals, but you have to account for the kilocalories in your diet. If you stop drinking alcohol, you can lose a significant amount of weight. For example, a person who consumes three drinks a night and stops can lose nearly 12 kilograms (26 pounds) in a year.

How alcohol helps prevent heart disease

When taken in moderation, alcohol has a number of effects that help prevent heart disease and heart attacks. Alcohol can do the following:

✔ Decrease insulin resistance

✔ Increase the level of the good cholesterol, called HDL cholesterol

✔ Decrease the tendency of blood platelets to form clots that block arteries in the heart

✔ Increase the tendency of chemicals in the blood to break down clots that do form

Alcoholic drinks tend to contain sugar too. Avoid sweet drinks such as sherry or port, and select dry red or white wine instead.

Excess alcohol causes cirrhosis of the liver, raises blood pressure, and can cause abnormal heart rhythms that are linked with sudden death. Alcohol also worsens diabetic neuropathy. Do you need any more reasons not to drink too much alcohol?

Avoiding tobacco

Whether you smoke, chew, or inhale it because someone else is smoking, tobacco shortens your life and makes you a prime candidate for many types of cancer. The connection between cancer and tobacco is a scientific fact. Just why tobacco isn't a banned substance like heroin or crack cocaine is a mystery (although the tobacco companies know the solution to that one).

Everything about tobacco is negative. It stains your teeth and fingers, gives you bad breath, causes wrinkles, and ruins your heart, lungs, and many other organs. And people are dumb enough to pay for it! People with diabetes who smoke are much more prone to amputations of their feet and legs.

Numerous ways are available to stop if you already smoke. Unfortunately many smokers quit only after the first major event, such as a heart attack or a cancer they're lucky enough to survive. Don't find yourself in that group. Give it up, now! Your doctor and pharmacist can help.

Staying away from illicit drugs

Do you really want to screw up your life and make your diabetes almost impossible to control by adding illicit drugs to the mix? Some of them interact with your diabetes drugs, causing high or low blood glucose levels. If you use needles to inject these drugs, you may get infections, hepatitis, and even HIV sooner or later.

You can get high without illegal drugs. Try exercise instead. Climb those steps up to your office and enjoy the feeling that comes when you're no longer carrying an extra 9 kilograms (20 pounds) of weight on your stomach. These highs benefit your diabetes at the same time.

Driving safely

Having diabetes means that you need to take special precautions before you drive. You need to test your blood glucose before driving and raise it to normal before you get behind the wheel. Always carry a source of glucose in your car to take if your glucose falls. When it falls much below 4 mmol/l while driving, your concentration is affected just as if you are drunk.

Wear a seat belt when you drive. Doing so prevents major injury if you get into an accident. Of course, _you_ never drive faster than the speed limit, but you need to worry about the other driver. You never know what he or she is going to do.

Benefiting from relationships

People in loving relationships live longer than those who live alone. This fact is especially true for people with diabetes, many of whom depend to some extent on support from someone else. Perhaps your spouse or significant other buys or prepares the food that you eat. Or perhaps he or she is your invaluable exercise partner, cajoling you along. On the rare occasions when your blood glucose falls very low, he or she is also the one that calls for help and gets the glucose that restores you.

Belonging to a special-interest group is also helpful. For example, perhaps you're a keen biker, stamp collector, or bridge player. Getting together with others who share your interest is a great stress reducer, which can benefit your diabetes.

People with diabetes also benefit from joining a diabetes support group. Here you discover that you're not alone in your troubles. In addition, others often have helpful suggestions on managing their diabetes that you can use.

Maintaining your sense of humour

If you have diabetes, or any other chronic disease for that matter, keeping a sense of humour makes the inconveniences and associated complications much easier to bear. Some people, such as author Norman Cousins, even claim that you can reverse a disease that's considered irreversible if you expose yourself to all kinds of funny experiences. He listens to audiotapes of the comedians he finds the most funny and reads humour books that keep him laughing. He also watches movies that make him roar with laughter.

Life is a human comedy. Surely you can laugh about some things in your life, even associated with your diabetes. If Woody Allen or the Marx Brothers don't do it for you, maybe Monty Python, Jo Brand, Billy Connolly, or Graham Norton can get you going. Like beauty, humour is in the eyes of the beholder.

Find your favourites and get their performances in any media available. Watch or listen to them regularly. Rather than an apple, 'a laugh a day keeps the doctor away'.

Chapter 2

Eating to Live with Diabetes

. . . .

. . . .

*T*he problem of obesity in the United Kingdom and throughout the world is continuing to explode. The incidence of diabetes has also reached epidemic proportions in a parallel fashion. Currently, 46 per cent of men and 32 per cent of women are overweight and, on top of this, 17 per cent of men and 21 per cent of women are classified as obese. Frighteningly, the percentage of adults who are obese is now double the figure for the mid-1980s, with the result that over half of all adults in the UK are not in the healthy weight range for their height. And children and adolescents are part of this epidemic too, with 13 per cent of 8-year-olds and 17 per cent of 15-year-olds being in the obese range.

We need to reverse this trend. Otherwise, millions of people are in danger of going blind, developing kidney failure, and requiring amputations. In addition, millions of people are queuing up for coronary heart disease, many of whom aren't going to survive their first heart attack.

For people with diabetes, a healthy diet is crucial to help control blood glucose levels. Eating healthily can lower the level of haemoglobin A1c – a measure of your average blood glucose over the last two to three months – by 1 per cent or more. This amount may not seem like much, but for every 1 per cent reduction in haemoglobin A1c, you enjoy a 20 per cent reduction in your risk of developing diabetes complications. See *Diabetes For Dummies,* 2nd Edition, by Dr Sarah Jarvis and Dr Alan Rubin (Wiley) for more information on haemoglobin A1c.

This chapter tells you how much to eat, what to eat, and when to eat. Because most people with diabetes are overweight, it provides advice to help healthy eating become a normal way of life for you. And don't forget the important value of exercise, particularly 'skipping' fizzy drinks, 'skipping' fatty foods, and 'skipping' desserts!

The first thing you need to know when you plan your diet is how much you can eat. To find out your ideal weight and how many *kilocalories* (commonly called *calories*) you need depending on your lifestyle and weight loss goals, just do some simple sums, as Chapter 3 explains more fully.

After you know your total kilocalorie intake objective, break it down into the three sources of energy: carbohydrates, protein, and fat.

Calculating Carbohydrates – Precursors of Glucose

When you eat a meal, the carbohydrates it contains provide the immediate source of sugar that enters your circulation and causes your blood glucose levels to rise. One group of carbohydrates is the starches, found in 'healthy' foods such as cereals, grains, wholemeal pasta, brown bread, crackers, starchy vegetables, beans, peas, and lentils. Fruits make up a second major source of carbohydrates, especially the fruit sugar, fructose. Milk and milk products contain not only carbohydrate (from milk sugar, lactose) but also protein and a variable amount of fat, depending on whether the milk is whole, skimmed, or semi-skimmed. Other sources of carbohydrate include 'unhealthy' foods such as cakes, biscuits, sweets, sugary drinks, and ice cream. These foods also contain a variable amount of fat.

To determine what else is found in food, check out *Diabetes for Dummies*, 2nd Edition (Wiley).

Determining the amount of carbohydrate

How much carbohydrate can you have in your diet? Some experts prescribe exact percentages of carbohydrate, protein, and fat kilocalories in your daily diet but this approach is rather out of fashion. Up-to-date experts are much more flexible and allow the percentage of carbohydrate to vary from 40 to 65 per cent of daily kilocalories. Experience shows that those who keep their carbohydrate intake on the lower side of that range have less trouble controlling their blood glucose levels and maintaining lower levels of blood fats. Your doctor or dietician may recommend a high percentage, which is fine as long as you maintain satisfactory blood glucose levels while not increasing your level of *triglyceride* – a type of harmful blood fat that is made in your body from excess dietary carbohydrate.

Considering the glycaemic index

Various carbohydrate sources differ in the degree to which they raise your blood glucose level. This difference is the basis of the *glycaemic index* (GI), which refers to the glucose-raising power of a food compared with pure glucose (which is given an arbitrary GI value of 100 to make calculations easier).

In general, choose foods with a low to moderate glycaemic index in order to keep the rise in your blood glucose to a minimum. Carbohydrate sources that are at the lower end of the glycaemic index scale are foods such as fruit, vegetables, wholegrain breads, unrefined cereals (such as oats and unsweetened muesli), and brown basmati rice. Biscuits, cakes, and muffins made with fruits and whole grains tend to have a lower glycaemic index as well. Predicting the glycaemic index of a mixed meal (one that contains an appetiser, a main dish, and a dessert) is nearly impossible, but you can make some simple substitutions to lower the glycaemic index of your diet, as shown in Table 2-1.

Table 2-1	Simple Diet Substitutions to Lower GI
High-GI Foods	*Low-GI Foods*
White bread	Wholemeal (brown) bread
Processed breakfast cereal	Unrefined cereals like oats or processed low-GI cereals
Plain biscuits and crackers	Biscuits containing dried fruits or whole grains like oats
Cakes and muffins	Cakes and muffins made with fruits, oats, and whole grains
Tropical fruits like bananas	Temperate-climate fruits like apples and plums
Potatoes	Wholemeal pasta or legumes
Rice	Wholegrain basmati or other low-GI rice

Many of these lower glycaemic index foods contain a lot of fibre. Fibre is a carbohydrate that isn't broken down by digestive enzymes, and therefore it doesn't raise blood glucose levels and adds no kilocalories. Fibre can reduce your risk of coronary heart disease and diabetes while also improving bowel function to help prevent constipation. For someone with diabetes, fibre also helps to reduce blood glucose levels.

The best sources of fibre are fruits, whole grains, and vegetables, especially legumes (beans). Animal food sources don't provide fibre. Aim to consume 25 grams (0.88 ounces) of fibre daily. Table 2-2 shows some foods that provide good amounts of fibre.

Table 2-2	Sources of Fibre	
Food, Amount	*Fibre (g)*	*Kilocalories*
White kidney beans, cooked, 100g	10.5	140
Bran cereal, 25g	8.8	78
Kidney beans, cooked 100g	9.3	123
Split peas, cooked, 100g	8.1	116
Lentils, cooked 100g	7.8	115
Black beans, cooked, 100g	8.7	132
Wholemeal English muffin	4.4	134
Pear, raw, small	4.3	81
Apple, with skin, 1 medium	3.3	72

Fibre exists in two main forms:

- **Insoluble:** This type of fibre doesn't dissolve in water but stays in the intestine as *roughage,* which helps to prevent constipation; for example, fibre found in wholegrain breads and cereals, and the skin of fruits and vegetables.

- **Soluble:** This form of fibre dissolves in water and enters the blood, where it helps lower glucose and cholesterol; for example, fibre found in barley, brown rice, and beans, as well as vegetables and fruits.

Wholemeal products, which are made from wholegrain flour, provide much more fibre than refined grains like white flour. When the grain is refined, it is cracked, crushed, or flaked. This process removes the parts of the grain that contain fibre as well as vitamins, minerals, and other essential nutrients. If a food is classed as 'wholemeal' or 'wholegrain', you know that it contains at least 51 per cent of the whole grain parts that contain those nutrients.

For years, doctors told people with diabetes not to eat sugar. Now we know that many foods, such as corn and potatoes, raise blood glucose almost as fast as table sugar, and because these foods would never be banned, the current recommendations are different.

You can now take the odd spoonful of sugar in your coffee and have a little sugar in your food, but keep count of the number of kilocalories you are adding with no micronutrients (that is, essential vitamins and minerals present in tiny amounts). See 'Monitoring Your Micronutrients', later in this chapter, for more information.

Choosing sugar substitutes

Although people with diabetes are allowed to have some sugar in their diet, sugar is more appropriate for those who are a normal weight – not those who are also obese. Preventing obesity is a matter of avoiding as little as 50 extra kilocalories a day over the years. If this target is accomplished using artificial sweeteners that provide sweetening power without kilocalories then so much the better.

Some of the recipes in this book originally called for 50 grams (1.75 ounces) or more of sugar. These recipes now suggest you use a granulated sweetener as a sugar substitute, to significantly lower the kilocalories from sugar. You can do the same with recipes from other sources too.

Kilocalorie-containing sweeteners

Several sugars besides sucrose (table sugar) are naturally present in food. These sugars have different properties to glucose, are taken up differently from the intestine, and raise the blood level at a slower rate (or not at all if they're not ultimately converted into glucose). These sugars can sometimes cause diarrhoea, however.

Although these kilocalorie-containing sweeteners are sweeter than sugar and you use them in smaller amounts, they *do* have kilocalories that you must count in your daily intake.

The following sweeteners contain kilocalories but act differently in the body than sucrose:

✔ **Fructose, found in fruits and berries:** Fructose (fruit sugar) is sweeter than table sugar and is absorbed more slowly than glucose. When it enters the bloodstream, the liver takes it up and here it is converted to glucose. This process takes time, and so fructose raises glucose levels quite slowly.

➤ **Xylitol, found in strawberries and raspberries:** Xylitol is also sweeter than table sugar and has fewer kilocalories per gram. Xylitol is absorbed more slowly than sugar. As a bonus, when used in chewing gum, it can reduce the occurrence of dental cavities (tooth decay).

➤ **Sorbitol and mannitol, sugar alcohols occurring in plants:** Sorbitol and mannitol are half as sweet as table sugar and have little effect on blood glucose levels as very little is absorbed from the gut.

Sweeteners without kilocalories

This group of non-nutritive or artificial sweeteners is much sweeter than table sugar and contains no kilocalories at all. Much less of these sweeteners provide the same level of sweetness as a larger amount of sugar. However, the taste of some of them may seem a little 'off' compared to sugar or honey. They include the following:

➤ **Acesulfame-K:** This sweetener is 200 times sweeter than sugar. Acesulfame-K is heat stable and is therefore used in baking and cooking.

➤ **Aspartame:** This sweetener is more expensive than saccharin (see below), but people often prefer its taste. Aspartame is 150 to 200 times as sweet as sugar, but loses its sweetening power when heated, and so is not used if food is cooked for longer than 20 minutes.

➤ **Saccharin:** This sweetener has 300 to 400 times the sweetening power of sugar. Saccharin is heat stable and is therefore used in baking and cooking.

➤ **Sucralose:** This sweetener, which is made from sugar, is 600 times sweeter than its parent, sucrose. It remains stable when heated and has become a favourite sweetener in the food industry. Because foods don't bake the same when made with sucralose, a combination of sucralose and sugar is often used to reduce kilocalories while providing the baking characteristics of sugar.

Appendix D shows the amount of these various sweeteners that provide the same sweetening power as a measured amount of sucrose (table sugar). Feel free to substitute kilocalorie-free sweeteners whenever sugar is called for in recipes. Over time, the sugar and kilocalories you save can make a big difference to your diabetes and weight.

Contrary to opinions that you may hear or read, no compelling scientific evidence exists that these sweeteners are harmful to health at normal intake levels – otherwise they are quickly banned.

Getting Enough Protein (Not Just from Meat)

Most people are already eating more than the recommended daily intake of protein. Protein comes from meat, fish, poultry, milk, and cheese, and is also found in beans, peas, and lentils, which are mentioned in the carbohydrate discussion of the preceding section. Meat sources of protein are low or high in fat, depending on the source. When you have diabetes you need to keep the fat content of your diet fairly low, and so select low-fat sources of protein, such as skinless white meat (chicken or turkey), flounder or halibut, and fat-free cheeses. Beans, peas, and lentils, which are very good sources of protein, don't contain fat but do contain carbohydrate and fibre.

How much protein should you eat? Ideally, aim for 40 per cent of your kilo-calories as carbohydrate, and limit your fat intake to 30 per cent of your kilocalories. The remaining 30 per cent is protein.

Protein doesn't cause an immediate rise in blood glucose, but it can raise glucose levels several hours later, after your liver processes the protein and converts some of it into glucose. Therefore, protein isn't a good choice if you want to treat low blood glucose, but a snack containing protein at bedtime may help prevent low blood glucose during the night.

Focusing on Fat

Fat comes in many different forms. The type everyone talks about is cholesterol, the type found in the yolk of an egg. However, most of the fat you eat comes in a chemical form known as triglyceride. This term refers to the chemistry of the fat, and we don't have to get into the details of it for you to understand how to handle fat in your diet. In the following sections, we start with a discussion of cholesterol and then turn to other forms of fat.

Zeroing in on cholesterol

These days, just about everyone knows his or her cholesterol level. Doctors routinely check cholesterol levels and you can request a test at pharmacies. You usually find out your total cholesterol level, and the breakdown into good *HDL (high-density lipoprotein)* cholesterol and bad *LDL (low-density lipoprotein)* cholesterol. If your total is high, and much of that cholesterol is the good HDL kind, you have little to worry about, but if it's mostly LDL cholesterol then you are potentially in trouble and need medical treatment to bring the level down. If you're interested in knowing the balance between good and bad cholesterol in your body, talk to your doctor who can request a blood lipid screen for you.

The Framingham Study, an on-going analysis of the health of the citizens of Framingham, Massachusetts, shows that the total cholesterol amount divided by the good HDL cholesterol figure gives a number that's a reasonable measure of your risk of a heart attack. People with a total/HDL cholesterol ratio that's less than 4.5 are at lower risk of heart attacks, whereas those with a ratio of more that 4.5 are at higher risk. The risk increases as the number rises.

The level of bad LDL cholesterol plays a very important role in causing heart attacks. For people at high risk of a heart attack, the recommended level for LDL cholesterol is less than 2.6 mmol/l (millimole per litre). (Refer to Chapter 1 for more on this measurement system.)

The daily recommendation for cholesterol is less than 300 milligrams, but your body makes significantly more than this amount from another type of fat in your diet – saturated fat. Although one egg almost supplies the recommended daily cholesterol intake, you can include eggs as a regular feature of your diet as long as you select the omega-3 enriched eggs that are now widely available. These eggs have a beneficial effect on your blood cholesterol balance.

Taking a look at other types of fat

Although cholesterol gets all the press, most of the fat you eat is in the form of triglyceride, the fat you see on fatty meats (and the type stored on your hips and around your waist). Triglycerides are found in whole-fat dairy products and in many processed foods. Several forms of triglyceride exist:

- ✔ **Saturated fat** is the kind of fat that comes from animal sources like rib-eye steak, butter, bacon, cream, and cream cheese. Saturated fat increases your bad cholesterol levels and is best eaten in moderation.

- ✔ **Trans fats** are an invention of food manufacturers to replace butter, which is more expensive. Unfortunately trans fats (often listed as partially hydrogenated oil on food labels) are significantly worse at causing coronary heart disease than saturated fat. Trans fats are found in margarine, cake mixes, dried soup mixes, many fast foods and frozen foods, doughnuts, biscuits, crisps, breakfast cereals, sweets and whipped toppings. Keep them out of your diet by reading food labels.

✔ **Unsaturated fats** come from vegetable sources such as olive oil and rapeseed oil. Here are the two forms of unsaturated fats:

- **Monounsaturated fats,** which don't raise cholesterol in the blood. Olive oil, rapeseed oil, and avocado are some examples. The oil in nuts is also monounsaturated.

- **Polyunsaturated fats,** which don't raise cholesterol but can lower good or HDL cholesterol. Corn oil, mayonnaise, and some margarines have this form of fat.

Curbing your fat intake

Fat is a concentrated source of kilocalories, so don't eat too much fat in your diet. However, monounsaturated fat seems to protect against heart disease. The increased intake of olive oil by people living around the Mediterranean Sea is one of the reasons for their lower incidence of heart disease.

Although vegetable sources of fat are generally better than animal sources, the exceptions are palm oil and coconut oil, which are highly saturated fats. However, virgin coconut oil (for example, Coconoil) is rich in *medium chain fatty acids,* which are used in the liver as a fuel and aren't converted into fat. For this reason, they increase energy levels and have an unexpected beneficial effect.

The bottom line recommendation is that no more than 30 per cent of your kilocalories should come from fat, and of that, no more than a third should come from saturated fat. For a person eating 1,500 kilocalories a day, this recommendation means 450 kilocalories from fat, and 150 of those kilocalories from saturated fat.

Use vegetable oils, preferably olive oil, as your primary source of fat, because this helps to lower your total cholesterol level.

Choose fish or poultry as your source of protein in order to avoid consuming too much fat. If you remove the skin from chicken, you get significantly less fat. Oily fish is fine because it contains omega-3 polyunsaturated fatty acids that help to lower cholesterol and have lots of other body-wide health benefits too.

Any products that claim to be 'reduced-calorie', however, must contain at least 25 per cent fewer kilocalories than the standard versions.

Demystifying label speak

If you're concerned about the amount of fat in your diet (and of course you are), you may be worried to know that, although health and nutrition claims on labels aren't allowed to mislead, no legally agreed definitions currently exist for terms such as 'low-fat', 'fat-free', 'lean', 'Lite', 'no added sugar', or 'unsweetened'. Therefore, you need to treat these sort of claims with caution. Check the nutrition information panel and the ingredients, which are listed in descending order, with the most abundant ingredient first. The following table contains a rough guide of what constitutes 'high' or 'low' content.

Per 100 grams (3.5 ounces) food or per serving, whichever is the least:

This is A LOT	This is A LITTLE
* 20g fat or more	* 3g fat or less
* 5g saturates or more	* 1g saturates or less
* 0.5g sodium or more	* 0.1g sodium or less
* 10g sugars or more	* 2g sugars or less

Figuring Out Your Diet

After you know how much to eat of each energy source (carbohydrate, fat, and protein), how do you translate this amount into actual foods? This section details the three basic approaches you can use.

Using the food plate

To help you picture the relative amounts of foods to eat in a day, imagine a plate divided into sections with one third for fruit/vegetables, one third for starchy foods such as bread, potatoes, cereals and grains, and one third for protein and fat-containing foods such as lean meat, fish, and cheese and other dairy products.

Aim to eat at least five portions of fruit and vegetables per day (and preferably eight to ten). A portion consists of:

✔ Three heaped tablespoons of vegetables such as peas, carrots, or sweetcorn

✔ One piece of larger fruit such as an apple, banana, pear, or orange

✔ Two pieces of smaller fruits such as plums or clementines

✔ A handful of grapes, cherries, or berries

✔ One tablespoon of raisins

✔ A cereal bowlful of mixed salad

✔ A small glass of pure fruit or vegetable juice or a smoothie

The Balance of Good Health

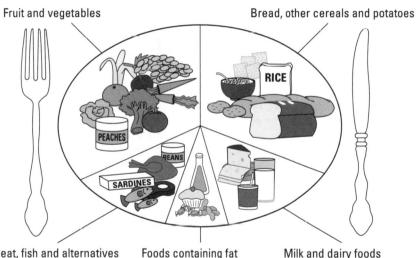

Fruit and vegetables

Bread, other cereals and potatoes

RICE

PEACHES

BEANS

SARDINES

Figure 2-1:
The food
plate guide
to a healthy
diet.

Meat, fish and alternatives

Foods containing fat
Foods containing sugar

Milk and dairy foods

You can only count juices, smoothies, and pulses (beans) as a maximum of one serving per day (for example, three glasses of juice count as only one serving, not three). And potatoes don't count towards your vegetable servings at all, because they are classed as a starchy food.

Aim to eat two portions of fish per week, one of which is oily such as sardines, salmon, mackerel, herring, or fresh tuna (tinned tuna doesn't count as oily, because the oil is removed during processing).

Select lower fat varieties of dairy products such as milk (go for skimmed or semi-skimmed), yoghurt, cheese, and mayonnaise: This approach is a relatively painless way to reduce your intake of both fat and kilocalories. Remember to check labels, however, because as the sidebar 'Demystifying label speak' explains, no legal definitions currently exist for phrases such as 'low fat' in the UK. Look at the sugar content too, because you don't want to eat products that have merely replaced the fat with extra sugar.

The food plate and general eating guidelines are probably a good tool for someone with type 2 diabetes who doesn't tend to gain weight, but someone with type 1 diabetes or the person who is obese with type 2 diabetes needs to know the specific number of kilocalories and particularly the carbohydrate kilocalories that he or she is eating. The next sections provide this information in the form of diabetic exchanges and carbohydrate counting.

Working with diabetic exchanges

Despite the huge variety of foods that you can make from the various ingredients available, all foods belong to one of several *exchange* groupings, which means that a given quantity of that food has approximately the same kilocalorie count and content of carbohydrate, protein, and/or fat. For example, half a small bagel can replace one slice of bread, half a hot dog bun, half a beefburger roll, a 15-centimetre (6-inch) tortilla, or 10 grams (0.35 ounces) of bran cereal. In Appendix B, all foods that contain the same kilocalorie count coming from the same amounts of carbohydrate, protein, and fat are shown in the various exchange lists.

The exchange lists consist of starches, fruits, milks, other carbohydrates, vegetables, meats and meat substitutes, fats, and *free foods* (those that contain no kilocalories and can be eaten 'freely'). When you know how many kilocalories of each energy source you can eat, you can create a diet for yourself. Because balancing all the information – and the foodstuffs – is a bit complicated, you may find that a training session with a dietician is helpful.

When choosing exchanges, try to follow the recommendations for more fibre, whole grains, and so forth by choosing exchanges that emphasise those nutrients. Someone who has diabetes and follows these guidelines enjoys much better blood glucose levels as a result.

Using the percentages from the preceding sections, here's how the exchange system works for a man who needs to eat 1,800 kilocalories per day:

✔ **Carbohydrate:** He can eat 40 per cent of his kilocalories as carbohydrate, which gives him around 720 kilocalories of carbohydrate. Because each gram of carbohydrate is 4 kilocalories, he can eat 180 grams (6.35 ounces) of carbohydrate. As you can see in the Appendix B exchange lists, one exchange of carbohydrate is 15 grams (0.53 ounces), and so he can eat 12 carbohydrate exchanges in a day.

Carbohydrate is found in milk, fruit, starch and vegetables.

✔ **Protein:** He can eat 30 per cent of his diet, or 540 kilocalories, as protein. A gram of protein is 4 kilocalories, and so he can eat 135 grams (4.75 ounces) of protein. Each meat or meat substitute exchange has 7 grams (¼ ounce) of protein in it. Therefore, he can eat about 19 protein exchanges each day.

Protein is found not just in meat but also in milk, starch, and some vegetables.

✔ **Fat:** He can eat no more than 30 per cent, or 540 kilocalories, of fat per day. A gram of fat is 9 kilocalories, and so he can eat no more than 60 grams (2.1 ounces) of fat per day. A fat exchange is 5 grams (0.17 ounces) of fat, and therefore he can eat 12 fat exchanges in a day.

Fat is found in milk, meat, and the other carbohydrate groups as well as pure fats like butter.

Table 2-3 provides a visual perspective of this 1,800-kilocalorie per day diet and the details of its exchange system.

Table 2-3	Exchange System for 1,800 Kilocalories Per Day					
Energy source	*Percentage of Daily Diet*	*Daily Amount of Kilo-calories*	*Kilo-calories Per Gram*	*Total Grams Per Day*	*Grams In One Exchange*	*Number of Exchanges Per Day*
Carbohydrate	40	720	4	180	15	12
Protein	30	540	4	135	7	19
Fat	30	540	9	60	5	12

The following sample of an 1,800-calorie diet shows proportions of 40 per cent carbohydrate, 30 per cent protein, and 30 per cent fat.

Breakfast:

One fruit exchange

One starch exchange

One medium-fat meat exchange

Two fat cxchanges

One semi-skimmed milk exchange

Lunch:

Three lean-meat exchanges

One vegetable exchange

Two fat exchanges

Two starch exchanges

Two fruit exchanges

Half a semi-skimmed milk exchange

Dinner:

Four lean-meat exchanges

Two starch exchanges

Two vegetable exchanges

One fruit exchange

Three fat exchanges

Snack:

Two starch exchanges

Two lean-meat exchanges

Half a semi-skimmed milk exchange

Using the exchange lists in Appendix B, you can select the foods you like to eat. For example, you can choose half a grapefruit, a third of a small cantaloupe, or half a glass of fruit juice as the fruit exchange for breakfast. And as thc four lean-meat exchanges for dinner you can eat 114 grams (4 ounces) of tuna, or 114 grams (4 ounces) of dark meat turkey or chicken, or 8 ounces of cottage cheese.

This technique of creating a diet gives you an infinite variety. In Part II of this book, which provides actual recipes, each recipe includes its food exchange value, so you can fit them into your exchange plan. Remember that you can take exchanges from one meal and move them to another. Therefore, a recipe that doesn't fit into a single meal can borrow some exchanges from other times of day, so long as the overall number of exchanges you eat during each day are correct for you. This approach makes for a very flexible diet programme.

Counting carbohydrates

People with type 1 diabetes and those with type 2 diabetes who take insulin may find that counting carbohydrates is the easiest technique for them. You still need to know how much carbohydrate you should eat in a given day. You divide the total into the meals and snacks that you eat and then, with the help of your doctor or a dietician, you determine your rapid-acting insulin needs based upon that amount of carbohydrates and your level of blood glucose when you measure it before that meal.

For example, suppose that a woman with diabetes is about to have a breakfast containing 60 grams (2.1 ounces) of carbohydrate. She knows from experience that each unit of rapid-acting insulin controls about 20 grams (0.7 ounces) of carbohydrate intake in her body. Figuring out the proper amount of rapid-acting insulin is accomplished through a process of trial and error, and consists of knowing the amount of carbohydrate intake and determining how many units are needed to maintain the blood glucose at the same level after eating the carbohydrate as it was before eating. (The number of carbohydrate grams that each unit of insulin can control differs for each individual, and for another person, one unit of rapid-acting insulin may only control 15 grams (0.53 ounces) of carbohydrate.)

In this example, the woman's measured blood glucose is 8.3 mmol/l. This result is about 3 mmol/l higher than she likes. She knows that she can lower her blood glucose by 3 mmol/l for every unit of insulin she takes. Therefore, she needs three units of rapid-acting insulin for the carbohydrate intake she is about to eat, and one unit for the elevated blood glucose for a total of four units. For more information on types of insulin, and figuring out insulin sensitivity, see *Diabetes For Dummies,* 2nd Edition (Wiley).

This woman then has a more active morning than she expected. When lunchtime comes, her blood glucose is down to 3.3 mmol/l. She's about to eat a lunch containing 75 grams (2.65 ounces) of carbohydrate. She takes four units of rapid-acting insulin for the food but reduces it by one unit to a total of three units because her blood glucose is low.

Later, at dinner, she eats 45 grams (1.6 ounces) of carbohydrate. Her blood glucose is 6.5 mmol/l. She takes two units of rapid-acting insulin for the food intake and needs no change for the blood glucose, and so she takes only two units.

To succeed at carbohydrate counting, you need to:

✔ Have an accurate knowledge of the grams of carbohydrate in the food you are about to eat.

✔ Measure your blood glucose and know how your body responds to each unit of insulin so you know how many units of insulin you personally need for a given number of grams of carbohydrate.

You can make this calculation a little easier by using *constant carbohydrates,* which means that you try to choose carbohydrates so that you are eating about the same amount at every meal and snack. This approach makes determining proper amounts of insulin less tricky; just add or subtract units based upon your blood glucose level before that meal. A few sessions with your physician or a dietician can help you feel more comfortable about counting carbohydrates.

Monitoring Your Micronutrients

Food contains a lot more than just carbohydrate, protein, and fat. Most of the other components are *micronutrients* (present in tiny or micro quantities), which are essential for maintaining the health of human beings. Examples of micronutrients include vitamins (such as vitamin C and vitamin K) and minerals (such as calcium, magnesium, and iron). Most micronutrients are needed in very small amounts, but even so the 2003 National Diet and Nutrition Survey found that significant numbers of men and women had low dietary intakes of vitamins A, B1, B2, C, and folic acid, and minerals iron, calcium, magnesium, zinc, iodine, and copper. If you eat a balanced diet you are more likely to meet your vitamin and mineral needs than if you eat lots of convenience foods and get little fruit and vegetables. In particular:

✔ Adults need to ensure that they obtain at least 1,000 milligrams of calcium each day. If you're a young person still growing, or you're pregnant or elderly, you need 1,500 milligrams daily. The best food sources of calcium are plain non-fat yoghurt, fat-free or low-fat milk, fortified ready-to-eat cereals, and calcium-fortified soy beverages.

✔ Some menstruating women lose more iron than their bodies can spare and need to ensure that they have a good intake of iron. The best sources of iron are iron-rich plant foods like spinach and low-fat meats. Vitamin C enhances absorption of iron, so wash down that lean steak with a glass of orange juice.

✔ Many people take in 20 to 40 times more salt (sodium) than they actually need, which contributes to high blood pressure and increases your risk of coronary heart disease and stroke. Avoid adding salt during cooking, or at the table, and avoid salty foods. Check food labels and go for brands containing the least amount of sodium.

✔ Aim to increase your intake of potassium to help flush excess sodium from your body via the kidneys, which can lower your blood pressure. The best sources of potassium are leafy green vegetables, fruit from vines, and root vegetables. For more information on micronutrients, check out *Diabetes For Dummies,* 2nd Edition (Wiley).

Recognising the Importance of Timing of Food and Medication

If you take insulin, the peak of your insulin activity should correspond with the greatest availability of glucose in your blood. To accomplish this aim, you need to know the time when your insulin is most active, how long it lasts, and when it's no longer active.

✔ **Rapid-acting insulin (insulin lispro, insulin aspart):** Starts to work rapidly, around 15 minutes after injection, and is injected or inhaled up to 15 minutes before or after a meal. You need to remember to eat within 15 minutes of administration. The greatest effect of rapid-acting insulin is from 45–90 minutes after injection, and its action finishes in three to four hours.

✔ **Short-acting insulin:** Also known as regular, or soluble, insulin, short-acting insulin starts to work within 30 to 60 minutes, peaks between two and four hours, and the effects last for up to eight hours.

✔ **Intermediate-acting insulin (lente insulin, isophane insulin, insulin zinc suspension):** Starts working around 1–2 hours after injection, has maximal action at 4–12 hours, and the effects last from 16–35 hours. Some intermediate-acting insulins are given twice a day together with a short-acting insulin, whereas others are used once daily, especially in older people.

✔ **Long-acting insulin (insulin glargine):** A relatively new development, this slow-release form of insulin starts releasing into your circulation 1.5 hours after injection, and diffuses constantly and evenly into your bloodstream over 24 hours, after just one daily injection. This system provides an even, basal level of insulin throughout the day, with no pronounced highs or lows, and may help to reduce the risk of hypoglycaemia. Most people use it at bedtime.

With twice daily regimes, intermediate-acting insulin analogues are usually prescribed. With a multiple injection regime, short- or rapid-acting insulin analogues are used to obtain the best glucose control.

When you go out to eat, you rarely know exactly when you're going to be eating. Using a rapid-acting insulin such as lispro, you can measure your blood glucose when the food arrives and take an immediate shot. This preparation really frees you to take insulin when you need it and adds a level of flexibility to your schedule that didn't exist before.

If you take regular insulin, keep to a more regular schedule of eating. If you have type 1 diabetes, or in some instances type 2 diabetes, you need to take a longer-acting preparation in addition to rapid-acting insulin. This approach ensures that some insulin is always circulating to keep your body's metabolism running smoothly.

Each person responds in his or her own way to different preparations of insulin. You will soon get a feel for how your blood glucose levels respond to your prescribed insulin regime.

An additional factor affecting the onset time of insulin is the location of the injection. Because your abdominal muscles are usually at rest, injection of insulin into the abdomen results in more even and consistent blood glucose levels than when injected elsewhere. If you inject into your arms or legs, however, the insulin is taken up at a more variable rate, depending on whether you exercise or not after injecting.

The depth of the injection also affects the onset of activity of the insulin. A deeper injection results in a faster onset of action. Always place your injection at the depth your doctor recommends.

You can see from the discussion in this section that a great deal of variation is possible in the taking of an insulin shot. No wonder people who inject insulin tend to have many more ups and downs in their blood glucose than those whose diabetes is controlled through diet alone, or via diet and blood-glucose-lowering drugs. But with proper education, these variations are readily evened out.

If you take oral medication, in particular the sulphonylurea drugs (such as glibenclamide, glyburide, gliclazide, glimepiride, glipizide, and gliquidone), the timing of food in relation to the taking of your medication is also important. For a complete explanation of this balance between food and medication, see *Diabetes For Dummies,* 2nd Edition (Wiley).

Chapter 3

Planning Meals for Weight Loss Goals

· ·

· ·

*Y*ou can eat wisely, get all the nutrients you need, and continue to eat great food, but you do have to limit your portions. In this chapter, we show you how to plan three different daily levels of *kilocalories* (the proper term for what most people call *calories* – refer to Chapter 1 for more on these measurements). You can lose weight rapidly, lose weight more slowly, or maintain your weight.

We prefer the slower approach to losing weight. With this method you're likely to feel less hungry, and cutting back a few hundred kilocalories a day doesn't cause a major upheaval in daily life. Also, maintaining a weight loss is easier if you lose the weight slowly.

Exercise can help speed up weight loss or permit you to eat more and still lose weight. Twenty minutes of walking burns up 100 kilocalories, and 30 minutes of walking burns up 150 kilocalories. Walk for 30 minutes a day, and you lose about 150 grams (5.3 ounces) per week (7 × 150 = 1,050 kilocalories, divided into 7,700, which is the number of kilocalories that make up 1 kilogram (2.2 pounds) of body fat) without reducing your kilocalories. That activity amounts to an annual weight loss of 7.8 kilograms (17.1 pounds) in a year. Who says you can't lose weight when you exercise but don't diet? Unfortunately things aren't always that simple, because your body can play tricks and become more efficient at using energy if you cut back on your food intake, or increase your activity levels too much. As a result, you don't lose as much weight as you may expect.

Considering the kilocalories you're storing

People often worry that they're going to feel hungry when they take in fewer kilocalories than they need. Does a bear feel hungry while it lives off its fat all winter long? No, it sleeps.

An interesting task is to work out how many kilocalories of energy are stored in the body of an overweight or obese person. Each kilogram of fat contains 7,700 kilocalories. If you're 10 kilograms overweight, you have 77,000 kilocalories (10 × 7,700) of stored energy in your body. Any idea what you can do with that much energy? You need 100 kilocalories to walk for 20 minutes at 6.5 kilometres an hour. So a walk of about 2.2 kilometres (roughly one third of 6.5 kilometres) burns 100 kilocalories. Your stored energy – 77,000 kilocalories – would take you about 1,700 kilometres (77,000 ÷ 100 × 2.2). Wow!

Unfortunately, you can't just stop eating and keep walking for any length of time in order to lose weight. But you can recognise that your stored energy, in the form of fat, provides all the kilocalories necessary to continue your daily activities without fatigue and often without hunger, as long as you tackle your weight loss in a sensible fashion without starving yourself.

Working Out How Many Kilocalories You Need

Before planning a nutritional programme, you need to know how much you need to eat on a daily basis to maintain your current weight. Then you can figure out how rapidly a deficit of kilocalories is going to get you to your goal.

Finding your ideal weight range

The ideal weight for your height is a range and not a single weight at each height, but the following examples use numbers that relate to a weight in the middle of that range. Because people have different amounts of muscle and different size frames, you're considered normal if your weight is plus or minus 10 per cent of this number. For example, a person who is calculated to have an ideal weight of 70 kilograms (11 stone) is considered normal at a weight of 63 (70 – 10 per cent) to 77 (70 - 10 per cent) kilograms (10–12 stones).

Because no two people, even twins, are totally alike in all aspects of their lives, only an approximation of your ideal weight and the number of kilocalories you need to maintain that weight is possible. You can test the accuracy of the approximation by adding or subtracting kilocalories. If your daily caloric needs are 2,000 kilocalories and you find yourself putting on weight, try reducing your intake by 100 kilocalories and see whether you maintain your weight on fewer kilocalories.

Table 3-1 shows the normal weight ranges for females and males from 1.47 metres to 1.88 metres in height.

Table 3-1	Normal Weight Range (Kilograms) at Each Height (Metres)	
Height	Male	Female
1.47	43–54	40–51
1.50	45–56	42–54
1.52	46–58	43–55
1.55	48–60	45–57
1.57	49–62	46–59
1.60	51–64	48–61
1.63	53–66	50–63
1.65	54–68	51–65
1.68	56–70	53–67
1.70	58–72	54–69
1.73	60–75	56–71
1.75	61–76	57–73
1.78	63–79	59–75
1.80	65–81	61–77
1.83	67–83	63–80
1.85	69–85	
1.88	71–88	

Now that you know your ideal weight for your height, what a surprise! Yes, okay, so you have big bones, but stick with the programme. Amazingly, those big bones often start to melt away as weight is lost!

Determining your caloric needs

After you know how much you should weigh, figure out how many kilocalories you need to maintain your ideal weight. Start by multiplying your ideal weight in kilograms by 22 (or your weight in pounds by 10). For example, if you're a male, 1.68 metres (5 feet, 6 inches) tall, your ideal weight is about 63 kilograms (midway between 56 and 70 kilograms). Your daily kilocalorie allowance is about 1,400 (1,386 if you want approximate exactitude!). But this number (considered to be your *basal* caloric need) is ideal only if you don't take a breath or have a heartbeat. You now need to increase your kilocalorie intake depending upon the amount of physical activity you do each day. Table 3-2 shows this graduated increase.

Table 3-2	Kilocalories Needed Based on Activity Level	
Level of Activity	*Kilocalories Added*	*1.68-Metre Male*
Sedentary	10% more than basal	1,540 kilocalories
Moderate	20% more than basal	1,680 kilocalories
Very active	40%+ more than basal	1,960+ kilocalories

The 'Very active' line displays a plus sign because some people doing hard manual labour need so many extra kilocalories that they lose weight if they stick to 'only' 40 per cent more than their basal kilocalorie intake. This requirement becomes clear as the person gains or loses weight on his or her food plan.

You gain weight when your daily intake of kilocalories exceeds your daily needs. Each kilogram (2.2 pounds) of fat has 7,700 kilocalories, so when the excess reaches that number of kilocalories, you're a kilogram (2.2 pounds) heavier. On the other hand, you lose weight when your daily expenditure of kilocalories exceeds your daily intake. You lose a kilogram (2.2 pounds) of fat each time you burn up 7,700 kilocalories more than you take in, whether you do it by burning an extra 100 kilocalories per day for 77 days or an extra 500 kilocalories per day for 16 days.

Now you can create a nutritional programme and fill in the blanks with carbo-hydrates, proteins, fats, and real foods.

Losing Weight Rapidly at 1,200 Kilocalories

If you're a moderately active male, 1.68 metres (around 5 feet, 6 inches) tall, you need 1,680 or approximately 1,700 kilocalories daily to maintain your weight. (Refer to Table 3-2.) If you eat only 1,200 kilocalories daily, you have a daily deficit of approximately 500 kilocalories. By dividing the kilocalories in a kilogram of fat (7,700) by 500, you can see that you lose a kilogram in 16 days on this programme (7,700 ÷ 500 = 15.4, so the loss takes just over a fortnight).

You can use the exchange system to create a nutritional plan providing 1,200 kilocalories per day with a breakdown of about 40 per cent carbohydrate, 30 per cent protein, and 30 per cent fat. You can find the various food exchange lists in Appendix B, and Chapter 2 explains the exchange system. You definitely need the help of a registered dietitian as you set up your plan.

Each item in an exchange list – for example, the fruits list – is considered to have the same nutrient content as any other item in that list and is, therefore, exchangeable for one another in the plan. For example, a small apple is the same as four apricots or twelve cherries or ½ cup of grape juice.

Table 3-3 shows the exchanges for a 1,200-kilocalorie diet. If you're a woman, you probably need to add some calcium in the form of tablets.

Table 3-3	Exchanges for a 1,200-Kilocalorie Diet
Breakfast	*Lunch*
1 fruit exchange	3 lean-meat exchanges
1 starch exchange	1 starch exchange
1 medium-fat meat exchange	1 vegetable exchange
1 fat exchange	1 fruit exchange
1 low-fat milk exchange	1 fat exchange
Dinner	*Snack*
3 lean-meat exchanges	1 starch exchange
1 starch exchange	½ semi-skimmed milk exchange

(continued)

Table 3-3 *(continued)*

Dinner	Snack
1 vegetable exchange	
1 fruit exchange	
2 fat exchanges	
½ semi-skimmed milk exchange	

The plan provides about 480 kilocalories of carbohydrate, 360 kilocalories of protein, and 360 kilocalories of fat.

After you know the various exchanges and the breakdown of exchanges in a specific nutritional plan, you can fill in the blanks with whatever food you prefer. Table 3-4 shows an example of a 1,200-kilocalorie diet.

Table 3-4   A Sample Menu for a 1,200-Kilocalorie Diet

Breakfast	Lunch
125ml apple juice	90g skinless chicken
1 slice toast	2 breadsticks
30g low-fat cheese	90g cooked green beans
1 teaspoon margarine	1 small pear
1 glass semi-skimmed milk	2 walnuts
Dinner	**Snack**
90g fresh salmon	3 tablespoons low-fat granola
1 slice wholemeal bread	½ glass semi-skimmed milk
90g of cooked broccoli	
1 slice honeydew melon	
¼ avocado	
½ glass semi-skimmed milk	

Because you can exchange many food items, you can make up an entirely different menu plan that provides the same number of kilocalories. Table 3-5 offers another 1,200-kilocalorie diet that uses entirely different selections.

Table 3-5	Another Sample Menu for a 1,200-Kilocalorie Diet
Breakfast	**Lunch**
½ grapefruit	90g fresh tuna
10g bran cereal	1 small roll
1 egg	1 bowl of salad greens
1 tablespoon sunflower seeds	1 peach
1 glass semi-skimmed milk	1 teaspoon margarine
Dinner	**Snack**
90g turkey	35g popcorn, no fat added
85g chips	½ glass semi-skimmed milk
90g cooked cauliflower	
½ bowl fruit cocktail	
½ glass semi-skimmed milk	

Notice that the dinner in the second sample menu (Table 3-5) doesn't contain two separate fat exchanges. The chips contain the fat, so it's not added separately. A chip is a simple example of a *combination food,* which is a food containing two or more energy sources (like fat and carbohydrate in this case). Understanding combination foods gets much more complex when you or a restaurant creates a dish containing multiple energy sources. Here are a few examples:

- Chow mein (average serving) with chicken, bean sprouts, mushrooms, pepper, and onions, plus a few noodles is one starch and two lean-meat exchanges.

- Pizza (two 25-centimetre – 10-inch – slices) with a meat topping is two starches, two medium-fat meats, and two fat exchanges.

- Turkey (300 grams – 10.5 ounces) with gravy, mashed potatoes, and dressing is two starches, two medium-fat meats, and two fat exchanges.

- Lasagne (225 grams – 8 ounces) is two starches and two medium-fat meat exchanges.

As Chapter 5 explains, this list shows why checking food labels is so important, to find out how much carbohydrate, protein, and fat the food actually contains.

The information on food packs that refers to *guideline daily amounts* (GDAs) are based on a 2,000-kilocalorie diet. Not one of the diets in this chapter allows you to eat that many kilocalories. Such a portion is much too large for a person on a 1,200-kilocalorie diet.

Losing Weight More Slowly at 1,500 Kilocalories

The smaller the deficit of kilocalories between what you need and what you eat, the more slowly you're going to lose weight. If your daily needs are 1,700 kilocalories and you eat 1,500, you're missing 200 kilocalories each day. Because just under ½ kilogram (a pound) of fat is 3,500 kilocalories, you lose that ½ kilogram in about 17 days (3,500 ÷ 200). You're going to lose just under a 1 kilogram (2 pounds) a month, or around 11 kilograms (24 pounds) in a year. You can accomplish this loss by reducing your daily intake by only the equivalent of a piece of bread and 2 teaspoons of margarine. Put that way, losing the weight doesn't seem difficult at all.

Table 3-6 shows the appropriate exchanges for a 1,500-kilocalorie diet. As you can see, it differs from the diet in the preceding section because this diet has two more lean-meat exchanges, one additional starch exchange, one additional vegetable exchange, one more fat exchange, and one more fruit exchange.

Table 3-6	Exchanges for a 1,500-Kilocalorie Diet
Breakfast	*Lunch*
1 fruit exchange	3 lean-meat exchanges
1 starch exchange	1 vegetable exchange
1 medium-fat meat exchange	2 fat exchanges
1 fat exchange	1 starch exchange
1 semi-skimmed milk exchange	2 fruit exchanges
Dinner	*Snack*
4 lean-meat exchanges	1 starch exchange
2 starch exchanges	½ semi-skimmed milk exchange
2 vegetable exchanges	1 lean-meat exchange

Dinner	*Snack*
1 fruit exchange	
2 fat exchanges	
½ semi-skimmed milk exchange	

In this plan, you're eating 600 kilocalories of carbohydrate, 450 kilocalories of protein, and 450 kilocalories of fat.

With the exchange lists in Appendix B in front of you, you can create an infinite number of daily menus.

As you create your meals, notice (in amazement) how small the portions really are: 120 grams (4.25 ounces) of lean meat isn't much compared to what most people are used to eating at home or in restaurants. Eating proper portions is very important because ultimately it makes the difference between weight gain and weight maintenance or loss. Portion size is often also the difference between controlling and not controlling your blood glucose. Check out Chapter 1 for more about portion sizes.

Think of the money you save if – each time you go to a pizza restaurant – your knowledge of portion sizes allows you to take home some of your pizza to eat the next day.

Maintaining Your Weight at 1,800 Kilocalories

Suppose that you finally reach a weight (not necessarily your 'ideal' weight as calculated in the earlier section 'Working Out How Many Kilocalories You Need') that allows your blood glucose levels to remain between 4 and 7 mmol/l (millimole per litre) all the time. Now, you want to maintain that weight. You want to eat about 1,800 kilocalories, up another 300 from the previous diet in this chapter. When you compare this to the 1,200-kilocalorie diet, it may seem like a lot of food.

The differences between this plan and the 1,500-kilocalorie diet are two additional fat exchanges, two additional starch exchanges, and one additional lean-meat exchange. The exchange list looks like Table 3-7.

Exercise for prevention

A study published in the 20 October 1999 edition of *The Journal of the American Medical Association* showed that walking may prevent the onset of diabetes. This research showed that, among a large group of nurses, the occurrence of diabetes was less in those who walked compared with those who were sedentary. The women who walk most briskly had the lowest incidence of diabetes.

Table 3-7	Exchanges for a 1,800-Kilocalorie Diet
Breakfast	**Lunch**
1 fruit exchange	3 lean-meat exchanges
1 starch exchange	1 vegetable exchange
1 medium-fat meat exchange	2 fat exchanges
2 fat exchanges	2 starch exchanges
1 semi-skimmed milk exchange	2 fruit exchanges
Dinner	**Snack**
4 lean-meat exchanges	2 starch exchanges
2 starch exchanges	2 lean-meat exchanges
2 vegetable exchanges	½ semi-skimmed milk exchange
1 fruit exchange	
3 fat exchanges	
½ semi-skimmed milk exchange	

This plan provides 180 grams (6.35 ounces) of carbohydrate, 135 grams (4.75 ounces) of protein, and 60 grams (2.1 ounces) of fat, maintaining the 40:30:30 division of kilocalories.

For people with type 2 diabetes, this plan is an excellent way to eat the right amount of kilocalories in the right ratios of energy sources. If you have type 1 diabetes, or you have type 2 and take insulin, you need to know the grams of carbohydrate in each meal in order to determine your insulin needs for that meal.

Checking Out Other Diets

If you go to the diet section of any large bookshop, you're inevitably over-whelmed by the options. You can find diets that recommend protein and no carbohydrate, carbohydrate and no protein, one type of carbohydrate and not another, all rice, all grapefruit, and so on. Do all these diets really work when many of them are exactly the opposite of others on the same shelf? The answer is they do and they don't. If you follow any diet closely, you can lose weight. But the most difficult part (as everyone knows) is keeping the weight off.

This section tells you about the most popular diets presently available from this or that brilliant 'scientist'. Which one's best? None of them, and all of them. If you find you can start losing weight successfully with one of these programmes, go ahead and do it, but remember that in the end you want to eat a balanced diet that's low in fat and protein and uses carbohydrates that emphasise whole grains and fibre. And remember that you're unlikely to succeed without exercise.

The low carbohydrate group

These diets are based on the claim that carbohydrates promote hunger. By reducing or eliminating carbohydrates, you lose your hunger as you lose your weight. The first of them, the Atkins Diet, promotes any kind of protein, including protein high in fat. Naturally, other diets quickly came out promoting very little carbohydrate but less fatty protein. Here are your options:

- **Atkins Diet:** This plan allows any quantity of meats, shellfish, eggs, and cheese but, initially at least, doesn't permit high-carbohydrate foods like fruits, starchy vegetables, and pasta. Small quantities of the forbidden foods are added in later. The programme does recommend exercise but doesn't suggest long-term changes in your eating behaviour.

- **South Beach Diet:** This diet restricts carbohydrates while recommending proteins that are lower in fat than the Atkins Diet. Daily exercise is an important component, but the plan doesn't suggest any changes in eating behaviour. Over time some carbohydrate is reintroduced into the diet.

- **Ultimate Weight Solution:** This plan recommends a lot of protein, which naturally results in a reduction in carbohydrate. This programme also advises you not to eat foods that are high in fat. Support groups in which you discover how to modify your eating behaviour are important, and you're supposed to stay in these groups throughout your life. The plan does emphasise regular exercise, such as walking.

✔ **Zone Diet:** This diet urges you to balance your food intake into exact amounts of carbohydrate, protein, and fat. You're not permitted to eat high-carbohydrate and high-fat food. Regular exercise is recommended, but the plan doesn't suggest changes in your eating behaviour. You have to continue with this balance throughout life to maintain your weight loss.

✔ **Low GI diet:** The best option for someone with type 2 diabetes is to select a less extreme, *low glycaemic index* (low-GI) diet. This type of diet reduces insulin needs in the body and improves glucose tolerance while still allowing you to eat so-called 'slow carbs', which have low to moderate impact on blood glucose levels. Full information is available at the 'home' of the glycaemic index, www.glycemicindex.com.

Low-fat diets

When your doctor or dietitian provides you with details of a diet, the chances are that the diet sheet is for a conventional low-fat diet. Although good for cholesterol levels, the evidence that low-fat diets help weight loss is conflicting. In fact, a recent government report admits that low-fat diets are no better than low-kilocalorie diets in helping people achieve long-term weight loss. The report suggests that the energy restriction is what helps the weight loss and not the diet being low in fat. Average weight loss is 5 kilograms (11 pounds) in people following a low-fat diet for six months, but after 18 months follow-up, those people tend to put all the weight back on – and more.

The portion control group

These diets recognise that how much you eat determines your weight rather than what you eat. They generally follow healthy eating guidelines. On average, people following a portion control/low-kilocalorie diet lose around 8 per cent of their body weight – that represents 8 kilograms (17.5 pounds) for someone weighing 100 kilograms (15 stones, 10 pounds) over a 6 to 12 month period. Studies looking at the ability of these diets to keep weight off, however, suggest that they are less effective in the long-term. After three to four years, the average weight loss is half that seen in shorter term trials, at around 4 per cent of body weight – equivalent to just 4 kilograms (8.8 pounds) for someone with a starting weight of 100 kilograms (15 stones, 10 pounds).

Here are some examples of portion control diets:

- **DASH Diet:** The emphasis of the DASH (*Dietary Approaches to Stop Hypertension*) plan is on grains, fruits, vegetables, and restricting the amounts of fat. A further modification for those with high blood pressure recommends very little salt. Animal protein, such as meat, fish, and poultry, is limited. An exercise programme is suggested but not defined. This diet includes suggested changes in eating behaviour. The DASH diet is a diet for life (and a very good one).

- **Weight Watchers:** This plan uses a point system in which foods are given points according to the amount of fat, fibre, and kilocalories in them. To get to and maintain a certain weight, you're given a daily number of points. As long as you stay within these points, you succeed. Therefore foods that have large amounts of kilocalories use up your daily points quickly. The programme suggests exercise and changes in your lifestyle.

Very low calorie diets

Although the medical profession once frowned on them, *very low calorie diets* (VLCDs) are now back into fashion and proving successful. On average, VLCDs allow people to lose 13–23 kilograms (28–50 pounds) of excess weight. After one year, however, little difference exists in the amount of weight loss between those following a VLCD and those following a low-kilocalorie/portion control diet. Analysis of 29 studies investigating how well people managed to keep the lost weight off, however, shows that VLCDs are significantly more successful and help people keep off significantly more weight at every year of follow-up – even up to five years – in comparison with a low-kilocalorie diet.

- **The Cambridge Diet:** This diet offers a number of flexible weight management programmes ranging from 411 kilocalories up to 1,500 kilocalories per day. Products include flavoured milk drinks, soups, and bars. When using the Cambridge Diet as the sole source of nutrition, you need to have no fewer than three full portions – four portions if you're male or a female over 173 centimetres (5 feet 8 inches) tall – with only one meal per day as a bar. You also need to drink at least 2.3 litres (4 pints) of kilocalorie-free liquid each day. After four weeks you usually add a meal per day.

  The Cambridge Diet is only available through independent Cambridge counsellors who provide a personal support service to help maintain motivation. A study presented at an Association for the Study of Obesity meeting shows that people with type 2 diabetes can safely achieve 10–30 kilograms (22–66 pounds) weight loss over three years, with preservation of lean body tissue, using a nutritionally complete VLCD such as the Cambridge Diet.

Proper medical supervision of VLCDs is *essential*, particularly at the lower end of the kilocalorie scale. Following diets with such low kilocalorie intakes can otherwise be very harmful.

✔ **Lighter Life:** This is a weight loss programme that combines a very low calorie diet with specialised counselling techniques such as cognitive behavioural therapy and transactional analysis. It is designed for people who are 20 kilograms or more overweight, and takes place in small, single-sex groups with a trained counsellor who helps you examine the thoughts, feelings, and behaviours that lead to overeating. You eat four food packs (shakes, soups, bars) a day, which supply around 500 kilocalories plus all the vitamins and minerals you need.

Losing 10 kilograms (22 pounds) of excess weight lowers your blood pressure, reduces fasting blood glucose levels, and improves blood fat levels enough to reduce your overall risk of premature death by 20 per cent, and the risk of a diabetes-related death by as much as 30 per cent. This weight loss also improves quality of life due to less back and joint pain and breathlessness, and improved fertility, sex drive, and sleep.

Chapter 4

Eating What You Like (Within Reason)

*H*aving diabetes doesn't mean giving up the foods you grew up with or the foods you love the most. Some parts of every ethnic diet fit well into a healthy eating regime for diabetes. Recipes that prove this point are in Part II of this book. You can also use all kinds of tricks to substitute good-for-you ingredients in place of those that are less helpful for diabetes. This chapter is all about eating what you like. Even foods that seemingly have no business on the plate of someone with diabetes are okay if eaten in small portions.

The fact that the word 'diet' even creeps into the diabetes vocabulary is a shame: Following a diet implies losing something or suffering somehow, and this is simply not the case. You can eat great food and enjoy the taste of every ethnic variety, as long as you concentrate on the amount you eat, and the way each food breaks down into different sources of energy, so that you keep your fat and carbohydrate intake under control. Perhaps the phrase 'nutritional plan' is better than 'diet'.

So, stop dieting and start eating delicious foods. It may take a lot of willpower, but you can give up dieting if you try hard enough!

Following Your Eating Plan

Creating an eating plan that provides the proper number of kilocalories from carbohydrate, protein, and fat is particularly important when you have diabetes. After you know how much of each food component you need, you can translate those numbers into exchanges and select your desired food: the delicious end point of all that calculating. (Food components and exchanges are covered in Chapter 2.) Make sure that your choices come from a variety of foods instead of eating the same thing over and over. You're much more likely to keep with the programme if your taste buds aren't bored with what you eat.

Before you cook, ensure that the recipe fits into your eating plan. If your carbohydrate portions for the day are already in your stomach, select a recipe that contains little carbohydrate. The same is true for protein and, of course, fat. If you think 'moderation' as you draw up your meal plan, keeping to the portions that you need to eat – and no more – is easier.

Wherever possible, try to select foods that are in season. These foods are usually the freshest available and the least expensive, as well as being grown locally and freshly harvested for maximum nutrient content. The recipes you can prepare with these fresh foods are also among the most delicious.

Time is an important factor in your eating plan. You may not have a great deal of time to prepare your food, and some of the recipes in this book may take more time than you can spare. Therefore, choose meals that fit into your schedule. But remember – after you prepare a recipe several times, preparation becomes much faster and easier. After a while, you may not even need to follow the recipe. Consider the time you spend preparing delicious healthy food as an investment in your wellbeing. Take the time to eat properly now so that in later life you don't waste precious time being unwell.

As a person with diabetes, especially if you have type 1 diabetes, considering the timing of your meals is also important so that you eat when your medications are able to balance your carbohydrates. This process is much easier with rapid-acting insulin, but if you still use regular insulin, you need to eat about 30 minutes after you take your shot.

Another essential part of your planning is what to do when you feel hungry but shouldn't eat. You can prepare a low-kilocalorie snack for these occasions, such as baby carrots, cherry tomatoes, a piece of fruit, or low-fat pudding.

Your diabetes medication may require you to have three meals a day, but if not, having three meals is still important. This approach spreads kilocalories over the day and helps you avoid coming to a meal extremely hungry. Try not to skip breakfast: It really is the most important meal of the day, because your reserves are running on empty after a night's sleep. Make your own lunch as often as possible as this gives you control over what you eat. The fast-food lunches served in restaurants and takeaways rarely provide the lower fat, lower glycaemic index nutrition you need. For example, salads are often covered with a lot of oil, and even healthy olive oil contains kilocalories that you need to consider when you're watching your weight. If your weight is perfect, by all means bring on the olive, walnut, almond, macadamia nut, or rapeseed oils, because they have beneficial effects on your cholesterol levels.

Eating the Best of Ethnic Cuisines

When you have diabetes you don't have to give up the kinds of food you love eating. You can eat the same foods but just decrease the portion sizes, particularly if you're overweight. People who are in the normal weight range for their height are doing things that you need to do as well: eating smaller portions, eating slowly, enjoying each mouthful, stopping eating when they are full, leaving some food on their plate, and keeping physically fit with exercise.

After you receive a diagnosis of diabetes, try to find a dietitian with experience in advising members of your ethnic group. This person is best trained to show you how to keep eating what you love, while altering your diet slightly to fit your needs. The alteration is often no greater than simply reducing the amount of food you eat each day. Or it may involve changing ingredients so that you exchange a high-fat source of energy with a low-fat source without affecting the flavour.

Valuing British food

Increasing numbers of the sedentary British population are overweight or obese and have related problems such as high blood pressure, diabetes, and coronary heart disease.

Traditional British foods include fish and chips, roast beef and Yorkshire pudding, Cornish pasties, Melton Mowbray pork pies, and Cheddar cheese. All these foods are delicious, but full of kilocalories, and rich in carbohydrate, fat, or both.

You don't have to abandon these foods but you do need to eat them carefully. Instead of deep-frying your fish, serve it grilled or baked, and replace a large portion of deep-fried chips with a small portion of low-fat oven-baked chips. Instead of a hand-held pasty, make a pasty pie that has only a small amount of pastry on top – and leave half of it on your plate. Have a small portion of pork pie rather than a large one and concentrate on eating the filling while leaving a lot of the pastry crust. Roast your beef joint on a rack so that the fat drips away, and have only a small Yorkshire pudding instead of a large one. If you must have roast potatoes, have one larger one rather than several small ones, which soak up proportionately more fat. And fill up on green vegetables and carrots. Stop eating when you're full, but if you fancy dessert have bio yoghurt or fresh fruit rather than trifle and custard.

Flavour your food with black pepper rather than salt, and select leaner cuts of meat. You can even make an omelette using just egg whites instead of the whole egg. And avoid deep-frying as much as possible.

Chewing on Chinese food

When you think of Chinese food, you think rice. White rice has a relatively high glycaemic index (GI), but you can use Basmati rice, which has a slightly lower GI. (Refer back to Chapter 2 for more on the glycaemic index.) You can also use brown rice in place of white, which has a lower GI because the outer rice bran remains intact.

Add vegetables to the rice, such as soybeans, peppers, onions, baby sweetcorn, pak choi, and beansprouts, plus lean sources of protein such as prawns, fish, chicken, or soybean curd (tofu). Then add flavour with ginger, garlic, black pepper, and low-sodium soy sauce.

Chinese food is traditionally cut into very small pieces and quickly stir-fried to conserve both fuel and cooking oil. Stir-fried vegetables are therefore served still crisp and brimming with nutrients.

Chinese cuisine is generally healthy and includes lots of vegetables, fruits, and seafood, while keeping sugar and desserts to a minimum. Chinese restaurants offer wonderful vegetable dishes, many with tofu as a protein source.

When you cook Chinese food, use as little sugar and fat as possible, steer clear of deep-fried dishes, and avoid eating too much rice.

Feasting with French food

French food is associated with the term *haute cuisine,* which means fine food prepared by highly skilled chefs. This kind of cooking includes the use of truffles and mushrooms and the preparation of rich, glazed sauces. Although these meals taste exquisite, they're often brimming with fat and kilocalories. Have only the smallest amount, and adopt another French fashion in *nouvelle cuisine* – a 'new' way of eating in which only small amounts of food are served. In nouvelle cuisine the emphasis is on the way the food is arranged on the plate.

The French way of eating also involves serving a series of dishes, one after the other, instead of a large buffet where you help yourself to everything at once. This sequential way of eating means that recognising when you feel full is easier, so that you can stop before you eat too much. Honest.

 French food can contain a lot of butter and cream, but some restaurants use these ingredients more sparingly. The essence of the new French food is very fresh ingredients cooked in light sauces (including fresh fish and shellfish), whole grains, and light oil. Don't eat too much of the delicious French bread or slather it with butter, and avoid using the bread to mop up the heavy French sauces, because this quickly takes you over the kilocalorie count you so cleverly calculated.

Currying flavour: Indian food

In some parts of India, the traditional meals include plenty of chicken, beef, fish, and lamb. However, many Indian dishes are vegetarian and are based around lentils, aubergines, okra, peppers, tomatoes, and onions among others.

Most meals are served with rice and/or breads such as naan and paratha. Many different varieties of rice are available (including long-grain rice, round-grain rice, polished rice, pressed rice, red rice, and beaten rice) as well as many kinds of lentils (such as yellow, red, small, large, round, flat, and so on). With such a wealth of ingredients, the possibilities are endless.

Fish, including shellfish, is popular in much of the coastal regions of southern India. In northern India, however, lamb is king. The varieties of lamb dishes are almost as numerous as the varieties of rice. Because of the Muslim influence, Indian people rarely eat pork (although pork and clam curry is a staple in Goa), and because Hindus consider the cow to be sacred, beef is usually shunned. Chicken dishes are available, but they don't compare in quality to those made with lamb.

Interestingly, research shows that some Indian spices such as cinnamon, ginger, chilli, and turmeric have beneficial effects in the body, reducing inflammation and improving glucose tolerance.

Indian food is good for someone with diabetes, so long as you don't eat too much of it. Overeating is easy to do because the food is so delicious. Watch out for too much white rice and the traditional naan bread. A vegetarian diet is especially conducive to good health.

Enjoying Italian food

Italy is divided into many different regions, each with its own individual cuisine. So, although we often sum up Italian food as pizzas, pasta, and risotto, several regional trends exist which include different farmhouse cheeses like ricotta, pecorino romana – made from sheep milk – and parmigiano reggiano (parmesan).

The food of northern Italy features more wild game, such as deer and rabbit, along with some farm animals, such as beef, chicken, and even goat. Seasonings include garlic, onions, rosemary, and bay leaves. Northern Italian cooking emphasises cream and meat sauces. Rice dishes like risotto and polenta made from yellow corn are enjoyed along with gnocchi, a potato dumpling.

In the south, seafood receives more emphasis. The olive also joins many dishes, along with wine for cooking. In southern Italy, the tomato is the basis of most cooking, particularly its use in pasta dishes. Here the Italian staple, artichoke, is widely cultivated too.

A person with diabetes doesn't have to avoid mouth-watering Italian dishes. The Mediterranean diet, with its emphasis on olive oil, fish, tomatoes, garlic, fruit, and vegetables, is undoubtedly healthy for your heart. One of the key changes you may need to make, however, is to reduce the amount of fat in your ingredients. Olive oil is a fat, and even though it's very good for you, the kilocalories climb rapidly as you add more to your dishes. When Italians traditionally worked hard in the fields all day, they needed those extra kilocalories to sustain them. But when you just potter around at home all day, the kilocalories end up on your hips and affect your glucose control. If you want to eat more of these delicious foods, you need to get more active.

A second important step is reducing the size of your portion of pasta or risotto, whether eating at home or in a wonderful Italian restaurant. If you look at the exchanges for various foods in Appendix B, you see that one start exchange is 70 grams (3 ounces) cooked pasta, or 65 grams (2¾ ounces) cooked rice, or two bread sticks. Compare that with the usual large portions that a restaurant serves, and you quickly discover what changes you need to make.

On the other hand, the great fresh fruits and vegetables in Italian cooking, like tomatoes, artichokes, and green beans, are just what the doctor orders. These ingredients fit perfectly into a healthy diet that emphasises more fibre and less fat.

Top off your meal with a glass of Chianti from Tuscany. (Chapter 1 tells you about the benefits of a moderate intake of alcohol.) But skip the rich Italian desserts, or perhaps share a dessert with three other people. These changes aren't too much of a hardship, and they take nothing away from the glory of Italian cooking.

Munching Mexican food

Traditional Mexican food features fish, wild game (such as rabbit and turkey – yes they were originally wild), plus beans and corn. Additional flavour is supplied courtesy of chocolate, vanilla, honey, and chilli peppers.

Chocolate is a great food because it's as rich in beneficial antioxidants as green tea and red wine. Select your chocolate carefully, however. Go for dark chocolate containing at least 72 per cent cocoa solids, because these provide the benefits without too much added fat or sugar. And only eat a few squares when you're watching your weight. You can even get 100 per cent cocoa solid chocolate but it's very much an acquired taste. You can add it to chilli con carne, however, for additional flavour.

True Mexican tortillas are made from cornmeal, not wheat, and like burritos they're stuffed with a combination of beans, chicken or beef, rice, and salsa. If you buy them ready-made they often contain a lot of salt, but when you make your own, you can control the amount of added salt – ideally none at all.

The ingredients in a burrito, minus the high salt content, make a great meal in a hurry. When you make burritos, however, avoid too much cheese or excessive rice and watch out, especially, for the hot chilli pepper.

Tasting Thai food

Thai food is a good option for people with diabetes: Stir-frying is the method of choice, and so little fat is used in the cooking. Also, Thai cuisine serves meat, fish, and poultry in small quantities, thus providing taste rather than bulk as in a Western diet. Thanks to the Chinese, the five basic flavours of Asian cuisine – bitter, salt, sour, hot, and sweet – are established, and Thai meals use them as their basis for a balance of flavours. Dishes made with soy and ginger provide good examples.

Choosing from familiar foods

Jennifer lives in Cornwall and loves all the foods she grew up with in her home town of Padstow. These foods include dinner-plate-sized Cornish pasties, fish and chips, pies, fried breakfasts, and home-made jam sponges – not to mention the delicious Cornish clotted cream she buys from a local farm.

Jennifer is 46 years old and weighs 70 kilograms (11 stone) even though she's only 1.6 metres (5 feet, 4 inches) tall. Thanks to her typical Cornish diet she gains at least 2 to 3 kilograms (4 to 6 pounds) each year and now takes little exercise as it leaves her too breathless.

After feeling tired and run down with recurrent infections, she visits her doctor for a check up because she thinks she's anaemic. Her doctor suspects what's wrong with her immediately and diagnoses type 2 diabetes because her blood glucose level is 14 mmol/l (millimole per litre). He refers Jennifer to a dietitian and a diabetes specialist, and tells her that she must start losing weight and exercising more. After all, she's still young and wants to maximise the quality and quantity of the years ahead of her.

The dietitian explains to Jennifer that she eats way too much fried food, too many kilocalories, and excessive amounts of carbohydrate and fat. She decides to manage her diabetes without giving up the staples of her native cuisine – and the dietitian understands because she loves Cornish food too. She recommends that Jennifer does the following:

✔ Trims off visible fat from her meats

✔ Reduces the amount of frying and begins grilling and baking instead

✔ Reduces the amount of fat she uses in cooking

✔ Switches to olive oil in place of lard for cooking

✔ Eats only half a small pasty, instead of a whole one, and keeps the rest for the next day, as well as eating less of the pastry

✔ Selects more fruit and vegetables

✔ Adds more fish and poultry to her diet

✔ Keeps clotted cream as an occasional treat on fresh fruit salad rather than serving with scones and jam

Jennifer finds that these alterations don't affect her diet too much. For example, one of her favourite dishes, an omelette made with three eggs, tastes just as delicious when made with two eggs – a smaller portion doesn't diminish the taste. And she discovers that she enjoys Cornish clotted cream even more when she adds a little to fresh strawberries rather than eating it in the classic way with scones and strawberry jam.

She starts to exercise more and instead of taking the free bus up the hill to the local supermarket, she walks up and back. She now regularly walks around the quay to admire the boats and scenery in the evenings rather than staying in just watching TV, and buys fresh fish such as mackerel directly from the local fishermen as their boats come in at dusk.

After discovering how to modify her lifestyle and diet – eating less, rather than giving up her favourite foods – Jennifer begins to lose weight. She gradually loses 5.5 kilograms (12 pounds) over the next six months, and her blood glucose rapidly falls into the normal range, and stays there, so that she doesn't need to take medication. Because she makes these changes for all members of her family, everyone benefits too.

Most Thai dishes also contain garlic, a condiment that grows all over Thailand, and which has a number of beneficial effects on the heart and circulation.

Coconut milk – a combination of the coconut flesh and the liquid inside the coconut – is widely added to Thai curries and soups and is something of a staple in delicious fragrant dishes such as Thai green chicken curry or prawn soup flavoured with coconut milk, lemongrass, Kaffir lime leaves, and the wicked little Thai red chilli peppers which are hot, hot, hot. However, you can always get dishes that aren't so spicy, and the subtle tastes of good Thai cooking make it tremendously popular in the United Kingdom and throughout the world wherever Thais are found. Rice is generally part of the meal, and vegetables are eaten in large quantities.

Fish is a major ingredient because the settled areas of Thailand tend to be close to the sea. Fish sauce, for example, made by fermenting shrimp, salt, and water together, takes the place of soy sauce in Thai cooking. Look for low-sodium versions, even though you only need a few drops of this pungent sauce when cooking. The dipping sauces tend to have strong tastes too, so that they're used in very small quantities, minimising the salt and sugar in the diet.

And, at the end of the meal, Thai people enjoy fruits like lychee, mango, pineapple, guava, and papaya, which provide fibre, vitamins, and minerals with relatively few kilocalories and low to moderate impact on your circulating glucose levels.

In Thai restaurants, a dish called pad thai is a favourite entrée. Pad thai means 'Thai-style stir-fried noodles' and, although not exactly representative of the finest Thai cuisine, you need to be aware of it because the sauce often contains a lot of sugar. A small portion of pad thai is fine for a person with diabetes, but leave at least half the serving on your plate or, if making it at home, cut back on the amount of sugar you add and leave some of the meal to freeze and eat another day.

Thai food is so nutritious that there's little else to warn you about. But, as always, avoid large portions and too much rice. And take care with those unusually hot chilli spices.

Eating the rest of the world's cuisine

Covering all the world's wonderful cuisines in detail isn't possible in this book, although this chapter tries hard to cover the most popular foods in the UK. We have, however, left out delicious cuisines that many of you love from other countries, such as Greece, Guatemala, Costa Rica, Argentina, and Brazil. But the message is, hopefully, clear:

✔ You don't have to give up the foods you love just because you have diabetes.

✔ You can reduce the fat in your food, and still eat delicious meals.

✔ You can reduce your salt intake to help lower your blood pressure.

✔ You can avoid the empty kilocalories in fatty, sugary desserts.

✔ You can solve one of biggest problems (the large size of the portions) by sharing or saving the food for another meal.

✔ You can take more exercise to help reverse the effects of just about any dietary indiscretion.

A nutritional plan is all about discovering how to eat to live – not living in order to eat. What you put in your mouth has a lot to do with your state of health, no matter where the food comes from.

Stocking Up with the Right Ingredients

Some common ingredients are used in many different recipes. Having them to hand is convenient, saving you needless trips to the shops and more exposure to foods you don't need. These ingredients can be divided into staple ingredients that can be frozen or stored, and fresh produce.

Storing up staples

Some of the foods that belong in every kitchen or store cupboard (if you're a vegetarian, make the appropriate substitutions) include the following:

For the freezer:

Chicken breasts	Fruit juices
Fish fillets	Lean minute steaks
Frozen fruit	Wholegrain bread

For the pantry:

Black pepper	Dried fruit, unsugared
Canned tomatoes	Fat-free salad dressing
Canned tuna, salmon in water	Fresh garlic

Fresh onions

Fruit spreads

Grains (brown rice, couscous)

Healthy oils (olive, peanut, walnut, rapeseed)

Ketchup

Legumes (peas, beans, lentils)

Mustard

Non-fat dry milk

Non-stick cooking sprays

Nuts: walnuts, almonds, Brazils

Pasta sauce

Red and white cooking wines

Reduced-kilocalorie mayonnaise

Reduced-sodium soy sauce

Sugar-free cocoa mix

Tomato purée

Vinegars

Worcestershire sauce

For baking:

Baking powder

Baking soda

Cocoa powder

Cornstarch

Cream of tartar

Dry breadcrumbs

Extracts (vanilla, lemon, almond)

Flour (all-purpose, wholemeal)

Rolled oats

Dark chocolate (at least 70 per cent cocoa solids)

Sugar-free gelatin

Sweeteners:

Artificial sweeteners

Honey

Light maple syrup

Molasses

Seasonings:

Dried herbs

Fresh herbs and spices

Pepper

Salt

Focusing on fresh produce

Buy fresh produce that is, where possible, in season and locally grown. Look for organic box schemes in your area so that you buy fresh, organic items direct from the growers, which works out cheaper. Buy as wide a range of fresh fruit, vegetables, and salad leaves as possible, and buy little and often to ensure maximum freshness. Here are some ideas to whet your taste buds:

Fruit:

Apples	Melons
Apricots	Olives
Bananas	Oranges
Blueberries	Pears
Dates	Pineapples
Figs	Pink or red grapefruit*
Grapes	Raisins
Kiwi fruit	Raspberries
Lemons	Strawberries
Limes	Watermelons
Mangoes	

* Check for interactions between grapefruit and any medication you are taking. Grapefruit affects the metabolism of some drugs used to treat high blood pressure, for example.

Vegetables:

Aubergines	Curly kale
Broccoli	Corn on the cob
Cannellini beans	Courgettes
Carrots	French green beans
Chickpeas	Jerusalem artichokes

Lentils	Potatoes (waxy, new)
Mangetout	Shallots
Okra	Spinach
Onions	Sweet potatoes
Pak choi	

Salad stuff:

Avocadoes	Mixed salad leaves
Bean sprouts	Mooli
Beetroot	Peppers (red, green, yellow, orange)
Celery	Rocket
Cos lettuce	Spring onions
Cucumber	Tomatoes (cherry, beef, sundried)

Watercress With these ingredients, you're ready for just about any of the recipes in this book. The exceptions are exotic ingredients, such as those used in Thai or Indian foods, which you can buy in specialty shops as you need them.

Prepare a list of these ingredients and make multiple copies so that you can check off what you need before you go shopping. Leave a little space for the perishables such as fresh fruits, vegetables, milk, meat, fish, and poultry. In Chapter 5, we tell you more about the process of shopping for these ingredients.

Using the Right Tools

Just as you wouldn't try to bang in a nail with a shoe (especially with your foot inside), don't try to cook without the right tools. Spending a little more at the beginning pays huge dividends later on. For example, get the best set of knives you can afford. They make all cutting jobs much easier, and they last a long time. Buy good non-stick pans; they make cooking without oils much easier.

Here's the basic equipment that all kitchens need in order to turn out delicious meals:

Chopping boards	Pots and pans
Food processor	Salad spinner
Knives	Scales
Measuring cups and spoons	Steamer with at least two different compartments
Microwave	
Mixer with dough hook	Thermometer (for roasting meat)

Making Simple Modifications

You can make all kinds of simple modifications that reduce kilocalories and the amounts of foods (such as those containing cholesterol) that you're trying to keep in check. You can easily do the following:

- ✔ Use semi-skimmed or skimmed milk instead of whole milk.
- ✔ Use low-fat cuts of meat rather than high-fat meats. Low-fat meats include lean beef, lean pork, and skinless white-meat poultry.
- ✔ Trim all visible fat off meats and poultry.
- ✔ Stay away from packaged luncheon meats, which tend to be high in fat.
- ✔ Select foods that are low in sodium and saturated fats (check the label on the food).
- ✔ Choose high-fibre foods like whole fruits, vegetables, and grains.
- ✔ Enjoy non-fat or low-fat yoghurt instead of sour cream.
- ✔ Have dressings, sauces, and gravies served on the side.
- ✔ Substitute lentils and beans for meat, fish, and poultry.
- ✔ Replace butter with olive oil, herbs, spices, or lemon juice.
- ✔ Prepare foods by baking, poaching, grilling, and so on – any method other than frying.

Use your imagination to come up with your own unique ways to cut down on kilocalories and fat.

Taking Holiday Measures

The heading to this section is particularly appropriate, because the key to maintaining good control of your diabetes while on holiday is to control the portions of everything you eat. Eating too much is too easy.

If you encounter a buffet table, vow to make only one trip. You're likely to fill your plate with more food than you need, so plan to leave a large portion on the plate. Focus on healthy foods and avoid high-fat and high-sugar foods, particularly desserts. Stick to fruits for high-fibre, low-kilocalorie desserts.

If you're planning a dinner party, make something that you know is going to work for your nutritional plan. You can certainly find something in this book that suits you. These recipes are all taste-tested and delicious, so you don't have to think that you're making something inferior. And if you're going out to a dinner party, have a snack before you go so that you don't arrive feeling hungry.

Most important of all, try to forget the all-or-nothing mindset. If you go off your nutritional plan once or twice, put the lapse behind you and get back to doing the things you know are right for you. The benefits are immediate in the form of a general feeling of wellbeing and, of course, you don't develop the long-term complications of diabetes.

Chapter 5

Stocking Up at the Supermarket

*E*very trip to the supermarket is an adventure. This chapter is about coping with the challenge of going food shopping, without being lured into buying items that aren't good for your diabetes nutritional plan, and overcoming your natural desire to take home what you know isn't good for you.

You deserve the best, and that holds true for the food you eat as much as anything else. Of course, you can always respond like the man whose doctor told him that the best thing to do for himself was to get on a really good diet, stop chasing women, and stop drinking so much alcohol. The patient replied: 'I don't deserve the best. What about second best?' But we hope you don't settle for second best.

Going in with a Plan – or at Least a Shopping List

When you have a hobby, you develop a series of steps to accomplish your chosen activity in the most efficient manner, whether you're painting pictures or raising tomatoes. If you paint pictures, you certainly don't start painting without deciding on a subject and buying the right paints, brushes, and canvas. If you raise tomatoes, you prepare the soil, add nutrients such as manure, and buy the seeds or, more likely, the plants. You use a watering system as well as canes to hold up your crop.

Try planning your excursion to the shops in the same careful manner. Decide in advance what items you need that comply with your nutritional plan. Chapter 4 gives you a list of recommendations for the staples you need at home. You can use these suggestions to make a shopping list that ensures that you purchase exactly what you need. To that list, add the perishables that you're going to use immediately, such as meat and poultry or fish, milk and other dairy products, and, of course, fruits and vegetables.

Eat something before you go shopping so that you aren't hungry as you walk down the aisles.

Most supermarkets are set up in the same way: like a huge menu to entice you. This setup is no accident, but is arranged to encourage you to buy. Unfortunately, what you buy on impulse is often the most kilocalorie-concentrated and expensive food that's least appropriate for your health. You find that all the perishable food is arranged around the perimeter of the supermarket. The high-kilocalorie foods are in the aisles in the middle of the shop. Unless you want to take the long way around, you're forced to pass through these aisles to get to the meat, milk, fruit, and vegetables. You pass the loose sweets, the biscuits, the high-sugar cereals, and all the other no-nos on the way. But, if you prepare a list and decide to stick firmly to it, so that you buy only from the list, you can avoid purchasing any of those bad-for-you foods. Walking into the supermarket hungry and without a list is dangerous both for your finances and your health.

Sometimes the larger supermarkets employ a person who is trained to help people with medical conditions avoid bad choices. Check with your super-market to find out if such a person is on staff, and spend some time touring the aisles with him or her. You're sure to pick up some valuable insights to help make your shopping choices easier.

Here are some keys pieces of advice on how to shop at the supermarket most effectively:

- ✔ Shop at the same supermarket each time.
- ✔ Shop as seldom as you can.
- ✔ Shop at the supermarket when it's not crowded.
- ✔ Don't walk down every aisle.
- ✔ Don't get tempted with free samples. They're usually high in kilocalories to appeal to your taste buds.
- ✔ Don't take your children along unless you have to, and if you do, make sure that they aren't hungry.
- ✔ Take care in the checkout lane, where supermarkets force you to run through a gauntlet of goodies – none of which are good for you.

Most supermarkets offer a variety of sections. Each one presents a different challenge and requires a different strategy. Try working your way around the shop so that you visit the healthiest sections first – choose lots of whole grains, fruits, vegetables, and salad stuff before moving on to the dairy and meat products, and try giving the fats and sweets a total miss. (Check out Chapter 2 for more about healthy eating.)

The supermarket isn't the only place to find good food. Check out your local farmer's market – especially the organic ones. Most areas have these markets, and many are open all year. Another option is to sign up for an organic box scheme, which delivers fresh fruit and vegetables directly to your door. Look out for specialty food shops that stock more exotic ingredients too.

The butcher

Look for low-fat cuts of meat. The best options for you are topside, sirloin, and flank steak. These cuts of meat are usually the leanest and are also very tasty. When buying minced meat (for home-made beefburgers, for example), consider how you plan to cook it. If you like meat cooked well done, you don't always have to choose the package with the lowest fat content, because you can cook out the fat and drain it off. Otherwise, look for lower-fat minced meat.

Try to buy skinless poultry to eliminate a major source of the fat in chicken. Or pull the skins off yourself. You need to cook skinless chicken for a shorter time, and you can barbecue it using an indirect method such as placing the coals along the sides of the chicken rather than underneath – this technique helps the meat stay juicier and helps prevent it from drying out.

Don't forget – lentils and other legumes (beans) provide protein too.

The baker

You can really make a dent in your diet in the bakery section, where all the desserts are on display. These foods usually contain too much fat and carbohydrate; however, you don't need to give up all your 'treats'. The key is to work a rich dessert into your meal plan, but only on an occasional basis. Remember to keep the portion small, in any case.

Muffins and pastries are traditionally high in fat, but in deference to the popular belief that fat makes us fat, shops now sell low-fat muffins and pastries. The problem is that these products still contain lots of kilocalories and carbohydrates, so don't overdo it. Try a smaller portion or share your muffin with a friend. A popular choice is angel food cake, but watch out: Even though it's totally fat-free, angel food cake is filled with kilocalories. You can enjoy a small portion, though.

Select wholegrain breads that have at least 2 grams of fibre per slice. Ensure that your muffins and rolls are wholegrain as well. Don't forget that individual buns are usually too large, so plan on eating a serving of half or less. (That goes for any bread.) If you eat too much, you consume too many kilocalories.

The greengrocer

Fruits, vegetables, and foods used in salads are so good for you that you should eat at least five servings per day – but make sure that each serving is different so you get plenty of variety. Although shops continue to offer the usual apples, pears, and bananas, more exotic fruits and vegetables are also now widely available. This area is where you can add some real variety to your diet. Try some of these new items, and you may discover that you can substitute them for the cakes, pies, and other concentrated kilocalorie foods that you now eat. For example, you may find that you like some of the new varieties of melons, which are sweet and have a great texture.

The other benefit to trying new fruits and vegetables is that you get a variety of vitamins and minerals from these different sources. Each differently coloured vegetable provides different nutrients, so aim for a rainbow of colour on your plate.

To prolong their season, you can freeze some of the fruit, especially the berries, and use as you need them.

Remember that dried fruits are a concentrated source of carbohydrate, so eat them sparingly.

Root vegetables need no refrigeration but you need to keep them in a cool, dry place. Store most other vegetables in the refrigerator – but eat them as fresh as possible as their nutrient content decreases the longer you store them.

The dairy

At the dairy counter, you can make some very positive diet modifications. Go for the lower fat items where possible – skimmed and semi-skimmed milk contains just as much calcium as full-fat milk (actually, a bit more) but wrapped in fewer kilocalories. Look for low-fat cheeses, yoghurt, and cottage cheese. You can even buy cheeses that aren't low fat if you use them sparingly.

The deli

A deli counter offers luncheon meats and prepared foods that often contain a lot of salt and fat. You want to avoid most of the foods in this area (with the exception of spit-roasted chicken, which is high in protein, low in fat and tasty too). Even the low-fat meats in this section are often rich in salt. Pickled foods also tend to contain a great deal of salt, even though they are low in kilocalories and free of fat.

If you choose salads from this area, pick out those that contain olive oil, or low-fat or fat-free dressing, instead of cream. If unsure, always ask deli assistants about the exact ingredients in these prepared foods and they can check labels for you.

The fishmonger

The fresh fish counter provides some good choices for your protein needs. Buy no more than a normal serving for each member of the family. Just because the fishmonger has cut a 340-gram (12-ounce) piece of swordfish doesn't mean that you have to buy the whole thing. You're entitled to buy just the piece you want. For convenience, you can get two servings at one time if you know you have the willpower to save the second serving for another meal. Ask the attendant to cut the fish in half so you aren't tempted to eat the whole thing.

Try to eat fish at least twice a week as it has positive effects on your blood fat balance. Remember that although oily fish such as salmon is especially good for you, it does add extra fat kilocalories, so serve with low-kilocalorie accompaniments such as a nice, large, mixed salad, or steamed greens.

The fresh fish counter usually offers breaded or battered fish to make your life easier, because you only have to put it in the oven, right? The problem is that the breading or batter often contains too much butter, fat, and salt. Ask the person serving you for a list of the ingredients in the breading or batter. Or better yet, skip the prepared fish and head for the fresh.

If you notice a very fishy smell, the fish isn't very fresh. Buy elsewhere.

Frozen foods and diet meals

When the season for your favourite fresh fruits and vegetables is over, the frozen food section may stock these items.

Food manufacturers produce a variety of frozen foods that you heat in the microwave oven. Although simple to prepare, these meals are often high in fat and salt. Always read the food label, as shown in the later section 'Deciphering the Mysterious Food Label'. Avoid frozen foods that have cream or cheese sauces.

Diet meals are a good option if you want to save time in preparation. Frozen diet meals are low in kilocalories and often low in salt and fat as well. Most diet meals have no more than 350 kilocalories and usually taste good. If you have type 1 diabetes and need to count carbohydrates, they're listed on the box.

Healthy Choice, Lean Cuisine, Weight Watchers, and Boots, for example, manufacture low-kilocalorie diet meals that taste good. Supermarkets usually have several brands on sale, including their own range, so you can choose the least expensive and the lowest in salt when you shop.

Are frozen diet foods a good option for you? Many people complain that they lack the time to prepare the 'right' foods. For these people, diet ready-meals work very well. However, for someone who likes to involve him or herself in food preparation – for example, people who bought this book for the wonderful recipes – this approach is not the way to go.

Low-glycaemic index foods are also available from many food manufacturers. Chapter 2 discusses how these foods can fit into your nutrition plan.

Canned and bottled foods

Canned and bottled foods are often healthy and can help you quickly make recipes calling for ingredients such as tomato sauce. Check the Nutrition Information label (see the later section 'Deciphering the Mysterious Food Label') to determine the kind of liquid in which a food is canned. Oil adds a lot of fat kilocalories, so look for the same food canned in water if possible – but avoid those canned in brine or syrup. Brine adds too much salt and syrup too much sugar.

Canned vegetables often contain too much salt, so look for low-salt varieties. Canned fruits often contain too much sweetener, so you're better off with fresh if possible.

Watch for this marketing trick: Supermarkets often display high-price canned foods at eye level and low-price products on lower shelves. Also remember that shops' own brands are often less expensive and just as good as name brands.

Bottled foods include fruit juice drinks, which are high in sugar and low in nutrition. You're better off drinking a small glass of pure fruit juice rather than a sweetened juice drink diluted with other artificial ingredients.

The same principle is true for bottled and canned fizzy drinks, which have no nutritional value and lots of kilocalories. Substitute water for this expensive and basically worthless food that really doesn't quench your thirst (soft drinks often leave an aftertaste, especially the diet drinks). Try adding a squeeze of fresh lemon or lime to a glass of sparkling water.

You can find low-fat or fat-free salad dressing and mayonnaise in this area. Better yet, try using mustard and some of the other condiments to spice up your salads without adding many kilocalories.

The best options for snacks

You probably frequently feel like eating a little something between meals. Your choice of foods may make the difference between weight gain and weight control, and between high blood glucose levels and normal levels. Here are the best selections to choose as you make your way around the supermarket:

- ✔ **Baked crisps:** Avoid fried crisps, which add lots of fat kilocalories. Even 30 grams (1 ounce) of baked crisps amounts to 110 kilocalories.

- ✔ **Flavoured rice cakes:** These items are filling without many kilocalories.

- ✔ **Fruit and fig bars:** These items can satisfy hunger without adding too many kilocalories.

- ✔ **Low-fat muesli:** Watch out for regular muesli, which is high in kilocalories. Depending on the brand, a small serving of low-fat muesli contains 220 to 250 kilocalories.

- ✔ **Plain popcorn:** If you prepare plain popcorn in a microwave oven, a 10 gram (⅓ ounce) serving contains only 38 kilocalories and is free from salt and fat.

- ✔ **Raisins and other dried fruit:** Stick to small portions. Thirty grams (1 ounce) of raisins is only 90 kilocalories – look for packs of miniature boxes.

The preceding list should give you enough options to satisfy your hunger without wrecking your diabetic control.

Deciphering the Mysterious Food Label

Most packaged foods have a food label known as the Nutrition Information label, which isn't really mysterious if you know how to interpret it. Figure 5-1 shows a typical food label.

The little 'g' after each amount means grams, 'kj' stands for kilojoules (you can safely ignore these), and 'kcal' is short for kilocalories.

NUTRITION INFORMATION		
Typical values	Per 100g	Per serving (207g)
ENERGY	309 kj 73 kcal	640 kj 151 kcal
PROTEIN	4.9 g	10.0 g
CARBOHYDRATE of which sugars	12.9 g 5.0 g	26.7 g 10.4 g
FAT of which saturates	0.2 g 0.1 g	0.4 g 0.2 g
FIBRE	3.8 g	7.9 g
SODIUM	0.3 g	0.7 g
SALT EQUIVALENT	0.8 g	1.7 g

Figure 5-1:
A Nutrition Information food label.

The label in Figure 5-1 is from a 415-gram (14.5-ounce) tin of baked beans. You can see the following information on the label: values for energy, protein, carbohydrate, fat, fibre, and sodium per 100 grams and values per serving (in this case, 207 grams or 7.25 ounces). Values per 100 grams are useful for comparing different labels to see which is the most healthy. Values per serving are useful for planning your personal nutritional intake.

> ✔ **Serving size:** Note that the serving size is probably not the same as an exchange (see Chapter 2 for an explanation of exchanges, and check out Appendix B for a comprehensive list). The serving size on this food label is 207 grams (7.25 ounces), but an exchange of baked beans is 65 grams (2.3 ounces) (which you can find in the 'Starch Exchanges' list in Appendix B). Therefore, one serving is around three exchanges. You may need to eat less than the suggested serving size on the tin to fit this amount into your daily nutrition plan.

At 415 grams, this tin of baked beans holds two servings. If you use the exchange list serving size of 65 grams, this tin contains over six exchanges.

✔ **Energy:** These numbers show the amount of energy in a serving, given as both kilojoules (you can ignore these) and kilocalories – in this case, 151 kilocalories.

✔ **Protein:** As a person with diabetes, knowing the grams of protein in a portion is important, because some is converted into glucose in your body.

✔ **Total carbohydrate:** As a person with diabetes, you definitely need to know the grams of carbohydrate in a serving, to fit it into your nutritional plan and determine your insulin needs if you use insulin.

✔ **Sugars:** The 10.4 grams of the 26.7 grams of carbohydrate that comes from sugar are rapidly absorbed into your circulation.

✔ **Fat:** These beans are low in fat, providing just 1.2 grams per 100 grams, or 2.4 grams of fat per serving. Half this amount is in the form of saturated fat (saturates).

✔ **Fibre:** These beans provide 7.9 grams of fibre per serving, which is a good amount.

✔ **Sodium:** At 0.7 grams of sodium per serving – equivalent to 1.7 grams of salt – these beans provide almost a third of the recommended maximum intake of no more than 6 grams of salt per day (and preferably less).

Calculating Exchanges from the Food Label

The Nutrition Information label doesn't provide information about the diabetic exchanges that make up the food. To determine the exchange value of a food (see Chapter 2 for more details on exchanges), follow these guidelines:

✔ If the food is mostly carbohydrate (cereals, grains, pasta, bread, dried beans, peas, and lentils), divide the grams of carbohydrate by 15, because each starch exchange contains 15 grams of carbohydrate. Remember that starch exchanges also contain 3 grams of protein. A fruit exchange also contains 15 grams of carbohydrate but no fat or protein.

✔ If the food is mostly protein (meat and meat substitutes), divide the grams of protein by 7, because each meat exchange contains 7 grams of protein. Remember that an exchange is a lean-meat exchange if it contains 3 grams or less of fat, a medium-fat meat exchange if it contains 4 to 5 grams of fat, and a high-fat meat exchange if it contains 8 or more grams of fat.

✔ If the food is mostly fat (avocado, cream, butter, nuts, and seeds), divide the grams of fat by 5 to calculate the fat exchanges.

✔ Milk exchanges contain 12 grams of carbohydrate, 8 grams of protein, and a variable number of grams of fat – 0 grams in the case of skimmed milk or non-fat yoghurt, 5 grams for semi-skimmed milk (2 per cent milk or plain low-fat yoghurt), and 8 grams for whole milk.

✔ Vegetable exchanges contain 5 grams of carbohydrate and 2 grams of protein per exchange.

Calculating the exchanges in food with several energy sources can get complicated, so get some help from your dietitian.

The best way to verify that your trip to the supermarket is a success is to evaluate the contents of your carrier bags. The division of the contents need to look similar to the food plate diagram in Chapter 1.

Part II
Healthy Recipes That Taste Great

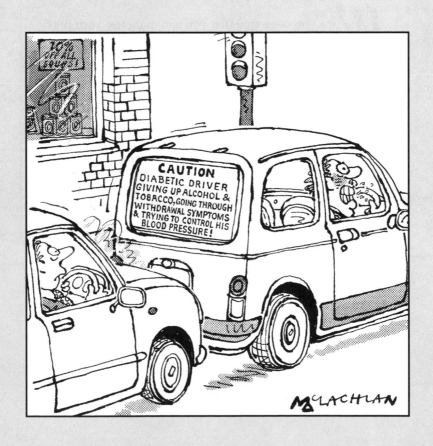

In this part . . .

When you were told that you had diabetes, your first impression probably was that you were doomed to bland, uninteresting food for the rest of your life. This part shows you that impression could not be more wrong. Starting with your breakfast and working through the day with lunch, snacks, main courses, desserts, and more, your food can be just as exciting, exotic, and full of taste as it always was, perhaps even more so.

You can choose from simple recipes, requiring few ingredients, or take it to the next level by trying recipes with more ingredients. We guarantee that all will be delicious, because we've tested all of them to make sure that you will enjoy them and can cook them yourself.

Chapter 6

Enjoying the Benefits of Breakfast

In This Chapter

▶ Updating classic breakfast mainstays

▶ Baking muffins and soda bread

▶ Munching delicious muesli

▶ Making the most of eggs

*E*ating regularly is a big part of keeping your blood sugar steady. Typically, the longest break without food occurs at night. While your body rests and revitalises itself, your blood glucose level takes a nosedive. Start the right way with a healthy, balanced breakfast each and every day. Never skip this important meal. Choose a quick scrambled egg and wholemeal toast if you're in a hurry. But for a change of pace, brush up on the recipes in this chapter. Planning ahead means breakfasts are delicious and never boring.

Balancing Your Breakfast

Breakfast is a critical meal for someone with diabetes. Getting your day off to a steady, balanced start sets you up successfully for the rest of the day. Check out Chapter 4 to help you plan your meals for the day based on your individual needs. The following sections help you to make the right breakfast choices.

Figuring out which fruit is right for you

Fruit isn't a dirty word when you have diabetes. Although fruit is full of natural sugar, much of that sugar is in the form of fructose, which has minimal impact on your blood glucose levels. Fruit is also rich in anti-ageing, antioxidant nutrients.

Select the whole fruit rather than the juice because the fibre in whole fruit slows down the digestion of fruit, resulting in a more gradual rise in your blood sugar level.

Here's a list of fruits with a lower glycaemic index (see Chapter 2 for more details about glycaemic index values):

- Apples
- Apricots
- Blueberries
- Cherries
- Grapefruit
- Kiwis
- Strawberries

And just for balance, here are a few fruits with a higher glycaemic index:

- Cantaloupe melon
- Dates
- Pineapple
- Raisins
- Watermelon

Just because a fruit has a higher glycaemic index doesn't mean that you can't eat it. Just take the higher GI value into consideration when deciding at what time of the day to eat that fruit and what you eat with it.

Putting together protein-packed punches

Eggs aren't the only breakfast protein, but do check out the 'Enjoying Egg-ceptional Dishes' section, later in this chapter, for smart ways to include eggs at breakfast. Consider other non-traditional options too. Here's a list of protein-rich foods that may make a good addition to your breakfast table:

- 1 slice of lean ham wrapped in a wholemeal tortilla or pitta bread
- Smoked mackerel or sardines on wholemeal toast
- 2 tablespoons of peanut butter on wholemeal toast
- 1 slice of ham wrapped around low-fat 'string' cheese
- Grilled, lean bacon with grilled tomatoes and mushrooms
- Small carton of low-fat cottage cheese with pineapple or chopped cherry tomatoes

Starting with Familiar Favourites

When you're told that you have diabetes, you may think that your days of eating toast and marmalade or a classic British fry-up are over. Although starting every day by downing white toast dripping with butter and very sugary marmalade isn't a good idea, you can still enjoy variations on old familiar themes, such as using brown bread, a healthy spread and selecting a high fruit (low sugar) conserve.

Skip the butter because the following recipes are delicious without it. If you don't feel like going totally without butter, look for low-fat spreads such as those made with olive oil that contain no partially hydrogenated (trans) fats.

What's so great about whole grains?

Refined grains are processed to remove the bran and the hull, and along with them, up to 90 per cent of the nutrients, including vitamins E and B. Whole grains have a lower glycaemic index than refined grains. So whole grains are less likely to send your blood glucose soaring and then dipping. The protein, fat, and fibre in whole grains slow their absorption into the bloodstream. In addition, whole grains make you feel fuller and stay fuller for longer.

Read labels carefully to ensure that the food you're getting is made from whole grains. Don't just look for 'wheat' bread; make sure that it says 'wholewheat' or 'wholemeal'. Some manufacturers add caramel colour or molasses to refined flour and sell the bread as 'wheat bread', potentially confusing hopeful healthy eaters.

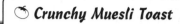 **Crunchy Muesli Toast**

Here's the crunchy cousin to French toast. The sweetness of the muesli makes honey or jam unnecessary. If you really need extra sweetness, try topping it with a ripe, sliced banana.

Preparation time: *5 minutes*

Cooking time: *6 minutes*

Serves: *4*

2 egg whites, lightly beaten	*100 grams low-fat muesli, crushed*
150 millilitres skimmed milk	*8 thin slices wholewheat or multigrain bread*
1 teaspoon grated orange zest	*1 tablespoon unsalted butter*
1 teaspoon vanilla extract	

1 In a bowl, whisk the egg whites, milk, orange zest, and vanilla extract until blended.

2 Place the muesli in another bowl. Dip each slice of bread into the egg mixture and then into the muesli.

3 Melt a quarter of the butter in a large frying pan over a medium heat. Place 2 coated bread slices in the pan; cook for approximately 3 minutes. Turn and cook on the other side until golden brown, for approximately 3 minutes.

4 Prepare the remaining bread slices in the same manner.

Per serving: *Kilocalories 254; Fat 6g (Saturated 2g); Cholesterol 10mg; Sodium 343mg; Carbohydrate 39g; Dietary Fibre 2g; Protein 11g.*

Exchanges: *2½ starch, 1 fat.*

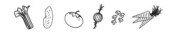

☙ *Wholemeal Waffles*

This recipe is reason alone to invest in a waffle maker. Look for one with nonstick coating for easy waffle removal. Make sure that you let the batter rest for the full 1½ hours before making the waffles. You get waffles with a much lighter texture and better flavour as a result.

Preparation time: *90 minutes*

Cooking time: *4 minutes per waffle*

Serves: *4*

240 millilitres 'light' evaporated milk

1 teaspoon active dry yeast

120 grams wholemeal flour

Grated zest of 1 orange

Drop of vanilla extract

4 teaspoons granular Splenda sweetener

Nonstick cooking spray

1 Warm the milk and dissolve the yeast in it. In a bowl, mix the yeast mixture with the flour, orange zest, vanilla, and Splenda granular sweetener. Let the mixture sit, covered, at room temperature for 1½ hours.

2 Using a waffle maker coated with nonstick cooking spray, prepare the waffles, following the manufacturer's instructions.

Tip: *Instead of syrup, serve these beauties with Warm Pineapple Salsa, using the recipe in Chapter 7.*

Per serving: *Kilocalories 157; Fat 1g (Saturated 0g); Cholesterol 3mg; Sodium 76mg; Carbohydrate 26g; Dietary Fibre 4g; Protein 9g.*

Exchanges: *1½ starch, ½ milk.*

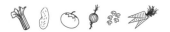

🍒 Blueberry and Almond Pancakes

Blueberries are one of the best sources of antioxidants compared with most other fruits. Almonds are also one the best nut sources of the antioxidant, vitamin E. Enjoy these tasty fruit and crunchy nuts in this breakfast favourite.

Preparation time: *10 minutes*

Cooking time: *5 to 7 minutes*

Serves: *4 (total 16 pancakes)*

125 grams plain flour

90 grams wholewheat flour

2 teaspoons apple juice concentrate

2 teaspoons baking powder

Pinch of salt (optional)

1½ teaspoons unsweetened apple sauce

300 millilitres low-fat milk

Drop of almond extract

3 egg whites

110 grams fresh blueberries, or frozen berries, thawed

1 tablespoon almond flakes, crushed

Nonstick cooking spray

1 In a bowl, combine the plain flour, wholewheat flour, apple juice concentrate, baking powder, and salt (if desired), and set aside.

2 In another bowl, combine the apple sauce, milk, almond extract, egg whites, blueberries, and almonds, and stir well. Add the flour mixture. Stir until you achieve a fairly smooth batter consistency, for approximately 2 minutes. Feel free to leave a few lumps, because over-mixing can result in a tougher finished pancake.

3 Coat a large frying pan with the cooking spray, and place over a medium heat until hot. Spoon in a small ladleful of batter for each pancake. When bubbles form on top of the pancakes, turn them over. Cook until the bottom of each pancake is golden brown.

Per serving: *Kilocalories 209; Fat 2g (Saturated 1g); Cholesterol 3 mg; Sodium 419mg; Carbohydrate 34g; Dietary Fibre 4g; Protein 10g.*

Exchanges: *2½ starch, ½ fat.*

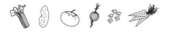

⚘ Blueberry Porridge

This recipe makes any morning special. Just as quick as 'regular' porridge, the added fresh blueberries give your antioxidant levels a boost and your taste buds a treat. If fresh blueberries aren't in season, you can substitute frozen. Choose blueberries that are frozen without additional sugars, and thaw them before adding to your oats.

Preparation time: *5 minutes*

Cooking time: *3 minutes*

Serves: *2*

40 grams rolled oats

480 millilitres water

2 teaspoons honey

145 grams fresh blueberries

1 In a microwave-safe bowl, combine the oats and water. Microwave on high for 3 minutes. Or, make in a saucepan according to the instructions on the packet.

2 Remove the bowl from the microwave and stir in the honey and then the blueberries.

Per serving: Kilocalories 218; Fat 3g (Saturated 0g); Cholesterol 0mg; Sodium 6mg; Carbohydrate 37g; Dietary Fibre 6g; Protein 7g.

Exchanges: 2 starch, 1 fruit.

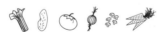

Stocking Up on Baked Goods

Having diabetes doesn't mean that you have to deprive yourself of the ease (and deliciousness!) of grabbing a muffin, or a quick slice of brown bread. Plan ahead and keep some healthy-heart options available for breakfast on the go.

Using a blend of plain (white) flour and wholemeal flour helps you ease into whole grains if you're not used to them. For information on the benefits of using whole grains in a healthy diet, check the earlier sidebar 'What's so great about whole grains?'.

☼ Irish Soda Bread

This traditional Irish breakfast bread is quick and easy to make, and is delicious served warm from the oven. You can also toast it. Spread with a little olive-oil based spread and high fruit, low sugar jam or marmalade. You can even drizzle it with olive oil and eat with cheese or ham for a more continental start to your day.

Preparation time: *15 minutes*

Cooking time: *45 minutes*

Serves: *8*

225 grams plain white flour
225 grams wholemeal flour
1 level teaspoon salt

1 level teaspoon bread soda
350 to 400 millilitres buttermilk, to mix

1 Preheat the oven to 230°C/450°F/Gas Mark 8.

2 Sieve the flour, salt, and soda into a bowl.

3 Make a 'well' in the middle and pour in most of the buttermilk. Mix in the flour from the sides, adding more milk if necessary to produce a soft dough that is not too wet and sticky.

4 Turn out onto a floured work surface. Pat the dough into a round about 3cm thick. Cut a deep cross into the top of the bread.

5 Bake in the hot oven for 15 minutes, then turn the temperature down to 200°C/400°F/Gas Mark 6 for a further 30 minutes or until the bread is cooked.

Tip: *Tap the bottom of the bread. It will sound hollow if cooked.*

Per serving: Kilocalories 201; Fat 1.5 g (Saturated 0.5 g); Cholesterol 1 mg; Sodium 412 mg; Carbohydrate 42 g; Dietary Fibre 3.5 g; Protein 8 g.

Exchanges: 3 starch.

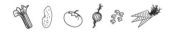

Carrot–Pineapple Muffins

The orange colour of carrots means that they're rich in carotenoids, which are powerful antioxidants. The body also converts some of these carotenoids, such as betacarotene, into vitamin A, which is essential for skin and eye health.

Preparation time: *10 minutes*

Cooking time: *20 to 25 minutes*

Makes: *16 muffins*

190 grams plain flour
180 grams wholemeal flour
1 teaspoon salt
150 grams sugar
2 teaspoons cinnamon
2 teaspoons baking soda
2 teaspoons baking powder
220 grams grated carrots
320 millilitres apple sauce
250 grams pineapple chunks (packed in own juice), including juice
8 egg whites
2 teaspoons vanilla extract
Nonstick cooking spray

1 Preheat the oven to 190°C/375°F/Gas Mark 5.

2 In a bowl, combine the plain flour, wholemeal flour, salt, sugar, cinnamon, baking soda, and baking powder. Mix well.

3 In another bowl, combine the carrots, apple sauce, pineapple, egg whites, and vanilla. Mix well.

4 Mix the flour mixture into the carrot mixture.

5 Coat muffin tins with nonstick cooking spray.

6 Spoon the mixture into the muffin tins, filling each two-thirds full. Bake for 20 to 25 minutes. To test whether they're done, insert a toothpick in the centre of one muffin (preferably one in the centre of the tray). When the toothpick comes out clean, the muffins are done.

Tip: *Use granular Splenda or fructose in place of sugar for a lower glycaemic index. For example, 28 grams of sugar is equivalent to 2 tablespoons of granular Splenda. Fructose is sweeter, so you generally use one-third less and cook at a lower temperature – always read on-pack conversion and cooking instructions for alternative sweeteners.*

Per serving (1 muffin): *Kilocalories 151; Fat 0g (Saturated 0g); Cholesterol 0mg; Sodium 384mg; Carbohydrate 30g; Dietary Fibre 3g; Protein 5g.*

Exchanges: *2 starch.*

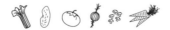

Musing Over Muesli

Muesli is a great way to start your day. It's full of healthy wholegrains but bought versions often have added sugar, milk powder, salt, and other unwanted ingredients. Select those that consist purely of unsweetened grains, nuts and dried fruit – or make your own. Here are a couple of recipes to get your taste buds going.

○ Traditional Muesli

This version includes apricots which are another one of those 'good for the eyes' foods as they are rich in carotenoids – especially betacarotene. They also supply dietary fibre, and a delicious flavour too.

Preparation time: *20 minutes*

Serves: *10*

100 grams rolled oats

100 grams toasted wheat flakes

100 grams bran flakes

100 grams dried apricots, chopped

50 grams walnuts, chopped

50 grams mixed seeds (sunflower, pumpkin, sesame)

1 Mix together all the ingredients and store in an air-tight container.

2 Shake well before weighing out each serving as the small seeds will tend to settle.

3 Serve with semi-skimmed or skimmed milk.

Tip: *It's easy to change this recipe and add other ingredients such as hazelnuts, macadamias, or pecans, plus different dried fruits such as raisins, cranberries, or even dried coconut. You can also top the muesli mix with fresh, chopped fruit for extra vitamins, minerals, antioxidants, and fibre. Try bananas, raspberries, strawberries, blueberries, nectarines – whatever is in season.*

Per serving: *Kilocalories 187; Fat 7.5g (Saturated 1g); Cholesterol 0 mg; Sodium 110mg; Carbohydrate 26g; Dietary Fibre 4.5g; Protein 6g.*

Exchanges: *2 starch, 1½ fat.*

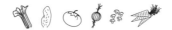

☞ *Swiss Bircher Muesli*

This style of muesli was originally invented by a naturopath, Dr Bircher, at his diet clinic in Zurich, during the 1880s. It's still one of the healthiest ways to breakfast – although his original recipe used sweetened, condensed milk. Bircher muesli contains grated apple, and apple juice, which are rich in a class of antioxidant called flavonoids. These help to protect against heart disease and asthma – suggesting that an apple a day really can keep the doctor away. Try varying the amount of juice you add to produce a thicker or thinner style of muesli if you want.

Preparation time: *10 minutes*

Serves: *4*

Dessert apple, grated	*200 millilitres unsweetened apple juice*
Juice and zest of one lemon	*4 tablespoons low-fat natural bio yoghurt*
100 grams rolled oats	*2 tablespoons raisins*

1 Remove the core and grate the apple into a bowl containing the lemon juice and zest to help stop it discolouring.

2 Add all the remaining ingredients and mix well.

3 Leave it in the fridge for at least 30 minutes until it is ready to eat. You can make it the night before and eat it the next morning, if you want.

Per serving: *Kilocalories 188; Fat 2.5g (Saturated 0.2g); Cholesterol 1.5mg; Sodium 51mg; Carbohydrate 38g; Dietary Fibre 2.5g; Protein 6g.*

Exchanges: *2½ starch, ½ fat.*

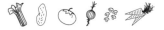

Enjoying Egg-ceptional Dishes

Choosing eggs gives you a protein power punch to start your day. This simple food is an ideal source of protein, containing all the essential amino acids. Eggs are also a source of B complex vitamins, vitamins A, D, and E, selenium, and zinc. Although egg yolks also contain a significant amount of cholesterol, select omega-3 enriched eggs for healthy benefits for your heart.

Facing facts about feta cheese

If you don't know this terrific Greek cheese, here's your chance to meet it. Feta cheese is a soft, salty cheese with a tangy bite. It crumbles easily, and is a great addition to salads, eggs, or stuffed in olives. The commercially available variety is made from cows' milk and sold in small squares. Find feta cheese in the gourmet or specialty cheese section of your local supermarket.

One of the best things about feta is its strong flavour. A little goes a long way. So if you're looking for flavour but don't want to weigh down your food with lots of cheese and fat, feta's a good choice. Look for flavoured feta cheese for a change of pace, blended with sun-dried tomatoes and basil, or peppercorns.

☜ Baked Eggy Tomatoes

Tomatoes are an excellent source of a red antioxidant pigment called lycopene. As well as being good for the eyes and heart, lycopene has been shown to protect against some forms of cancer. Cooking tomatoes releases even more lycopene to increase the amount your body can absorb. Here, tomatoes are teamed up with omega-3 enriched eggs. Serve with warm Irish Soda Bread (see earlier in this chapter) or on toast.

Preparation time: 15 minutes

Cooking time: 15 minutes

Serves: 4

6 large, firm tomatoes	Spring onion, chopped
4 omega-3 enriched eggs	Garlic clove, crushed
Freshly ground black pepper	Handful chopped parsley

1 Preheat the oven to 180°C/350°F/Gas Mark 4.

2 Cut lids off the top of 4 tomatoes, and set aside. Scoop out the interiors of each tomato and reserve separately.

3 Carefully break an egg into each hollowed tomato shell. Season with black pepper, replace the tomato lid, and bake for 15 minutes.

4 Meanwhile, finely chop the tomato insides and the 2 remaining whole tomatoes. Place in a saucepan with the spring onion and garlic, and simmer gently for 10 minutes to make a tomato sauce. Season with black pepper to taste.

5 Serve each eggy tomato with some of the sauce drizzled over. Garnish with freshly chopped parsley.

Per serving: *Kilocalories 126; Fat 7.5g (Saturated 2g); Cholesterol 234mg; Sodium 105mg; Carbohydrate 7g; Dietary Fibre 2.5g; Protein 10g.*

Exchanges: *1 protein, 1½ fat, 1 vegetable.*

🍅 Greek Omelette

You can get creative with this recipe. The essential Greek ingredients are the feta and spinach. But add any vegetables you like – the more the better! Good choices include artichoke hearts, red peppers, onions, courgettes, or asparagus. Just throw them in at Step 2 and cook them until they're tender. Enjoy!

Preparation time: *5 minutes*

Cooking time: *10 minutes*

Serves: *2*

Nonstick cooking spray

75 grams diced green peppers

35 grams sliced mushrooms

Pinch of dried marjoram, crumbled

150 grams chopped spinach

2 whole eggs

4 egg whites

75 grams crumbled feta cheese

Small plum tomato, seeded and chopped

1 Coat a large frying pan with the cooking spray and place over a medium heat. Sauté the peppers, mushrooms, and marjoram until the vegetables are tender – for approximately 6 minutes. Add the spinach and cook until wilted (roughly 4 minutes).

2 In a bowl, mix together the eggs and egg whites. Pour the egg mixture over the spinach mixture in the pan. Cook over a low heat, stirring occasionally until the eggs are almost cooked. Top with the feta cheese and tomato and cover until the eggs are puffy (approximately 5 minutes). Fold the omelette in half and serve.

Per serving: *Kilocalories 230; Fat 13g (Saturated 7g); Cholesterol 246mg; Sodium 607mg; Carbohydrate 6g; Dietary Fibre 2g; Protein 20g.*

Exchanges: *3 medium-fat meat, 1 vegetable.*

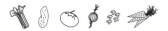

Chapter 7

Starting Well: Hors d'Oeuvres and First Courses

Appetisers help to stimulate your appetite and prepare you for the meal ahead. But for someone with diabetes, they also help you to squeeze in a quick nutritious bite, keeping your blood glucose levels stable until the main event. Healthy appetisers are the best way to get you started on a great eating path for the evening.

This chapter gives you many great options for healthy eats, whether you're having a party, an intimate dinner with friends, or a casual night in with the family. Look here for enticing new ways to enjoy seafood as a first course, and for terrific salsas – no, not the Spanish dance, but the spicy Mexican sauce – complete with tips for creating your own varieties. We also include a great selection of dips and dippers. This chapter contains lots of recipe ideas for you to enjoy, and shows that you don't need to skimp on taste: Just remember to choose appropriate portion sizes and pace yourself.

Appetising Seafood Starters

Most people don't get enough seafood in their diet. Rich in omega-3 fatty acids, protein, calcium, and many other nutrients, seafood is an excellent part of any well-rounded (or at least nicely-proportioned) diet. This delectable food is lower in cholesterol than beef and chicken and has so many varied flavours and textures that you can't get bored with it.

If your experience of seafood is limited to fish sticks or battered cod, here are some great ideas for getting you going with seafood appetisers. You can experiment with new flavours without committing yourself to a full seafood meal. Take a look at Chapter 12 for even more taste-tempting seafood recipes.

Sizing up shellfish

Shellfish, such as scallops and prawns, are sold according to weight and size. Make friends with a local fishmonger who can advise you on the best seasonal buys.

Always clean prawns properly before cooking them. If you buy prawns from a supermarket, the head is often already gone but they're probably not *deveined,* which means that the dark 'vein' running down the back of the tail is still present. This vein-like object is actually the prawn's intestinal tract, so it really needs removing before you start cooking. Using a sharp knife, run it along the back of the prawn to open it up so you can remove the 'vein'. Or, if you can find one, use a shrimp deveiner, which cracks the shell and removes the vein in one easy step. You can buy these online via the Internet. Then rinse the prawn in cool water. Check out Figure 7-1 to see the deveining process.

Cleaning and Deveining Shrimp

Figure 7-1:
You can use a special tool to clean and de-vein prawns safely and properly.

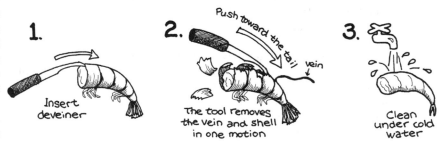

The following recipes are delicious ways to include shellfish in appetisers.

Prawn Quesadillas

This recipe puts a nice twist on a classic Mexican dish. Although shellfish contain some cholesterol, they're low in total and saturated fat – a great alternative to high-fat meats.

Preparation time: *15 minutes*

Cooking time: *10 minutes*

Serves: *4*

80 grams low-fat natural yoghurt

2 medium plum tomatoes, seeded and chopped

Nonstick cooking spray

4 × 25 centimetre (1½ × 10 inch) diameter wholewheat tortillas

450 grams prawns, cooked

2 teaspoons fresh coriander or parsley, chopped

120 grams grated Monterey Jack or mozzarella cheese

1 In a small bowl, combine the yoghurt and tomatoes. Set aside.

2 Coat a large frying pan with the cooking spray. Place the pan over a medium heat until hot. Add one tortilla to the pan. Top the tortilla with half of the prawns, 1 teaspoon of the chopped coriander, and half of the grated cheese. Place a second tortilla on top of the mixture. Cook the quesadilla until the cheese begins to melt and the bottom tortilla becomes golden brown. Flip the quesadilla over, and continue to cook until the cheese is fully melted and the tortillas are lightly browned. Remove from the pan and place on a chopping board.

3 Repeat Step 2 with the remaining tortillas, prawns, coriander, and cheese.

4 Slice each quesadilla into 6 pieces. Place 3 pieces and a quarter of the tomato mixture onto each of 4 plates.

Per serving: *Kilocalories 364; Fat 13g (Saturated 6g); Cholesterol 204mg; Sodium 1,653mg; Carbohydrate 27g; Dietary Fibre 6g; Protein 29g.*

Exchanges: *2 starch, 1 high-fat meat, 3 very lean meat.*

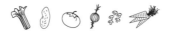

Crab Puffs

Crab puffs are an ideal finger food for parties. For this recipe, use the best quality Parmesan cheese you can find – its strong flavour is a terrific complement to the delicate crab and artichoke without adding many kilocalories or much fat. If you're a fan of spicy food, feel free to bump up the horseradish in this recipe for a sinus-clearing experience.

Preparation time: *20 minutes*

Cooking time: *6 to 7 minutes*

Serves: *6 (4 pieces each)*

3 tablespoons freshly grated Parmesan cheese

400-gram can artichoke hearts, drained and chopped

225 grams picked crabmeat

1 egg white

60 millilitres low-fat sour cream

60 millilitres low-fat mayonnaise

1 teaspoon fresh squeezed lemon juice

1 teaspoon prepared horseradish

½ teaspoon Worcestershire sauce

Small garlic clove, crushed

3 muffins, halved

1 Preheat the grill.

2 In a small bowl, reserve 2 tablespoons of the Parmesan cheese. In a medium bowl, combine the remaining 1 tablespoon of Parmesan cheese, the chopped artichokes, crabmeat, egg white, sour cream, mayonnaise, lemon juice, horseradish, Worcestershire sauce, and garlic.

3 Place the muffin halves on a baking tray and spread the crab mixture equally onto each muffin. Sprinkle the reserved Parmesan cheese on top.

4 Place the pan in the freezer for 10 minutes, or until the crab mixture holds its form.

5 Remove the pan from the freezer and place the pan under the grill for 6 to 7 minutes, or until the muffin topping is lightly browned and bubbling. Cut each muffin into quarters.

Per serving: *Kilocalories 180; Fat 5g (Saturated 2g); Cholesterol 41mg; Sodium 536mg; Carbohydrate 19g; Dietary Fibre 1g; Protein 13g.*

Exchanges: *1 starch, 1½ very lean meat, 1 fat.*

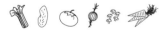

Putting a new twist on seafood favourites

If you love the taste of classic seafood appetisers, you're in luck – updating these dishes is a snap, as shown in the following recipe for Salmon Mousse.

Prawn cocktail is an easy classic seafood appetiser. Don't settle for the bland, mushy, pre-cooked cocktail prawns at the seafood counter. Make your own quickly and easily. Bring water to a gentle boil in a saucepan. Add generous amounts of seasonings such as ground black pepper and chopped herbs. Drop in some fresh prawns and cook for just a few minutes, until the tails curl and the prawns become opaque: Take care not to overcook them. Serve with a low-fat, cocktail sauce.

If you want to pre-peel prawns for your guests, do so just after cooking them, when they're cool enough to handle. Make sure that you wash your hands well and then use your sharp knife or handy de-veining tool (as shown in Figure 7-1) to clean them.

Salmon Mousse

In this recipe, the 1960s classic hostess mousse gets a 21st-century update. Vary your spices to change the flavour profile: Substitute coriander and red pepper flakes for the paprika and dill, or throw in a little prepared horseradish to kick up the spice quotient. Choose a fun silicon mould (such as a fish or shamrock) or look for more sophisticated mini-moulds to make individual portions of this great starter. If you use metal or glass moulds, dip them in warm water for a minute or so before removing the mousse from the mould, to help them come out easily.

Preparation time: *10 minutes, plus 3 to 4 hours chilling time*

Serves: *8*

1 tablespoon unflavoured gelatin	*425-gram can red salmon, drained*
2 tablespoons lemon juice	*Pinch of paprika*
1 slice of onion	*Handful chopped fresh dill*
120 millilitres boiling water	*240 millilitres low-fat sour cream*
120 millilitres mayonnaise	

1 In a food processor, combine the gelatin, lemon juice, onion, and water. Blend for 45 seconds.

2 Add the mayonnaise, salmon, paprika, and dill, and blend until smooth (approximately 45 seconds).

3 Add the sour cream and blend. Pour the mixture into a mould or loaf tin. Refrigerate until set (approximately 3 to 4 hours).

Per serving: *Kilocalories 213; Fat 18g (Saturated 4g); Cholesterol 45mg; Sodium 293mg; Carbohydrate 5g; Dietary Fibre 0g; Protein 11g.*

Exchanges: *1½ lean meat, 3 fat, ½ milk.*

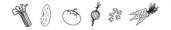

Savouring Salsas

Salsa is a tasty Mexican treat that's easy to fall in love with. Most shop-bought versions contain too much sugar and vinegar, and aren't nearly as good as the home-made variety, so why not create your own? Although *salsa* simply means 'sauce', these salsa recipes taste anything but simple.

Stocking essentials for scrumptious salsas

Add the standard salsa seasonings to any healthy grains or legumes for a tasty and nutritious treat anytime. Try flavouring cooked brown rice, quinoa, or cooked beans with any of these tasty additions:

- Coriander leaf
- Garlic
- Lime or lemon juice
- Onions
- Peppers (especially spicy jalapeños and other types of chilli)
- Tomatoes

Check out the following salsa recipes, which use these delicious ingredients.

Lentil Salsa

This recipe includes high-fibre lentils with such tasty ingredients that you hardly notice you're eating healthily. Serve this salsa with wholegrain crackers or thick slices of red pepper.

Preparation time: 15 minutes

Cooking time: 35 to 40 minutes

Serves: 6

450g brown lentils	½ green pepper, seeded and chopped
1 litre low-sodium chicken broth	Small carrot, peeled and chopped
Bay leaf	1 teaspoon chopped fresh garlic
2 tablespoons olive oil	2 tablespoons chopped fresh parsley
½ small red onion, chopped	1 tablespoon finely chopped walnuts

1 In a medium saucepan, cook the lentils in the broth with the bay leaf, for about 35 minutes. When cooked, drain the lentils and remove the bay leaf.

2 Heat a small frying pan over a medium to high heat. Add the olive oil, onion, pepper, carrot, and garlic and sauté for 1 to 2 minutes. Don't allow the vegetables to cook so long that they're tender.

3 Remove the vegetables from the heat and mix them together with the lentils. Add the parsley and walnuts. Serve the salsa chilled.

Per serving: Kilocalories 331; Fat 7g (Saturated 1g); Cholesterol 3mg; Sodium 80mg; Carbohydrate 29g; Dietary Fibre 18g; Protein 22g.

Exchanges: 3 starch, 3 very lean meat, 1 fat.

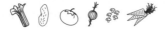

☞ Mexican Salsa
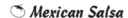

Mexican salsa is a great way to get a good helping of lycopene, because tomatoes are one of the best sources. *Lycopene* is an antioxidant that helps fight heart disease, helps prevent prostate cancer, and is also important for maintaining eye health. If you're a fan of coriander, toss in even more. Why use a teaspoonful when you can use a handful? Serve the salsa with pittas, tortilla chips, crispbread, or rice cakes.

Preparation time: 10 minutes

Serves: 4

½ teaspoon lemon juice

Pinch of salt

450 grams fresh tomatoes, cored and chopped

½ medium onion, diced

1 tablespoon fresh chopped jalapeño pepper

Small garlic clove, finely chopped

1 teaspoon fresh chopped coriander

1 In a mixing bowl, combine the lemon juice and salt, and stir to dissolve.

2 Add the tomatoes and coat them with the juice. Add the onion, jalapeño, garlic, and coriander, and stir together.

Tip: If you like a smooth rather than a chunky salsa, toss all the ingredients in a food processor and process the mixture in pulses until it reaches the consistency you desire.

Per serving: Kilocalories 30; Fat 0g (Saturated 0g); Cholesterol 0mg; Sodium 301 mg; Carbohydrate 5g; Dietary Fibre 2g; Protein 1g.

Exchanges: 1½ vegetable.

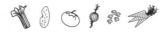

Use caution when slicing and dicing hot chilli peppers such as jalapeños. Use your knife, not your fingers or fingernails, to remove the super-spicy ribs and seeds, and consider wearing gloves if you have sensitive skin. The pepper oil can get stuck under your nails, making it painful to touch, for example, your eyes or nose later. And if your skin is exposed to sunlight with residual pepper oil, you can get a nasty burn.

Adding citrus and other fruits to salsas

To give your salsa a fruity twist, don't bother with bottled lemon or lime juice. Fresh fruit is definitely the way to go. Squeezing the juice out is easy to do, and the flavour is far superior.

Here's how to get the most out of your citrus fruit – see Figure 7-2 for details.

1. **Roll the fruit on a hard, flat surface, pressing down fairly hard to break up the juice sacs.**

2. **Cut the citrus fruit in half widthwise.**

3. **Holding one half in one hand, stick the tines of a fork into the fruit pulp and squeeze the fruit.**

   Twist the fork as necessary to release as much juice as possible.

Juice your fruit over a separate bowl, not into other ingredients. Doing so helps you catch any errant pips that may try to sneak their way into your delectable dishes.

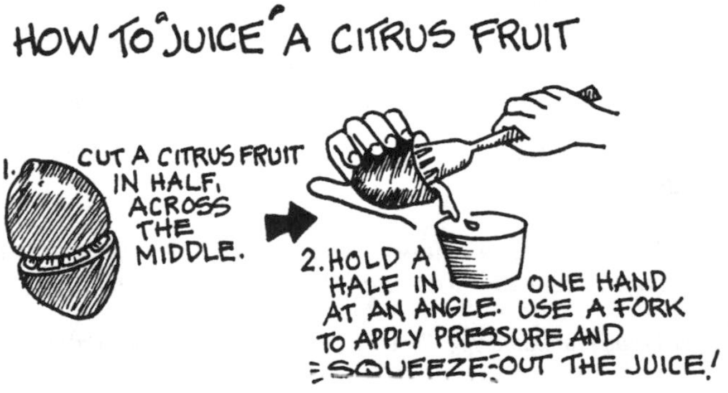

HOW TO "JUICE" A CITRUS FRUIT

Figure 7-2:
A fork is a handy tool to juice a lemon.

1. CUT A CITRUS FRUIT IN HALF, ACROSS THE MIDDLE.
2. HOLD A HALF IN ONE HAND AT AN ANGLE. USE A FORK TO APPLY PRESSURE AND SQUEEZE OUT THE JUICE!

Lemon and lime aren't the only fruity flavours you can add to your salsas. Try the following yummy salsas featuring mango and pineapple.

Warm Pineapple Salsa

Fruit salsa is a terrific sauce for fish, vegetables, or pitta wedges. Or you can use it like a jam or syrup on top of deserts, waffles, or pancakes. With cooked fruit salsa, you heat the ingredients until they almost form a glaze. Fruit salsa has a more syrupy consistency than a tomato-based salsa. Experiment and enjoy.

Preparation time: *20 minutes*

Cooking time: *15 minutes*

Serves: *4*

1 tablespoon olive oil	*1 tablespoon cider vinegar*
1 tablespoon flaked almonds	*Pinch of salt*
Small onion, thinly sliced	*1 tablespoon honey*
2 teaspoons curry powder	*1 tablespoon seedless raisins*
450 grams pineapple chunks, drained	

1 In a small saucepan, heat the oil over a medium heat. Add the almonds and gently toss in the oil.

2 Add the onion and cook until tender and until the almonds are golden brown.

3 Add the curry powder, pineapple, vinegar, salt, honey, and raisins. Bring the mixture to a boil, reduce the heat, and simmer for 10 minutes. Remove the salsa from the heat and serve warm.

Vary It! *Try this recipe with canned mandarin oranges, apricots, or peaches instead of the pineapple, depending on your accompaniments and your taste buds on a given day. Avoid fruit packed in heavy syrup – select fruit canned in spring water whenever possible.*

Per serving: *Kilocalories 114; Fat 5g (Saturated 1g); Cholesterol 0mg; Sodium 148mg; Carbohydrate 19g; Dietary Fibre 1g; Protein 1g.*

Exchanges: *1 fruit, 1 fat.*

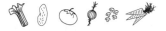

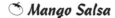

♋ *Mango Salsa*

This mango salsa recipe is similar to the Mexican Salsa earlier in this chapter but offers sweet, firm mango as a perfect partner to the peppers. Feel free to add less mango or more tomato as you experiment with this versatile recipe. With these great ingredients, it's hard to go wrong!

Preparation time: *15 minutes*

Serves: *4*

Large ripe mango, peeled, pitted, and chopped

½ small red pepper, seeded and chopped

Medium tomato, seeded and cubed

Spring onion, green and white parts, chopped

2 tablespoons finely chopped fresh ginger

Juice of 1 lime

3 tablespoons chopped fresh coriander

In a mixing bowl, combine all the ingredients and mix well. Cover and refrigerate until ready to serve.

Per serving: *Kilocalories 50; Fat 0g (Saturated 0g); Cholesterol 0mg; Sodium 4mg; Carbohydrate 11g; Dietary Fibre 2g; Protein 1g.*

Exchanges: *1 fruit.*

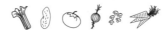

Discovering Delicious Dips

Dips aren't always fat-laden, creamy concoctions that add inches to your waistline and bags to your saddle. With a little creativity, you can create delicious dips that don't adversely affect your glucose levels.

Whipping up dips with kitchen staples

Dips are among the quickest and easiest (not to mention tastiest!) appetisers around. Keep your store cupboards and fridge stocked with a few dip-making essentials to make sure that you're never stuck wondering what to whip up when unexpected guests call round.

Here are some good, quick, dip-making essentials to keep on hand:

✔ **Any of the ingredients listed under 'Stocking essentials for scrumptious salsas', earlier in this chapter:** Adding salsa ingredients to many staples makes for a terrific dip. For example, try blending a can of black beans (rinsed and drained, of course) with 125ml of salsa. Whip the mixture in a food processor, and you have an instant party treat.

✔ **Beans:** Puréed beans make a great base for a dip, because they're high in fibre and low in fat. Blend them in a food processor and season with your favourite spices. Look out for fat-free, low-sodium canned beans, such as cannellini beans, black beans, pinto beans, black-eyed peas, garbanzo beans, chickpeas, navy beans, and kidney beans.

Unless a recipe says otherwise, rinse and drain canned beans before adding them to a dip. Often, the liquid they're canned in is salty or flavoured in some way. Rinse, drain, and season them your own way. Always check to see if the beans need additional cooking before use to destroy toxins – especially red kidney beans.

✔ **Fancy olives:** Olives impart great flavour and texture to dips. Blend some of the olive juice into the dip too – but avoid those stored in brine. If olives perk up a martini, just think what they can do for your dips!

✔ **Fresh herbs:** Fresh herbs make an instant impression on an otherwise bland dip base. Dill, basil, and coriander are excellent options to keep on hand.

✔ **Low-fat sour cream:** Use sour cream or crème fraiche to add a little body and creamy texture to your dips.

✔ **Natural yoghurt:** This ingredient is a natural partner for fresh herbs and a touch of lemon juice. Keep it handy to mix into a soon-to-be bean dip.

✔ **Spice blends:** Look out for prepared, salt-free spice blends. These healthy spices can take the guesswork out of seasoning.

◯ White Bean Dip

Here's a great dip that takes advantage of a well-stocked store cupboard. Add a handful of fresh baby spinach leaves during Step 1 to boost your vitamin and leafy greens quotient. Delicious!

Preparation time: *10 minutes, plus 3 to 4 hours chilling time*

Cooking time: *5 minutes*

Serves: *4*

Nonstick cooking spray	½ teaspoon chopped fresh sage
80 grams chopped onions	1 teaspoon balsamic vinegar
2 garlic cloves, crushed	1 tablespoon water
425-gram can cannellini beans, drained and rinsed	Pinch of salt
	Ground black pepper

1 Place a medium frying pan over a medium heat and coat it with nonstick cooking spray. Add the onions and cook until they're soft and translucent (about 1 minute).

2 Add the garlic and continue to cook for about 30 seconds.

3 Place the beans in a food processor and add the cooked onions and garlic, sage, vinegar, water, salt, and plenty of ground black pepper. Process until smooth (approximately 1 to 2 minutes).

4 Transfer the mixture to a bowl, cover, and refrigerate for 3 to 4 hours before serving.

Per serving: Kilocalories 65; Fat 0g (Saturated 1g); Cholesterol 0mg; Sodium 161mg; Carbohydrate 9g; Dietary Fibre 3g; Protein 3g.

Exchanges: ½ starch, ½ very lean meat.

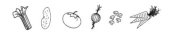

Tuna Pâté

This pâté is tasty and much lighter than the typical liver-and-oil-based spread that many people are familiar with. Using a food processor makes for quick prep work. Feel free to add more or fewer jalapeños, depending on your taste. Serve this dip with pitta bread, crispbread, rice cakes, or bagel chips, or spread it in celery sticks.

Preparation time: *10 minutes, plus 3 to 4 hours chilling time*

Serves: *6*

¼ small onion

2 teaspoons fresh coriander

1 tablespoon chopped jalapeño pepper

350 grams canned tuna, packed in water, drained

120 millilitres low-fat mayonnaise

Ground black pepper

1 In a food processor, combine the onion, coriander, and jalapeño, and process until chopped (approximately 1 minute).

2 Add the tuna and process for approximately 1 minute.

3 Slowly add the mayonnaise and process until smooth (approximately 30 seconds).

4 Add the pepper and process for 1 minute. Check for lumps and process until smooth. Transfer the dip to a serving bowl, chill for 3 to 4 hours, and serve.

Per serving: Kilocalories 195; Fat 16g (Saturated 3g); Cholesterol 30mg; Sodium 283mg; Carbohydrate 1g; Dietary Fibre 0g; Protein 11g.

Exchanges: 2 very lean meat, 2 fat.

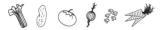

Choosing healthy dippers

A good dip's nothing without something to dip into it, right? Instead of dipping fried crisps, and ruining all that hard work making a healthy dip, here's some healthy alternatives to keep you moving in the right direction:

✔ **Bagel chips:** Look for these chips in the specialty bread section of your deli or supermarket, but read the label because some are high in fat and sodium. Slice slivers from a bagel and bake until they're crisp to make your own bagel chips.

- **Fresh veggies:** Choose broccoli florets, cauliflower florets, carrot sticks, celery sticks, courgette slices, red pepper spears, endive scoops, or any similar favourites. Any vegetable is a potential dip delivery system.

- **Pitta wedges:** Quarter some pittas and then bake until they're crisp to make your own wedges.

- **Vegetable chips:** These chips are becoming more and more popular, and use sweet potatoes, carrots, parsnips, and beetroot as an alternative to potato crisps. A recipe to make your own follows this list.

- **Wholewheat crackers:** Look for these in healthfood shops, delis, and supermarkets. Crispbread and rice cakes are also a filling and tasty option.

⟳ *Vegetable Crisps*

Carrots, parsnips, and beetroot are root vegetables that make healthy snacks with more nutrients – especially antioxidants – than traditional potato crisps.

Preparation time: *10 minutes*

Cooking time: *45 minutes*

Serves: *4*

Pinch of salt	*100 grams parsnip, peeled and cut into slices*
Ground black pepper	*2 tablespoons extra-virgin olive oil*
100 grams carrot, peeled and cut into slices	*Nonstick cooking spray*
100 grams beetroot, peeled and cut into slices	

1 Preheat the oven to 190°C/375°F/Gas Mark 5.

2 In a small bowl, combine the salt and pepper. Place the vegetable slices into a large bowl with the olive oil, and then toss them with the salt and pepper.

3 Coat a baking sheet with cooking spray and arrange the slices on the sheet. Bake for about 45 minutes, or until the slices are cooked through and lightly browned.

Per serving: *Kilocalories 90; Fat 7g (Saturated 1g); Cholesterol 0mg; Sodium 270mg; Carbohydrate 7g; Dietary Fibre 2g; Protein 1g.*

Exchanges: *1 starch, 1½ fat.*

Are sweet potatoes for you?

If you haven't yet tried sweet potatoes, buy some next time you see them in the supermarket. You use them just like potatoes, in that you peel them before boiling, making mash, or adding them to soups and stews. You can also bake them in the oven, or roast and fry them – but just occasionally, because of all that extra fat.

So why are they so special? Their flesh is a lovely yellow-orange colour, as they are teeming with antioxidant pigments – so much so, that their juice is used to dye cloth in South America. These antioxidants make sweet potatoes an excellent choice for people with diabetes as researchers have recently found they may help to stabilise blood glucose levels and lower insulin resistance.

Sweet potatoes are also a good source of vitamins C and B6, plus the minerals manganese and copper, while providing useful amounts of potassium and iron.

Chapter 8

Sipping Simply Divine Soups

Soups are the ultimate comfort food. Who doesn't feel better (even with a cold) after a bowl of warm chicken soup? And you can choose a soup for every different occasion. No matter what the weather, the state of your health, or who's coming for dinner, one of the soups in this chapter is perfect for you.

This chapter gets you started on the soup-making basics, taking you through each step to ensure that your soups turn out just right. We tell you about different types of stock, give tips on watching your salt intake, and help with getting your cupboards stocked with soup-making staples. This chapter also contains tips on making healthy, creamy soups that are full of flavour, but low in fat. And finally, you can even make delicious chilled soups to serve on hot summer days.

Whizzing Through Soup-Making Basics

In many soup recipes, the first few steps ask you to sauté some vegetables to bring out their flavour and soften them. Typically, you start cooking a combination of vegetables, such as onions, carrots, and celery, along with herbs and spices, in a small amount of fat.

You may sauté your vegetables in a small amount of low-fat cooking oil spray, olive oil, or butter, or even a bit of fatty, smoked meat such as bacon. You can also brown minced or cubed meats at this stage. As the ingredients cook, they begin to turn brown and *caramelise,* developing a rich and complex flavour.

Next, you add liquid, perhaps some vegetable, chicken, or beef broth, milk, wine, or water. Initially, add just a few splashes of liquid to *deglaze* the pot. During this procedure, use a wooden spoon or spatula to gently dislodge any bits of caramelised vegetables stuck to the bottom of the pot. You want these flavourful morsels to blend in with the other flavours of the soup. Now, you can pour in the remaining liquid.

In the final, and longest, steps of cooking, you place all vegetable chunks, beans, grains, or meats, into the simmering liquid and cook to perfection. But not everything cooks at the same rate. Therefore, use Table 8-1 to help you decide when to add ingredients so that you don't boil them to death or, conversely, serve them under-done.

Table 8-1	Cooking Times for Soup Add-Ins
Ingredient	*Cooking Time*
Beans, dried (pre-soaked 8 hours)	1½ hours to 2 hours
Beef, cubed	2 to 3 hours
Chicken, bone in, pieces	40 minutes
Chicken, boneless	15 to 20 minutes
Fresh vegetables	10 to 15 minutes (45 to purée)
Greens (spinach and others)	3 to 5 minutes
Lentils, dried	15 to 30 minutes
Pasta, dried	8 to 12 minutes
Pearl barley	50 minutes to 1 hour
Potatoes, white or sweet (diced)	30 minutes
Rice, brown and wild	45 to 55 minutes
Rice, white	15 to 20 minutes
Root vegetables (beetroot, turnips, and so on)	15 to 35 minutes
Seafood, shelled or boneless	5 to 15 minutes

These cooking times are only guidelines, so adjust them as you see fit. Experiment and decide what works best for you.

Serving Up Soups with Stocks and Other Essentials

Although you can begin a soup using water, real depth of flavour calls for stock. Basically, *stock* is a liquid in which solid ingredients, such as chicken meat and bones, vegetables, and spices, are cooked and then usually strained out. The flavours of these ingredients end up in the final broth.

Look for *stock bases,* the secret ingredient of many a restaurant, near the bouillon and broth shelves in the supermarket. Usually sold in large containers, you can make as much as five gallons of stock from a single jar or tub. Keeping a container in your cupboard (or fridge) is more convenient than keeping five gallons of canned broth.

Steering clear of salt in stock-based soups

Most supermarkets carry various brands of chicken and beef broth that offer good flavour. These products are adequate for making everyday soups and are well worth keeping on hand. Always choose the low-sodium versions as stock and resist the temptation to add more salt to your soup during cooking.

People with diabetes need to steer clear of salt as much as possible, because excess sodium quickly increases your blood pressure. If your doctor or dietitian tells you to watch your salt intake, you're probably trying to keep your daily intake under 6 grams of salt (sodium chloride) per day, or even to no more than 3 grams per day if you're on a strict sodium-restricted diet. That amount of salt adds up surprisingly quickly. Some foods are more salty than seawater, which contains 2.5 grams of salt per 100 grams of water.

Ready-made soups often contain a lot of salt, and so knowing how to calculate the amount of salt present in a serving is useful when checking labels.

To convert sodium to salt, you need to multiply the amount by 2.5: So, if the label says that Mr Dummy's Tomato Soup contains 0.4 grams of sodium per 100 grams, that's equivalent to 1 gram of salt per 100 grams.

You then need to know the weight of the serving portion in grams, so that you can divide the concentration of salt per 100 grams by 100 and multiply by the serving size.

For example, if Mr Dummy's Tomato Soup contains 0.4 grams of sodium per 100 grams and the suggested serving size is 200 millilitres (which weighs 200 grams):

0.4 grams sodium per 100 grams × 2.5 = 1 gram salt per 100 grams

1 ÷ 100 = 0.01 grams salt per 1 gram

0.01 × 200 = 2 grams salt per 200 millilitres serving

If you're on a 6-grams-of-salt per day diet, one serving of Mr Dummy's Tomato Soup contains a third of the maximum amount of salt you can eat in a single day.

Table 8-2 shows that selecting the low-sodium version of bought soup is worthwhile, wherever possible, to make salt savings. You can save even more if you make your own version with absolutely no added salt – just the natural amount of salt present in the vegetables and meat you use.

Table 8-2	Typical Salt Content of Different Bought Chicken Soups	
Soups	*Sodium Per 100g Serving*	*Salt Per 200g Serving*
Canned low-sodium chicken broth	60mg (0.06g)	0.3g
Canned low-kilocalorie chicken soup	370mg (0.37g)	1.85g
Canned cream of chicken soup	400mg (0.4g)	2g
Packet chicken soup (made-up)	470mg (0.47g)	2.35g
Instant chicken soup stock powder (made-up)	560mg (0.56g)	2.8g

Avoid any food when its labels show that it contains more than 1.25 grams of salt (or 0.5 grams of sodium) per 100 grams – this amount is the Food Standards Agency's cut-off point to class a food as high in salt.

For a low-salt vegetable stock alternative, simmer together aromatic vegetables such as onion and celery with carrots (which add sweetness) plus some parsley and a bay leaf. Simmer this mixture gently for about 20 minutes, and then strain to obtain a delicious, fragrant stock.

The posh term for this classic combination of vegetables (onions, celery, and carrots) is *mirepoix* (pronounced *meer*-pwa) and it's the basis of many soups and stocks. When you're chopping mirepoix for stocks, you can roughly chop the vegetables and even skip the peeling if you prefer. But when getting the veggies ready for soup, take the time to prep them as the recipe suggests.

Add strong-flavoured vegetables, such as broccoli, cauliflower, and aspara-gus, with caution, or they overpower your other ingredients. Instead, make a basic stock and add strong-flavoured vegetables as necessary for particular soups (curried parsnip, for example).

The following recipe takes advantage of low-sodium chicken broth as stock but is still full of great flavour.

Vichyssoise Leek Soup

This soup is a great basic comfort food. Slice the leeks and then soak and wash them thoroughly to remove dirt and sand deep down in the bulb. Check out Figure 8-1 to see how to cut up leeks. Swish the sliced leeks around in a bowl of cold water. Soak them for a few minutes until the dirt and grit settle to the bottom of the bowl. Lift the leeks out of the water and drain on a paper towel. Repeat the procedure again with fresh water.

Preparation time: *20 minutes*

Cooking time: *25 minutes*

Serves: *4*

Nonstick cooking spray

Large leek, chopped and rinsed (don't use the dark green part of the leek)

300 grams potatoes, peeled and cut into small cubes

475 millilitres low-sodium chicken broth

Ground black pepper

1 Coat a large pot with cooking spray and place over a medium heat until hot. Add the chopped leek. Sauté until soft and translucent.

2 Add the potatoes and chicken broth. Bring to a boil and simmer for 10 to 15 minutes, until the potatoes are cooked. Add black pepper to taste. Continue to simmer for 2 minutes. Remove from the heat.

3 Place half of the contents of the pot into a blender, cover, and process until smooth.

4 Carefully pour the blender mixture back into the pot with the remaining broth and potatoes. Stir together with a wire whisk. Bring back to a simmer.

Per serving: Kilocalories 87; Fat 1g (Saturated 0g); Cholesterol 2mg; Sodium 94mg; Carbohydrate 15g; Dietary Fibre 2g; Protein 3g.

Exchanges: 1 starch, ½ vegetable.

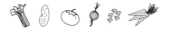

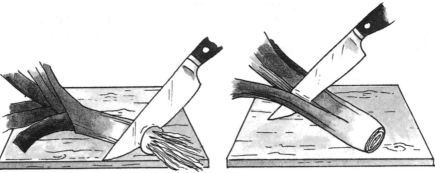

Figure 8-1:
Cutting up
a leek.

ON A CUTTING BOARD, USING A
CHEF'S KNIFE, CUT OFF THE ROOT
ENDS OF THE LEEKS.

SLICE THE LEEK LENGTHWISE,
WITH THE TIP OF THE KNIFE.

Aim to eat at least five servings of fruits and vegetables every day to ensure that you obtain an adequate intake of vitamins, minerals, and fibre. Enjoying a bowl of vegetable soup such as the one in the following recipe is a delicious way to meet your quota.

Hearty Vegetable Soup

When you prepare vegetable soup, first add the items that require longer cooking (such as beetroot and carrots) and later add quick-cooking ingredients (such as spinach and tomatoes). This procedure ensures that you have all your vegetables just where you want them, done to perfection when your soup is finished, but it does require time and attention. Another way to make sure that all the vegetables finish cooking about the same time is to cut the longer-cooking ones (such as potatoes) into smaller pieces and the faster-cooking types (such as squash) into larger chunks.

Preparation time: *15 minutes*

Cooking time: *30 minutes*

Serves: *4*

Nonstick cooking spray	*Courgette, chopped*
Large onion, chopped	*Bay leaf*
2 sticks celery, chopped	*Sprig fresh thyme*
Medium carrot, chopped	*Sprig fresh oregano*
Medium sweet potato, chopped	*480 millilitres low-sodium chicken broth*
Fresh tomato, chopped	*Ground black pepper*

1 Choose a large pot with a tightly fitting lid. Coat the pot with the nonstick spray and cook, stirring constantly, the onions, celery, and carrots until the onions are translucent – about 5 to 7 minutes. You can spray the pot with additional cooking spray or add a little stock or water if the vegetables begin to stick or burn. Add the sweet potato, tomato, courgette, bay leaf, thyme, oregano, and chicken broth, and stir to combine.

2 Bring the vegetable soup to a boil over a high heat, uncovered, and then simmer, covered, for 20 minutes.

3 Remove the bay leaf, season with black pepper, and serve immediately as a light lunch or mini meal.

Per serving: Kilocalories 128; Fat 1g (Saturated 1g); Cholesterol 2mg; Sodium 85mg; Carbohydrate 15g; Dietary Fibre 2g; Protein 3g.

Exchanges: 1 starch, 2 vegetable.

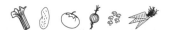

Stocking up with soup supplies

Different types of stocks aren't the only items that you need when craving soup. Keep the following ingredients at home for an impromptu soup-making session:

- ✔ **Canned evaporated milk:** Use this item in your creamy soup recipes, such as the Creamy Vegetable Soup later in this chapter. Evaporated milk is *not* the same as sweetened condensed milk (a syrupy milk-based concoction with lots of added sugar). Evaporated milk, which is milk from which 60 per cent of the water is removed, is concentrated and enhances the flavour of soups and other dishes.

  Choose whole evaporated milk rather than evaporated skimmed milk for soups and sauces. Evaporated skimmed milk has a tendency to curdle and break when heated. If you still want to save the kilocalories, purée the soup with the skimmed milk before serving.

- ✔ **Canned beans, lentils, and chickpeas:** These items are a great source of fibre and protein, but the dried varieties can take time to prepare. Therefore, keep the canned variety available, to toss in a soup pot in just seconds. You can use these hearty staples in the Indian Lamb and Bean Chilli recipe later in this chapter.

Always drain and rinse the liquid from canned beans and vegetables. This removes excess sodium and helps to keep your blood pressure down.

✔ **Canned tomatoes:** Whether chopped, puréed, whole, or stewed, these tomato products make for a quick soup (roast whole tomatoes first for extra flavour).

✔ **Dried herbs and spices.** Oregano, basil, pepper, salt, dill, and just about anything in your spice cabinet can work in a soup recipe. But for best flavour, use fresh rather than dried herbs whenever you can.

✔ **Dried mushrooms:** Rehydrate the mushrooms in hot water, steeping them for about 30 minutes, and then strain the liquid to remove any grit. Roughly chop the mushrooms and add the strained liquid for an extra punch of flavour.

✔ **Garlic:** Garlic adds an amazing flavour to just about anything. You can roast it, sauté it, or crush and purée it, whatever works for your soup. Garlic is great in creamy soups, tomato-based soups, or brothy soups (keeps vampires at bay too).

✔ **Grains:** Rice, pasta, and barley are great for making a soup heartier and more filling. Just ensure that you count the right starch exchanges for the amount you add to your soup. Check out Chapter 10 for the full story on cooking with grains.

✔ **Olive oil:** This terrific monounsaturated fat helps make an already nutritious soup heart healthy too. Keep some on hand at all times.

✔ **Onions:** These fragrant bulbs add their terrific flavour and aroma to anything you cook.

✔ **Potatoes:** These starchy vegetables cook up quickly and can add body to your soups. Choose them for puréed soups because they help thicken soups almost instantly, as in the Vichyssoise Leek Soup earlier in this chapter.

✔ **Salt-free seasoning mixes:** Salt-free herb seasoning blends provide many delicious flavour combinations and take the guesswork out of seasoning your soups.

The following unusual recipe features a low-sodium vegetable stock as its base as well as several of these handy pantry essentials.

Pea Soup with Crabmeat

Pea soup is one of those well-known, warming, comfort foods that are very welcome in wintertime. This one is different from the traditional version, though, but just as good – and better for you! The onions are sautéed in olive oil, making it heart-healthy, the peas ensure a good fibre level, and the crabmeat rounds out the dish with lean protein, making a complete meal. Remember that crab already contains a good amount of natural salt, so you don't need to add more.

Preparation time: *2½ hours*

Cooking time: *45 minutes*

Serves: *6*

2 onions, diced

2 tablespoons olive oil

4 large potatoes, peeled and diced

2 litres low-sodium vegetable broth

Ground black pepper

450 grams cooked peas

1 teaspoon ground nutmeg

450 grams fresh crabmeat, picked and cleaned

1 teaspoon truffle oil (optional)

1 In a large saucepan, sauté the onion in olive oil for 1 minute, and then add the potatoes. Cover with the vegetable broth, season with ground black pepper, and cook on a low heat for 30 minutes.

2 Remove the pan from the heat and set it aside to cool for about 1 hour.

3 When the soup has cooled, add the cooked peas. Place the mixture in a food processor or blender and pulse several times (this can be done in batches). Strain the mixture through a colander.

4 Reheat the thickened soup over a medium heat, and stir in the nutmeg. Ladle into serving bowls. Heat the crabmeat in a warmed frying pan, until heated through (approximately 3 minutes). Drizzle some truffle oil over each dish (if desired) and divide the crabmeat between each soup bowl.

Per serving: Kilocalories 496; Fat 12g; Cholesterol 129mg; Sodium 899mg; Carbohydrate 40g; Dietary Fibre 10g; Protein 34g.

Exchanges: 2½ starch, 2½ very lean meat, 1 fat.

Soups are part of every cuisine. And you can give virtually any soup a little ethnic flavour if you change the spices and seasonings (which can be found in most kitchens). In the next recipe, a traditional Indian spice blend called garam masala gives this chilli a taste of India. You can find this tasty spice blend in the spice section of most supermarkets. If you want to alter the flavour to match another culture's cuisine, just change the seasonings.

Try these substitutes for the garam masala, to change the flavour while keeping the same basic recipe:

- ✔ Basil, marjoram, oregano, thyme, and rosemary, for a taste of Italy
- ✔ Chilli powder and cayenne, for a traditional south-western American chilli
- ✔ Chinese five-spice powder, ground ginger, and a touch of sesame oil stirred in at the end of cooking, for a Chinese-inspired chilli
- ✔ Cinnamon, for a more Indian-flavoured chilli
- ✔ Cumin, coriander seed, and cloves, for a taste of North Africa
- ✔ Thyme, cinnamon, ginger, allspice, cloves, garlic, and onions, for a little Jamaican jerk flavour

Indian Lamb and Bean Chilli

This recipe is an easy, one-pot meal that's full of good nutritional benefits. The beans are a wonderful source of dietary fibre and, in this recipe, meet about a third of your daily fibre needs. Increased fibre can help with blood sugar control as well as keeping you fuller for longer. Lamb is a good source of iron and vitamin B12, which can help prevent and improve anaemia. Lamb is a higher-fat meat, however, so ensure that you drain off any excess fat during the cooking process.

Preparation time: *10 minutes*

Cooking time: *2½ hours (largely unattended)*

Serves: *8*

700g lean ground lamb

Large red onion, chopped

3 garlic cloves, crushed

2 400-gram cans no-salt-added chopped tomatoes, with juice

240 millilitres dry red wine

1 tablespoon chilli powder

1½ teaspoons ground coriander

1½ teaspoons garam masala

2 hot chilli peppers (serrano, for example), deseeded and chopped

400-gram can black beans, drained and rinsed

400-gram can lentils, drained and rinsed

400-gram can chickpeas, drained and rinsed

1 Combine the lamb, onion, and garlic in a large stockpot. Cook over a medium heat until the lamb is brown (about 5 minutes). Stir as needed. Drain in a colander to remove excess fat. Return drained meat mixture to the stockpot.

2 Stir in the tomatoes, wine, chilli powder, coriander, garam masala, and chillis. Bring to the boil. Cover, reduce heat, and cook for 2 hours, stirring occasionally.

3 Stir in the black beans, lentils, and chickpeas. Simmer for an additional 30 minutes. Serve immediately.

Per serving: Kilocalories 311; Fat 14g (Saturated 6g); Cholesterol 61mg; Sodium 213mg; Carbohydrate 29g; Dietary Fibre 6g; Protein 29g.

Exchanges: 1 starch, 2½ medium-fat meat, 1 vegetable, 1 lean meat.

Creating Creamy Concoctions

Who doesn't love a delicious creamy soup? But as you probably know, putting cream in soups adds kilocalories *and* saturated fat, neither of which is good for someone with diabetes. If you love creamy soups, however, here's some good news. You can enjoy a great creamy texture – without the stuff you don't need.

One great way to get the creamy texture without the bad stuff is to substitute semi-skimmed milk for cream in your favourite soups. It gives plenty of the creaminess you expect, because it does have some fat and body, but also cuts down on the fat and kilocalories. Try the following great alternative soup recipe.

Soups are a great way to work in your vegetables, as well as try out new ones. The following list includes some terrific veggies that make excellent soup add-ins:

- ✔ Beetroot
- ✔ Celeriac
- ✔ Greens (spinach, cabbage, chard, and pak choi among others)
- ✔ Herbs (chervil, dill, and coriander, or whatever you want)
- ✔ Mushrooms (morels, chanterelle, and wild mushroom blends)
- ✔ Parsnips
- ✔ Squash (pumpkin and butternut)
- ✔ Sweet potatoes
- ✔ Turnips and swede

Try sweet potatoes – rich in antioxidant carotenoids – in the following creamy soup. If they're not already on your favourite list, you're sure to add them soon.

☺ Cauliflower and Parmesan Soup

This soup is warm, hearty, and perfect for a cool day. Instead of cream, it uses semi-skimmed milk, which has just enough fat to prevent curdling. The milk reduces this soup's fat content considerably. Always try to use a low-fat version of dairy products.

This dish is reminiscent of a creamy potato soup, with far fewer kilocalories and starch. Cauliflower, a vegetable high in vitamin C and fibre, is a great substitute for potatoes in many traditional recipes. Try using cauliflower next time you're about to whip up a batch of mashed potatoes. You may find the taste surprisingly pleasant as well as benefit from the more modest effect on your blood sugar level.

Preparation time: *15 minutes*

Cooking time: *40 to 45 minutes*

Serves: *4*

600-gram medium head cauliflower, chopped	*2 tablespoons lemon juice*
2 shallots, chopped	*2 tablespoons honey*
720 millilitres semi-skimmed milk	*Ground black pepper*
50 grams grated Parmesan cheese	

1 Place the cauliflower, shallots, and milk into a large saucepan, and bring to the boil. Reduce the heat to a simmer until the cauliflower is tender (about 35 minutes).

2 Transfer to a blender and purée until smooth (always take care when blending hot liquids), or use a rotary beater to achieve a smooth consistency. While the soup is blending, add the cheese and process until smooth. To finish, add the lemon juice, honey, and plenty of ground black pepper.

Per serving: *Kilocalories 216; Fat 7g; Cholesterol 23mg; Sodium 251mg; Carbohydrate 20g; Dietary Fibre 3g; Protein 14g.*

Exchanges: *1½ vegetable, 1 lean meat, 1 reduced fat milk.*

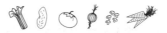

☺ *Corn and Sweet Potato Chowder*

A chowder is a thick soup that usually contains potatoes. This chowder contains the added health benefits of sweet potatoes, and is perfect for early autumn days when the temperature's just cool enough for something warm. The recipe is also a nutritional powerhouse, rich in antioxidants, vitamins, fibre, and protein. Enjoy it with dinner or as a meal in itself!

Preparation time: *15 minutes*

Cooking time: *35 minutes*

Serves: *8*

Large onion, chopped	*250 grams sweet potatoes, chopped*
1 tablespoon olive oil	*650 grams sweetcorn kernels (frozen)*
1 tablespoon cold water	*½ tablespoon cornflour mixed with ½ tablespoon cold water*
3 garlic cloves, crushed	*1 tablespoon white vinegar*
½ tablespoon curry powder	*Ground black pepper*
120 millilitres dry white wine	*2 tablespoons chopped fresh parsley*
1 litre semi-skimmed milk	

1 Heat a large saucepan over a medium heat and add the onion, oil and 1 tablespoon of cold water. Cook for 5 minutes or until the onions are soft and translucent. Stir in the garlic and curry powder, and then cook for an additional minute. Pour in the wine and reduce until all the wine has evaporated (about 3 to 5 minutes).

2 Add the milk and the sweet potatoes. Bring to a simmer and cook for 20 to 30 minutes, or until the sweet potatoes are cooked. Then add the corn and bring back to a simmer. Pour in the cornflour mixture while stirring. Add the white vinegar, plenty of ground black pepper, and the parsley. Serve immediately.

Tip: *This soup freezes well, so make extra.*

Per serving: *Kilocalories 192; Fat 5g (Saturated 2g); Cholesterol 10mg; Sodium 86mg; Carbohydrate 30g; Dietary Fibre 2g; Protein 8g.*

Exchanges: *1½ starch, ½ fat, ½ reduced-fat milk.*

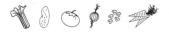

Top your soup with beautiful garnishes to make a simple weeknight supper as delicious for your eyes as for your taste buds. Favourite fresh garnishes include:

- ✔ Chopped olives
- ✔ Chopped red pepper
- ✔ Dollop of light sour cream and chopped coriander leaves
- ✔ Finely grated lemon zest
- ✔ Grated or shaved Parmesan cheese plus finely chopped parsley
- ✔ Julienned radishes, or daikon radish
- ✔ Thinly sliced green onions
- ✔ Torn basil leaves

Garnish this next creamy soup with grated Parmesan cheese and chopped parsley to add both freshness and richness.

☞ *Creamy Vegetable Soup*

This recipe's full of nutritional benefits as well as being super-tasty. One serving provides more than 100 per cent of your daily vitamin C needs, more than 50 per cent of your vitamin A needs, and more than 25 per cent of your potassium, calcium, and vitamin D needs – great for bone health! This soup's also a tremendous source of beta-carotene and lycopene. You can enjoy this dish by itself – the kilocalorie, carbohydrate, protein, and fat contents are just enough for a light meal.

Preparation time: *20 minutes*

Cooking time: *30 minutes*

Serves: *4*

2 tablespoons olive oil	*Pinch of ground thyme*
Medium onion, finely chopped	*Pinch of black pepper*
Large carrot, thinly sliced	*2 400-gram cans fat-free reduced-sodium vegetable broth*
Stick celery, thinly sliced	
2 garlic cloves, crushed	*175-gram can tomato purée*
200 grams sliced fresh mushrooms	*120 millilitres evaporated skimmed milk*
Medium red pepper, chopped	*250 grams cooked mini penne pasta*
1 teaspoon ground sage	*2 tablespoons chopped fresh parsley*

1 Heat the oil in a large saucepan over a medium heat until hot. Add the onion, carrot, celery, and garlic. Cook for 3 to 4 minutes, until the vegetables begin to 'sweat' and give off a bit of liquid.

2 Add the mushrooms, red pepper, sage, thyme, and black pepper. Cook and stir for 5 minutes or until the vegetables are crisp yet tender.

3 Add the beef broth and tomato purée; bring to a boil over a medium-high heat. Cook for 15 minutes.

4 Place half the soup in a food processor and purée (always use caution when processing hot liquids). With the food processor running, slowly pour in the evaporated skimmed milk.

5 Return the soup–milk mixture to the saucepan. Stir to combine. Add the cooked pasta and heat through. Serve immediately sprinkled with parsley.

Per serving: Kilocalories 281; Fat 8g (Saturated 1g); Cholesterol 40mg; Sodium 327mg; Carbohydrate 33g; Dietary Fibre 4g; Protein 16g.

Exchanges: 1 starch, ½ non-fat milk, 3 vegetable, 1½ fat.

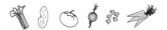

Choosing Chilled Soups

Chilled soups make great appetisers, light lunches, or even desserts. Choose any taste (sweet, spicy, savoury) or ethnic flavour (Spanish, Thai, French, you name it) and you can find a chilled soup to match. Because you serve these soups cold, they're great all summer long.

Don't feel that you need to wait for a special occasion to serve these chilled soups: They're so easy you can serve them any time.

Cooling off with veggies

Get started with this easy Chilled Cucumber Soup. Spice it up as you see fit, and substitute fresh mint or coriander for the dill to change the flavour.

♻ Chilled Cucumber Soup

Cucumber soup is even more refreshing if you add natural yoghurt. Yoghurt, plus the non-fat sour cream in this recipe, makes this soup a substantial and satisfying starter for lunch or dinner. Or add a pinch of lemon zest to create a tangy palate cleanser between courses.

Preparation time: *20 minutes*

Cooking time: *15 minutes*

Serves: *4*

Nonstick cooking spray

1 large or 2 small cucumbers, peeled, seeded, and cut into chunky slices

2 shallots, chopped

60 millilitres dry white wine

240 millilitres low-sodium vegetable broth

Pinch of ground black pepper

120 millilitres non-fat sour cream

120 millilitres plain low-fat yoghurt

4 fresh dill sprigs

1 Coat a large frying pan with the cooking spray and place over a medium heat until hot. Sauté the cucumber and shallots, tossing or stirring frequently until soft and translucent (about 5 minutes).

2 Stir in the wine and chicken broth. Bring to the boil and simmer for 10 minutes. Add the pepper and continue simmering for 2 minutes. Remove from heat.

3 Place the contents of the pan in an electric blender or a food processor, cover, and process until smooth.

4 Pour the mixture into a bowl and allow to cool slightly. With a wire whisk, stir in the sour cream and yoghurt. Cover and chill. Garnish with the dill sprigs.

Per serving: *Kilocalories 66; Fat 1g (Saturated 0g); Cholesterol 3mg; Sodium 87mg; Carbohydrate 6g; Dietary Fibre 1g; Protein 5g.*

Exchanges: *½ vegetable, ½ non-fat milk.*

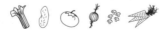

Focusing on fruit

Fruit soups are among the most popular chilled soups, probably because people often eat fruit cold and so puréeing and eating it isn't a stretch. Fruit soup recipes aren't always that simple, but they're not all that tough either.

Carrot and Orange Soup

This classic soup is a gorgeous sunny orange colour and brimming full of eye-friendly antioxidants. As a bonus, it's also low in kilocalories. You can vary the amount of freshly-squeezed orange juice you add to give a stronger or weaker fruit flavour, according to your taste.

Preparation time: *20 minutes*

Cooking time: *60 minutes plus 1 hour of chilling time*

Serves: *4*

Nonstick cooking spray

Medium onion, chopped

800 grams carrots, peeled and chopped

1 litre low-sodium vegetable stock or water

2 tablespoons fresh coriander leaf, chopped

Juice and zest of one large orange

Freshly ground black pepper

1 Coat a large saucepan with the cooking spray and place over a medium heat until hot. Sauté the onions, stirring frequently until soft (2 to 3 minutes).

2 Add the carrots to the saucepan, cover, and sweat the vegetables for a further 10 minutes.

3 Next add the stock, coriander, and the orange juice and zest. Bring to the boil and simmer for 40 minutes.

4 Let the soup cool, and then liquidise thoroughly so that it's completely smooth. Season well with freshly ground black pepper and serve chilled (or hot if you prefer).

Per serving: *Kilocalories 89; Fat 1g (Saturated 0g); Cholesterol 0mg; Sodium 52mg; Carbohydrate 20g; Dietary Fibre 5g; Protein 2g.*

Exchanges: *2½ vegetable.*

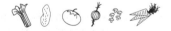

☙ *Watermelon Gazpacho*

Gazpacho is the fancy word for a cold, uncooked soup. Try this unusual and refreshing soup that's not only cool and invigorating, but also full of good nutrition. Watermelons are a great source of the antioxidants lycopene, betacarotene, and vitamin C. This soup is quite low in kilocalories, which is a good thing for your waistline. But before you go for a second scoop, remember that fruit has sugar and is best eaten in moderate amounts.

Preparation time: *45 minutes, plus 1 hour of chilling time*

Serves: *4*

Flesh of a watermelon, cubed and deseeded	4 tablespoons finely chopped parsley
120 millilitres cranberry juice	1 tablespoon sherry vinegar
Small red pepper, chopped	2 tablespoons lime juice
Small red onion, chopped	Small cucumber, thinly sliced
2 sticks celery, chopped	8 fresh mint leaves, torn

1 Place the watermelon and cranberry juice in a blender and pulse until just blended. (Over blending causes the watermelon to froth and lose its colour.) Pour through a sieve into a bowl and press on the pulp to extract all the juice. Discard the pulp.

2 Add the red pepper, onion, celery, parsley, vinegar, and lime juice to the watermelon juice. Cover and refrigerate for 1 hour to chill and allow the flavours to blend together.

3 Ladle the soup into chilled bowls (or martini glasses) and garnish with cucumber slices and mint.

Per serving: *Kilocalories 116; Fat 1g (Saturated 0g); Cholesterol 0mg; Sodium 17mg; Carbohydrate 18g; Dietary Fibre 3g; Protein 2g.*

Exchanges: *1½ fruit, 1 vegetable.*

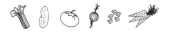

Chapter 9

Taking a Leaf from the Salad Bar

In This Chapter

▶ Exploring salad greens

▶ Trying out tomatoes and nuts

▶ Slipping in some fruit

▶ Including protein to complete your meal

Salads are among the most flexible items in a healthy diet. They're chock-full of delicious and nutritious vegetables with complex carbohydrates that help people with diabetes to manage their glucose levels. Depending on what you add to them, or dress or pair them with, salads can make a snack, appetiser, meal, or even a terrific last course. Stuff them in a pitta pocket for a quick sandwich, pile them into a portable plastic container for an easy lunch box, or toss them in a light vinaigrette for an easy meal.

This chapter shows you how to make the most from your salad choices, with excellent ideas for veggie-only salads and tips for whipping up great home-made dressings to match your nutritional needs. You can even add fruit to your salads for a sweet, refreshing twist. Read on for recipes to make entrée-style, protein-packed salads; the perfect meal solution for just about any nutritional quandary.

Feasting on Great Salad Leaves

You can make your salad really stand out by using special and novel greens, whether those greens are an important part of the salad or added just as garnish. Skip the pale green iceberg lettuce and buy some darker green lettuces instead, such as romaine and mixed exotic baby leaves (see Figure 9-1 for a sampling). The greener the leaf, the more nutrients it contains, especially magnesium, an important mineral for heart and bone health.

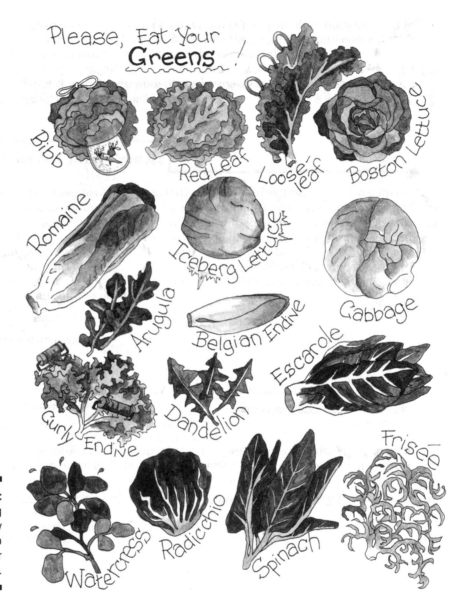

Figure 9-1:
A sampling
of tasty
greens to
try for your
next salad.

Picking fresh greens in the shop

When you go shopping, consider picking up some of these types of greens:

- Boston or butter lettuce
- Endive
- Escarole, also known as chicory
- Frisée
- Radicchio
- Red leaf lettuce
- Rocket
- Romaine
- Spinach
- Swiss chard
- Watercress

Store your salad greens in the vegetable bin of your fridge. Store romaine and radicchio with the head intact because the outer leaves keep the inner leaves moist. However, loose leaves such as rocket and baby spinach have a shorter shelf life. To store this type of lettuce, remove the leaves and wash and drain them. Gather and wrap them in a clean, damp paper towel or two and then store in a plastic bag. The leaves stay fresh for a couple days, but not much longer.

☙ Watercress Salad

During the summer months, take advantage of all the fresh, seasonal produce that's available. Forget about iceberg lettuce, which offers little in the form of good nutrition. Watercress, on the other hand, is a deep green leafy lettuce with lots of carotenoids, which are great for eye health. This green leafy vegetable also happens to provide nearly a quarter of your daily calcium needs, so eat 'em up for your bones.

The following recipe goes easy on the Gorgonzola cheese to keep the kilocalorie and fat levels at an acceptable level. Gorgonzola is a great cheese to use because it lends lots of good flavour in a small amount. Try sticking with sharper cheeses such as this one, Parmesan, or cheddar instead of the milder ones – you need less and get more punch!

Preparation time: *30 minutes*

Serves: *4*

Vinaigrette dressing:

½ onion, finely chopped	120 millilitres olive oil
1 teaspoon chopped fresh thyme	60 millilitres sherry vinegar
1 teaspoon chopped fresh oregano	Ground black pepper

Salad:

2 small Granny Smith apples	115 grams Gorgonzola blue cheese, crumbled
250 grams watercress, rinsed, de-stemmed, and patted dry (purchase ready-to-use watercress if time is limited)	Handful of dry roasted pecans (see the tip at the end of the recipe)

1 To prepare the vinaigrette, place the onion, thyme, and oregano into a large bowl. Add the olive oil and vinegar. Whisk the mixture together until everything is well combined. Add ground black pepper to taste.

2 Prepare the apples just before serving to maintain their freshness and colour. Leaving the skin on, slice the apples in half and core them. Julienne (slice into long strips) the cored apples.

3 Place the watercress in a large bowl and add the dressing. (You probably aren't going to need all the dressing, so add carefully to taste). Divide between four plates and sprinkle the blue cheese and pecans over the greens. Arrange the apples on top and serve.

Tip: *To prepare the roasted pecans, preheat the oven to 180°C/350°F/Gas Mark 4. Place a piece of parchment paper on a baking sheet and spread out the pecans in one even layer. Bake for 10 minutes and then remove from the baking sheet. Set aside to cool.*

Per serving (with 2 tablespoons vinaigrette): Kilocalories 368; Fat 32g (Saturated 8g); Cholesterol 25mg; Sodium 300mg; Carbohydrate 12g; Dietary Fibre 4g; Protein 9g.

Exchanges: *2 vegetable, ½ fruit, 1 high-fat meat, 4 fat.*

○ Mediterranean Salad

Also known as 'Panzanella', this classic Italian bread salad is a light and fresh dish that's perfect on a summer's day. Use vine-ripened tomatoes for the best flavour. This salad offers great nutrition, from the antioxidant-rich tomatoes to the olive oil's heart-healthy monounsaturated fats.

Preparation time: *20 minutes*

Serves: *4 to 6*

Dressing:

3 garlic cloves, chopped

1 tablespoon Dijon mustard

2 tablespoons capers

1 tablespoon Worcestershire sauce

2 tablespoons balsamic vinegar

6 large basil leaves

240 millilitres extra-virgin olive oil

Pinch of ground black pepper

Salad:

3 medium sized tomatoes, chopped

60 grams croutons (baked, not fried)

60 grams thinly sliced red onion

12 large basil leaves, chopped

75 grams crumbled feta cheese

2 tablespoons capers (optional)

Heart of one head of romaine lettuce, sliced thinly

1 To make the dressing, place the garlic, Dijon mustard, capers, Worcestershire sauce, balsamic vinegar, and basil leaves in a blender.

2 While the blender is running, drizzle in the olive oil in a slow steady stream. Season with pepper and put to one side. The dressing keeps for up to 1 week in the refrigerator.

3 In a large mixing bowl, combine the tomatoes, croutons, red onion, basil, feta cheese, and capers (if desired). Toss with 4 tablespoons of dressing and taste. Add more dressing if necessary, up to 6 tablespoons.

4 Arrange the romaine lettuce on the bottom of a large platter. Top with the mixed salad ingredients and serve.

Per serving (with 2 tablespoons dressing): *Kilocalories 349; Fat 31g (Saturated 6g); Cholesterol 11mg; Sodium 354mg; Carbohydrate 9g; Dietary Fibre 3g; Protein 5g.*

Exchanges: *2 vegetable, ½ starch, 1 medium-fat meat, 4 fat.*

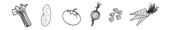

☙ Fresh Mushroom Salad

Mushrooms are a popular and versatile vegetable with numerous health benefits. They're a great source of dietary fibre as well as B vitamins, which help support good energy levels.

This salad, from Piemonte in Italy, is traditionally made with wild porcini mushrooms and white truffles. If you can't get fresh porcini, any cultivated mushroom still gives you a delicious salad. On top of the mushrooms drizzle the quite luxurious porcini olive oil into which the porcini mushrooms steep their flavour as they marinade together. If you don't have time to make your own olive oil, use a bottle of the ready-made porcini oil – or white or black truffle oil – that's readily available in delicatessens.

Preparation time: 20 minutes, plus several days for steeping the olive oil

Serves: 4

30 grams dried porcini mushrooms	*Bunch of oak leaf lettuce*
1 litre extra-virgin olive oil	*Juice of 1 lemon*
300 grams fresh porcini mushrooms	*Ground black pepper*
Bunch of Lolla Rossa lettuce (or substitute red leaf lettuce)	

1 Prepare your own porcini olive oil by steeping the dried porcini mushrooms in the olive oil. Let it stand for a few days so that the oil acquires the flavour of the mushrooms. Save the oil you don't need in this recipe for future use to give any number of dishes a fabulous taste.

2 Put 8 mushrooms aside and slice the remaining mushrooms very thinly.

3 On 4 medium-sized plates, place a few leaves of Lolla Rossa over a few oak leaf lettuce leaves. Place 1 whole mushroom on either side of the lettuce leaves to look as if the mushrooms are growing between the lettuce leaves. Place the sliced mushrooms in the remaining space on the plate.

4 Drizzle the porcini olive oil and lemon juice over the mushrooms and lettuce, and season with ground black pepper to taste.

Tip: Drizzle your extra porcini olive oil on steamed or roasted vegetables, add a touch to risotto during the final stages of cooking, or to pasta, or use it to give a punch of flavour to a marinade.

Per serving (with 2 tablespoons porcini olive oil): Kilocalories 286; Fat 28g (Saturated 4g); Cholesterol 0mg; Sodium 43mg; Carbohydrate 6g; Dietary Fibre 3g; Protein 4g.

Exchanges: 3 vegetable, 3 fat.

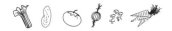

Buying bagged salads

Fortunately, produce manufacturers are taking convenience foods to a healthy level for a change. Look in your fruit and veg section for prewashed, ready-to-use salad greens and blends. You can open a bag and have a delicious meal in a matter of minutes. For super easy and quick salads, pick up prewashed salad blends such as the following:

- **Baby leaf mix:** This tasty blend of baby greens is a staple at most fine restaurants and usually includes baby spinach, radicchio, frisée, rocket, mizuna, and other aromatic leaves. This blend makes a gorgeous garnish or bed for serving fresh fish or steak.

- **Catalan blend:** This usually includes iceberg lettuce, carrot shreds, escarole/chicory, red pepper and red cabbage.

- **Crispy salad:** A great blend to try if your salad experience stops at iceberg lettuce. This blend includes mild green lambs lettuce, frisee, iceberg, and a bit of radicchio, and goes well with just about any dressing, toasted nuts, and any kind of cheese, including blue cheese and goats' cheese.

- **Italian blend:** This blend is terrific for simple protein-based salads, light Caesar dressing, or a traditional Italian vinaigrette, and usually consists of a blend of romaine and radicchio.

Different manufacturers use different trademarked names for their mixes. Many blends also include other vegetables, such as radishes, carrots, and even snow peas. Simply check the label to discover what tasty leaves are included in the package, find out what suits your fancy, and get munching! You really can't overdo these leaves, so fill up on them.

Although these blends of salad leaves are great, many manufacturers also sell kits that include the salad leaves plus things such as dressing, cheese, and croutons. Watch the fat and unnecessary kilocalories that these convenience kits can provide. And remember that you don't have to eat it just because it comes in the kit. Feel free to toss that full-fat Caesar dressing in the bin.

Growing your own greens

Growing fresh baby greens is incredibly simple, no matter where you live. Their shallow root systems make them ideal for indoor gardening. All you need is a shallow bowl or planter, high-quality potting compost, lettuce seeds, and a nice sunny window.

Here's how you do it:

1. **Fill a shallow container that has good drainage with high-quality potting compost.**

2. **Gently press seeds into the soil.**

   Because you're planning to harvest your baby greens when they're, well, babies, you don't need to space out the seeds. Go ahead and just sprinkle them around rather than making nice neat rows.

3. **Water your seeds.**

   Keep the seeds moist but not soggy. Light but frequent watering produces the best leafy greens.

4. **Set the container in a sunny window.**

   Most greens *germinate,* or sprout seeds, within a few weeks. Feel free to start harvesting when the greens are a few inches tall. Just trim off what you need with kitchen shears, and cut and cut again and again as the leaves regrow. Instant salad!

To keep a constant supply of greens on hand, sow a second container two weeks later. Use a mixture of different seeds to create your own spring mix. For more information on growing lettuce or other vegetables in containers, check out *Container Gardening For Dummies,* by Bill Marken and the editors of the National Gardening Association (Wiley).

Creating sensational homemade dressings

Until recently, bottled salad dressings didn't offer much in the way of flavour unless they also came with lots of fat, salt, and sugar. A new generation of delicious, light dressings is now available, but no substitute really exists for making dressings yourself. Believe it or not, the process is pretty simple. To make basic healthy vinaigrette, follow these steps:

1. **Measure equal parts oil (usually extra-virgin olive oil), acid (such as balsamic vinegar or lemon juice), and stock (for example, low-sodium chicken stock) and whisk them together.**

2. **Blend desired herbs, garlic, and other seasonings into the dressing and whisk some more.**

For a truly professional touch, combine all your ingredients (except the oil) in a food processor or blender. With the appliance running, slowly pour the oil into the other ingredients and the dressing *emulsifies,* or blends, really well.

○ *Truffle Vinaigrette*

Top chefs use truffles in their vinaigrettes to create a truly luxurious, distinctive flavour. Truffles are similar to mushrooms in that they're actually a fungus – but don't let that fool you; they taste wonderful. You can find truffles in most fine food stores – and they're worth searching out, though beware: They usually cost a frightening amount of money. A cheaper alternative is to use porcini mushrooms instead. You can drizzle this vinaigrette over steamed vegetables or mixed greens. It contains no cholesterol and only a trace of saturated fat – olive oil is one of those heart-healthy sources of mono-unsaturated fat that has beneficial effects on your cholesterol levels.

Preparation time: *5 minutes*

Serves: *18 to 20 (2 tablespoons per serving)*

30 to 60 grams truffles, cleaned and finely chopped

Small shallot, peeled and finely chopped

3 to 4 thyme sprigs, picked and chopped

80 millilitres balsamic vinegar

240 millilitres olive oil

Black pepper to taste

Drizzle of truffle oil

Combine all the ingredients in a bowl and whisk them together well, or combine all the ingredients in a jar with a lid and shake vigorously.

*Per serving (**2 tablespoons**): Kilocalories 105; Fat 11g (Saturated 2g); Cholesterol 0mg; Sodium 1mg; Carbohydrate 1g; Dietary Fibre 1g; Protein 0g.*

Exchanges: 2 fat.

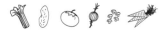

Often, a simple dressing is best. Steeping herbs, garlic, and dried mushrooms in oil gives you an excellent base to make your own tasty dressings. Add a little lemon juice or vinegar, and you're on your way.

Going Beyond Greens with Tomatoes and Nuts

For many people, salad and lettuce are synonymous. Although salad greens are amazingly nutritious, trying your hand at other salads can be fun; for example, ones that highlight other terrific vegetables, such as tomatoes and cucumbers. Flavour these ingredients up with extras, such as toasted nuts and freshly made dressings, and you have a great alternative to a traditional salad. For another great salad without greens, check out the Olive and Lentil Salad in Chapter 10.

🍎 Summer Tomato Salad

Although summertime is great for vibrantly red, juicy, sweet tomatoes, you can (and should!) enjoy them all year round. Tomatoes are packed with lycopene and beta-carotene, two antioxidants known for their disease-fighting actions. This dish is low in saturated fat and contains no cholesterol but is still full of intense flavour thanks to the fresh basil and garlic. In all your cooking, try using fresh herbs and spices for flavouring instead of high-fat spreads and salt.

Preparation time: *10 minutes*

Serves: *4*

4 medium tomatoes, diced small	*2 tablespoons olive oil*
Garlic clove, crushed	*1 tablespoon balsamic vinegar*
6 leaves basil, chiffonade (the sidebar 'Flavouring salads with fresh herbs', later in this chapter, explains chiffonade)	*Black pepper to taste*

Combine all the ingredients in a large bowl and serve the salad at room temperature.

Tip: *Try a combination of tomatoes in this salad to add colour and flavour. Look for green, yellow, orange, plum, vine-grown, and everyone's first favourite tomato, the cherry. So many choices, so little time!*

Per serving: Kilocalories 99; Fat 7g (Saturated 1g); Cholesterol 0mg; Sodium 8mg; Carbohydrate 3g; Dietary Fibre 1g; Protein 1g.

Exchanges: 1 vegetable, 1½ fat.

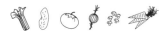

Nuts have an undeserved reputation as fattening. Not so! In moderation, nuts are an excellent source of fibre, antioxidants, and 'good' monounsaturated fat. Plus, they provide long-lasting protein that helps to stabilise your blood glucose level.

Here's a list of seeds and nuts to try in your next salad:

- ✔ Almonds
- ✔ Brazils
- ✔ Cashews

Flavouring salads with fresh herbs

Fresh herbs are an excellent addition to almost anything, especially salad. Their robust flavours can help you cut down the need for adding fat and salt to your foods. You can chop or even mince herbs, but some recipes, such as the one for Summer Tomato Salad, earlier in this chapter, call for a herb *chiffonade*. Chiffonade literally means 'made of rags', and pretty well describes what the final product looks like. Leafy lettuce or herbs are rolled together tightly and then thinly sliced widthwise to form long, stringy strips.

Here are descriptions of a few popular salad herbs:

✔ **Basil:** Technically a member of the mint family, this herb has a sweet peppery flavour that's the cornerstone of most pesto sauces. Look for basil varieties such as lemon basil and cinnamon basil to spice up your everyday salads.

✔ **Coriander:** Use the tender stems and leaves of this herb to give a pungent push to any Latin- or Asian-inspired dishes. Coriander pairs extremely well with citrus flavours.

✔ **Dill:** The feathery leaves of this pungent herb are the main ingredient in many a salad dressing and fish sauce. Dill is great paired with citrus.

✔ **Mint:** Sometimes thought of as only the dessert garnish, mint is used worldwide in both sweet and savoury dishes. This herb is incredibly aromatic and can lend its fragrance and flavour to salad dressings, dips, condiments, and beverages.

✔ **Parsley:** Whether you prefer flat-leaf or curly parsley, this herb is familiar to most people. The best way to describe its flavour is fresh. Some people use it as a natural breath freshener. Chop it up and throw it into a salad along with your greens to brighten the salad's flavour.

✔ Macadamias

✔ Pecans

✔ Pine nuts

✔ Pumpkin seeds

✔ Sunflower seeds

✔ Walnuts

Whenever possible, toast nuts before adding them to any dish. Toasting really brings out the flavour of nuts, making them much more satisfying to eat. Simply place them in a sauté pan over a medium-high heat, shaking them occasionally to ensure that they don't burn. They're done when they become fragrant and slightly darker in colour.

↻ Cucumber–Tomato Salad with Tahini and Toasted Pine Nuts

Enjoy a taste of the Middle East in your home with this easy-to-prepare fresh cucumber–tomato salad. The pine nuts and olive oil offer heart-healthy monounsaturated fats. Add all the cucumbers and tomatoes you want – they're full of fibre and fill you up for relatively few kilocalories. The fat and protein from the feta and pine nuts keep you satisfied until your next meal, and your blood glucose barely notices a thing!

Preparation time: *35 minutes*

Serves: *4*

Tahini (sesame seed) dressing:

120 millilitres tahini (sesame seed) paste

60 millilitres hot water

2 garlic cloves, chopped

80 millilitres fresh squeezed lemon juice

Ground black pepper

Salad:

4 vine-ripened tomatoes, quartered

2 seedless cucumbers, peeled and medium diced

60 grams flat-leaf parsley, washed and leaves picked

75 grams crumbled feta cheese

4 sprigs fresh mint, chiffonade (the earlier sidebar 'Flavouring salads with fresh herbs' explains chiffonade)

60 grams toasted pine nuts

60 millilitres extra-virgin olive oil

Ground black pepper

1 To make the dressing, combine the tahini paste, water, and garlic in a blender and process until smooth.

2 Add the lemon juice and blend again until smooth. If the mixture is too thick, add a little more hot water – up to 60 millilitres. (The dressing is thick, but not the consistency of peanut butter.) Season with ground black pepper to taste and set the dressing aside.

3 To make the salad, combine the tomatoes, cucumbers, and parsley in a large bowl and toss. Add the feta cheese.

4 Add the mint and pine nuts, toss with the olive oil and tahini dressing, and season with black pepper to taste. Serve on salad plates.

Per serving: *Kilocalories 498; Fat 42g (Saturated 8g); Cholesterol 17mg; Sodium 290mg; Carbohydrate 16g; Dietary Fibre 6g; Protein 15g.*

Exchanges: *3 vegetable, 1 medium-fat meat, 9 fat.*

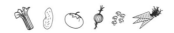

Adding Fresh Fruit to Your Salad

Everyone knows how refreshing a fruit salad tastes, made with three or four of the season's best crops. If you have diabetes you must carefully count fruit, which is full of natural sugars, in your daily meal plan. Most fresh fruit, however, has a low glycaemic index, meaning that it doesn't affect your blood glucose levels too much. Create meals with small amounts of fruit and combine with other foods, as in the following Blood Orange, Avocado, and Fennel Salad. Blood oranges are combined with crunchy liquorice-flavoured fennel, and the avocados and olive oil add fat to balance the carbohydrate in the fruit.

🍎 Blood Orange, Avocado, and Fennel Salad

This recipe creates a delicate salad of contrasts, making a beautiful presentation with the contrasting blood red oranges, green avocados, and white fennel. All at once, the taste is crunchy and soft, sweet and savoury. And another thing makes this recipe a winner: Avocados are rich in monounsaturated fats, which, in moderation, offer heart-healthy benefits.

Preparation time: *20 minutes*

Serves: *6*

4 blood oranges	*2 fennel bulbs*
3 ripe avocados	*Juice of 1 lemon*
Ground black pepper	*2 tablespoons extra-virgin olive oil*

1 With a sharp knife, cut a thin slice off the top and bottom of each orange. Set the oranges on a flat surface and remove the skin and pith in strips, following the curvature of the fruit. Slice the oranges into ½-centimetre pieces. Lay the slices in a single layer on a large platter.

2 Halve the avocados and remove the pits with a knife. Spoon out chunks of avocado, season them with black pepper, and place them over the orange slices.

3 Remove the outer layers of the fennel and slice the bulbs thinly. Place the slices in a large bowl. Pour lemon juice over the fennel and drizzle with the olive oil. Toss the fennel and place it over the orange slices.

4 Drizzle the lemon juice and olive oil remaining at the bottom of the bowl over the whole salad. Serve immediately.

Per serving: *Kilocalories 251; Fat 17g (Saturated 3g); Cholesterol 0mg; Sodium 17mg; Carbohydrate 13g; Dietary Fibre 12g; Protein 4g.*

Exchanges: *2 vegetable, 1 fruit, 3 fat.*

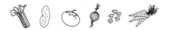

Enjoying Entrée Salads

For many people, salads are a main attraction. These days you can even get entrée salads at your local fast food outlets (which you don't often frequent, right?). Eating salad is so easy and healthy that here's some tasty entrée salads for you to try.

Surveying simple seafood salads

Most seafood is naturally delicious, and so turning it into something special doesn't take much effort. A little bit of seasoning, a light dressing, and some tasty greens, and you have yourself a meal. Marinate sea scallops in a little olive oil and lemon juice and grill them. Or steam your favourite white fish with herbs and seasonings and then serve on a bed of greens. Just about any seafood item (perhaps with the exception of sea slugs?) can take the main stage in your mostly salad meal. For more terrific seafood recipes, make sure you turn to Chapter 12.

Prawn Salad

The prawns and mayonnaise in this salad provide enough fat and protein to really stick with you and get you through to your next meal. Enjoy the extra crunch of the red and yellow peppers, and choose your favourite mixed greens. See 'Feasting on Great Salad Leaves', earlier in this chapter, for more information on salad greens.

Preparation time: *15 minutes*

Serves: *4*

450 grams, cooked, shelled prawns

40 grams chopped red pepper

40 grams chopped yellow pepper

2 tablespoons chopped fresh coriander

Handful of chopped fresh chives

60 millilitres low-fat mayonnaise

1 teaspoon Dijon mustard

1 teaspoon lemon juice

Ground black pepper

250 grams fresh mixed salad leaves

1 Rinse the prawns to remove excess sea salt. In a bowl, combine the prawns, red and yellow peppers, half of the coriander, and chives.

2 In another bowl, whisk together the mayonnaise, mustard, lemon juice, and black pepper. Spoon over the prawn mixture and toss together.

3 Arrange the salad greens on 4 large plates. Top the greens with equal portions of the prawn mixture.

4 Sprinkle with the remaining coriander.

Per serving: Kilocalories 154; Fat 3g (Saturated 0g); Cholesterol 221mg; Sodium 1,440mg; Carbohydrate 5g; Dietary Fibre 2g; Protein 25g.

Exchanges: 1 vegetable, ½ fat, 3 very lean meat.

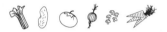

The typical Japanese diet gets a lot of attention in the media as a healthy way of eating. In general, Japanese populations tend to have fewer incidences of heart disease, cancer, and diabetes. Their diets tend to focus on seafood as the main protein, plant-based foods, such as soy products and rice, rather than dairy products, and tons of vegetables. The following recipe gives you a chance to sample the flavours of this healthful cuisine.

Using leftovers to your advantage

'Leftovers' is not necessarily a dirty word. In fact, think of them as a life simplification strategy. When you're marinating and grilling chicken for dinner, double your recipe and reserve the extra for quick salads later in the week. Stop at the greengrocers on your way home for a fresh bag of greens, and your healthful dinner is literally in the bag.

Here's a list of great 'leftovers' that can make an excellent next-day salad if you cook more than you need for a single meal:

- Lean baked ham
- Lean roast beef
- Poached salmon
- Roast chicken breast (remove the skin)
- Roast pork tenderloin

Teriyaki Salmon Salad

Salmon, nature's wonder food, is full of those omega-3 fatty acids, one of the good fats. Including them in your diet can help delay signs of ageing and wrinkles, treat arthritis and skin eruptions, and prevent cancer, heart disease, and Alzheimer's. Yes, omega-3s can do all that!

Preparation time: *15 minutes*

Cooking time: *10 to 12 minutes*

Serves: *2*

1 tablespoon Dijon mustard	*½ teaspoon garlic powder*
1 tablespoon dry white cooking wine	*Pinch of black pepper*
1 tablespoon low-sodium teriyaki sauce	*2 small, skinless salmon fillets*
1 teaspoon low-sodium soy sauce	*125 grams mixed salad leaves*
1 teaspoon honey	*¼ small red onion, thinly sliced*
1 teaspoon lemon juice	

1 Preheat the oven to 180°C/350°F/Gas Mark 4. In a medium bowl, combine the mustard, wine, teriyaki sauce, soy sauce, honey, lemon juice, garlic powder, and black pepper. Place the salmon in the bowl and coat thoroughly.

2 Place the salmon in a baking dish, pour the remaining liquid over the salmon, and place the dish in the oven. Bake for 10 to 12 minutes.

3 Arrange halve the salad leaves on each of two plates and place a salmon fillet on top. Sprinkle with red onion slices.

Per serving: Kilocalories 256; Fat 7g (Saturated 1g); Cholesterol 97mg; Sodium 559mg; Carbohydrate 6g; Dietary Fibre 2g; Protein 39g.

Exchanges: 1 vegetable, 5 lean meat.

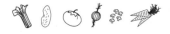

Punching up your salad with protein

Pairing salads and protein is a natural fit for someone with diabetes. Most of the meal is actually made up of the healthy vegetables, accented with a small but satisfying portion of protein.

Canned legumes, such as chickpeas and kidney beans, are an excellent and inexpensive way to make sure that you get enough protein. Plus these protein powerhouses are cholesterol free, making them an all-around excellent choice.

⚘ Chickpea Salad

This great, all-purpose salad is easily stuffed in a pitta pocket with mixed lettuce leaves for a quick, well-rounded meal. Vary the recipe with different vegetables, such as tomatoes, or different spices, such as cumin or curry powder. Make this salad your own.

Preparation time: _10 minutes_

Serves: _2_

360 grams canned chickpeas, drained and rinsed

40 grams celery, chopped

40 grams red pepper, chopped

4 tablespoons red onion, chopped

Ground black pepper

2 tablespoons low-fat mayonnaise

Pitta bread or mixed greens

_1_ In a bowl, coarsely mash the chickpeas. Add the celery, red pepper, onion, pepper, and mayonnaise and toss well.

_2_ Serve over pitta bread or mixed greens.

Per serving (without pitta or greens): _Kilocalories 206; Fat 3g (Saturated 0g); Cholesterol 0mg; Sodium 550mg; Carbohydrate 26g; Dietary Fibre 9g; Protein 10g._

Exchanges: _1½ starch, 1½ very lean meat, ½ fat._

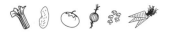

Crunchy Chicken Stir-Fry Salad

Here's a great way to enjoy a chicken salad that's not the same old leaves-topped-with-grilled-chicken-breast thing. This salad's loaded with interesting vegetables (such as pak choi and sugarsnap peas) and other tasty titbits (such as almonds) that give a terrific flavour and texture.

Preparation time: 15 minutes

Cooking time: 25 minutes

Serves: 2

1 tablespoon sesame oil

325 grams boneless, skinless chicken breasts, sliced into strips

60 grams baby carrots

Pinch of garlic powder

Pinch of onion powder

Pinch of black pepper

1 teaspoon sesame seeds

40 grams broccoli florets

Stick of celery, sliced small and diagonally

30 grams sugarsnap peas (or mangetout)

1 tablespoon low-sodium teriyaki sauce

1 teaspoon low-sodium soy sauce

120 millilitres low-sodium chicken broth

100 grams blanched and roughly chopped Chinese pak choi (see Chapter 11 for more about blanching)

2 tablespoons slivered almonds

1 Heat a large frying pan over a medium-high heat. Add the oil. Add the chicken strips, carrots, and garlic powder. Sauté until the chicken is lightly browned (about 7 minutes). Add the onion powder, black pepper, sesame seeds, broccoli, and celery. Cook and continue stirring until the vegetables are soft.

2 Lower the heat and add the sugarsnap peas, teriyaki sauce, soy sauce, and chicken broth. Continue stirring. Simmer until the liquid has reduced slightly.

3 Divide the pak choi between two plates. Spoon the chicken mixture over the pak choi. Sprinkle the almonds on top.

Per serving: Kilocalories 352; Fat 15g (Saturated 3g); Cholesterol 95mg; Sodium 403mg; Carbohydrate 7g; Dietary Fibre 5g; Protein 40g.

Exchanges: 2 vegetable, 6 very lean meat, 2 fat.

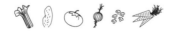

Oriental Beef and Noodle Salad

If you love Chinese takeaway, satisfy your hunger with this healthy, low-fat version, full of Asian flavour. Using a minimum of meat with lots of vegetables is typical of Chinese cooking. Although this style of cooking evolved from necessity, due to a scarcity of meat, the result of this hardship was the creation of an exceptionally healthy cuisine. A good example is this beef and noodle salad, made with lean meat and a minimum of cooking oil.

Preparation time: *15 minutes*

Cooking time: *15 minutes*

Serves: *4*

225 grams thin spaghetti

4 teaspoons sesame oil

Nonstick cooking spray

450 grams boneless top sirloin steak, trimmed of fat, cut into thin slices

2 teaspoons low-sodium soy sauce

2 teaspoons red wine vinegar

1 teaspoon Dijon mustard

Pinch of ground ginger

Garlic clove, crushed

Pinch of ground black pepper

2 tablespoons thinly sliced spring onion

2 tablespoons finely chopped red bell pepper

2 teaspoons chopped fresh coriander

1 Bring a large pot of water to boil and cook the spaghetti according to package directions, typically 5 to 6 minutes. Drain, rinse under cold running water, and drain again. Transfer to a large bowl and toss with the sesame oil and set aside.

2 Coat a large cast-iron or nonstick frying pan with the cooking spray and place over a medium-high heat until hot. Add the steak slices and cook until medium rare, about 1 minute per side. Add the steak to the bowl with the pasta.

3 In a small bowl, whisk together the soy sauce, vinegar, mustard, ginger, garlic, and black pepper. Add the spring onions and red pepper and toss well. Add to the bowl with the spaghetti and steak and toss well.

4 Divide among four serving plates, sprinkle with the coriander, and serve.

Per serving: *Kilocalories 435; Fat 14g (Saturated 4g); Cholesterol 71mg; Sodium 140mg; Carbohydrate 42g; Dietary Fibre 2g; Protein 34g.*

Exchanges: *3 lean meat, 3 starch, 1 fat.*

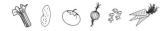

Chapter 10

Being Full of Beans
(and Grains and Pasta)

People with diabetes need to take note of their carbohydrate intake because carbs have a direct impact on blood glucose levels. A big source of carbohydrates is grains, one of the major categories of starch exchanges (refer to Chapter 2 for more about food exchanges). And yet grains form part of a healthy eating programme, so don't cut them out altogether. Instead, make sure that you choose whole grains (whose carbs have a slower impact on blood glucose levels) rather than processed grains (which quickly affect your glucose balance). Talk to your doctor and dietitian about the best options for your health situation.

This chapter shows you how to use rice and other grains to brighten up any meal. We also provide you with recipes and information on using pasta as part of your eating plans, and give you tips on how to use beans – or if you want the posh word, *legumes* – in many different ways. Grains and beans offer lots of new and tasty options.

Relishing Rice and Other Grains

Grains are truly the food that changed the world. Early farmers cultivated these little packets of nutrition, such as rice and quinoa, helping our ancestors to evolve into settled, non-nomadic peoples, building stable civilisations the world over.

Eating rice the right way

Rice is a worldwide staple, but often gets a bad reputation because so many people eat the bland, processed, white version, slathering it with fat-heavy sauces. Instead, try less processed, flavoured rice that stands on its own or is enhanced with a few simple seasonings or cooking techniques. And always remember to eat in moderation. A single serving of cooked rice is 65 grams (around 2 ounces) and represents 1 starch exchange.

Here are a few rice varieties to help give you a range of options, along with ideas on how to use them:

- ✔ **Arborio:** An Italian short- to medium-grained rice used in making risotto. The rice gives off starches as it cooks to add to the creaminess of this popular Italian dish. Try it for yourself in the recipe for Herby Risotto with Extra-Virgin Olive Oil in this section.

- ✔ **Basmati:** The name means 'fragrant' in Hindi, from its distinct nutty aroma during cooking. This fragrance is enhanced because the rice is aged after harvesting. True basmati rice is grown in the foothills of the Himalayas, but a few new basmati-like varieties are grown elsewhere, such as Texmati and Kasmati rice from America.

- ✔ **Brown:** This rice has the whole rice grain intact, with only the inedible outer husk removed. Because the bran coating is intact, brown rice is higher in fibre but has a shorter shelf life (around six months). Use it in any recipe that calls for white rice, but give it a bit more time to cook (about 45 minutes). To get you started, try the Middle Eastern Brown Rice Pilaf in this section.

- ✔ **Jasmine:** An aromatic long-grain rice from Thailand, this rice is highly prized but less expensive than basmati. Try it in the Black Bean Pie recipe later in this chapter.

- ✔ **Long-grain:** A broad (as well as long!) category of rice. This rice has long, evenly shaped grains that are usually drier and less starchy than short-grained varieties. Long-grain rice separates easily after cooking. Basmati, jasmine, and wild rice are all long-grain rice.

- ✔ **Medium-grain:** As the inspired name implies, medium-grain rice is longer than short-grain rice and shorter than long-grain rice.

- ✔ **Short-grain:** This rice has short, almost round grains and a higher starch content than long-grain rice, giving it a sticky, clumpy consistency after cooking.

- ✔ **Wild rice:** This 'rice' is actually the grain of a wild marsh grass and has a chewy texture and nutty flavour. Wild rice is often combined with other rice for a more exotic taste and appearance.

Middle Eastern Brown Rice Pilaf

Sometimes people complain that brown rice doesn't taste quite right or that it doesn't achieve a good consistency. Here's a dish that combines this whole grain with many other textures and flavours that leave you loving brown rice forever! This recipe also provides a good lesson in creativity and risk taking! Seek out new and different recipes that change the flavours until you find one you like. If you're hesitating about eating brown rice again, try this recipe before you swear off this healthy food forever.

Preparation time: *10 minutes*

Cooking time: *1 hour*

Serves: *6*

2 tablespoons olive oil	*140 grams uncooked brown rice*
240 grams chopped onion	*480 millilitres chicken broth*
Garlic clove, crushed	*2 spring onions, chopped*
2 carrots, sliced	*Ground black pepper*
140 grams fresh sliced mushrooms	

1 Heat the olive oil in a saucepan with a tight-fitting lid over a medium heat. Sauté the onions, stirring frequently until they soften. Add the garlic and carrots and continue stirring for 5 minutes. Add the mushrooms and rice and cook until the mushrooms soften, after about 7 to 8 minutes.

2 Add the chicken broth and bring to a boil. Cover and reduce the heat. Continue cooking until all the liquid is absorbed (approximately 45 to 50 minutes). Fluff with a fork. Toss with the spring onions. Season with freshly ground black pepper to taste.

Per serving: *Kilocalories 174; Fat 7g (Saturated 1g); Cholesterol 2mg; Sodium 69mg; Carbohydrate 22g; Dietary Fibre 3g; Protein 4g.*

Exchanges: *1 starch, 1 fat, 1 vegetable.*

☽ Herby Risotto with Extra-Virgin Olive Oil

Here is a wonderful risotto dish. Note the importance of stirring the risotto constantly! Cooking this dish is not a moment for TV-watching or telephone-answering if you want the risotto to come out smooth and flowing. And, once made, you must eat this dish immediately. The following Italian saying tells the story: 'You must wait for risotto, but risotto cannot wait for you.'

Making risotto with olive oil is certainly a healthy change from the traditional method, which calls for butter. Essentially, risotto is made from Italian rice, and for people with diabetes, rice is falsely accused of belonging on the list of 'bad' foods. Too many carbs are 'bad' (for that matter, too much of anything is 'bad'), but this risotto dish, served in moderation, can certainly form part of a balanced, healthy diet: It's absolutely delicious and worth every bite. Pair the risotto with some protein, such as fish or poultry, and fibre, from non-starchy vegetables, to keep your blood sugars on an even keel.

Preparation time: *45 minutes*

Cooking time: *20 minutes*

Serves: *6*

Bunch fresh sage	*½ medium onion, finely chopped*
Bunch fresh rosemary	*Ground black pepper*
Bunch fresh parsley	*200 grams Italian arborio rice*
Bunch fresh basil	*240 millilitres dry white wine*
1½ litres water	*50 grams grated Parmesan cheese*
5 tablespoons extra-virgin olive oil	

1 From the fresh sage, rosemary, parsley, and basil, chop equal parts (roughly 3 tablespoons) of each type of herb and set aside.

2 Using kitchen string, tie together one stem each of the sage, rosemary, parsley, and basil herbs to resemble a bouquet of flowers. Place the bouquet in a saucepan with the water and bring to the boil. Remove from the heat. Allow the bouquet to steep for 30 minutes. Strain and keep warm. This bouquet serves as your herb stock. Bring the stock back to a low simmer before adding to the risotto in Step 5.

3 In a 3-litre (5½-pint) saucepan, heat 3 tablespoons of oil over a medium heat.

4 Add the chopped onions and a good twist of freshly ground black pepper. Cook for 1 minute. Add the rice, wine, and chopped herbs. Immediately stir and continue to stir every 15 seconds until the risotto absorbs the wine. Keep the heat at medium to high.

5 When the wine has evaporated, begin to add the simmering stock, around 120 millilitres at a time, stirring continuously. Add a bit more pepper depending on your taste. After the first amount of stock is absorbed and the rice looks dry, add another 120 millilitres, and so on. Repeat until you've added roughly 700 millilitres to 1 litre of the herb stock, and the rice is soft but *al dente,* or firm to the bite. If the rice tastes hard and starchy, continue adding stock. This step takes about 25 to 30 minutes total. Note: You must continue to stir the risotto during this stage of cooking. Stirring helps to bring out the starchy creaminess in the rice and ensures the proper texture and consistency.

6 When the risotto is cooked, its consistency should resemble thick porridge. Remove the pot from the heat. Add the grated Parmesan cheese and the remaining 2 tablespoons of oil. Stir very well. Allow to rest for 2 minutes. Stir once more before serving. Season with ground black pepper to taste.

Per serving: Kilocalories 278; Fat 14g (Saturated 3g); Cholesterol 5mg; Sodium 98mg; Carbohydrate 30g; Dietary Fibre 1g; Protein 7g.

Exchanges: 2 starch, 2½ fat, ½ lean meat.

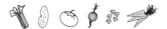

Kicking it up with quinoa

Quinoa (pronounced *keen-wah*) is one of the most nutritious whole grains, but isn't a popular food simply because few people know about it. As well as being high in protein and fibre, and providing 25 per cent of your daily iron needs, this miracle grain is a tremendous source of magnesium, potassium, and phosphorus. Quinoa is more nutritious than white rice, is easily substituted for it in most dishes, and should have a place in every larder!

For optimal results, prepare 2 parts of quinoa with 1 part low-sodium vegetable or chicken broth for added flavour or when using as a side dish such as a stir-fry. You can also serve this grain as a hot cereal for breakfast with fresh berries.

Moroccan Quinoa

Moroccan spices, such as turmeric, ginger, and cinnamon, combine with almonds and dried fruits to give this quinoa recipe a delicious North African flavour that keeps your taste buds perky and your blood glucose stable. This dish is a great way to get started with quinoa if you haven't already discovered this amazing grain.

Preparation time: *20 minutes*

Cooking time: *40 minutes*

Serves: *4*

170 grams quinoa	Pinch of turmeric
240 millilitres water	½ teaspoon cinnamon
240 millilitres low-sodium chicken broth	Pinch of ground ginger
2 teaspoons olive oil	25 grams flaked almonds, toasted
160 grams diced red onion	40 grams raisins
½ teaspoon cumin	Fresh mint (optional)

1 Rinse the quinoa and place in a fine mesh strainer. Run cold water through the grains until the water runs clear. Drain the water off, stir the grains around a bit, and then rinse again to ensure that you remove all the bitter outer coating. Don't even think of skipping this step! Even if your quinoa is processed, which removes much of the *saponin,* or protective outer covering, the dust still remains. This dust can add a nasty bitter flavour to your finished dish, so don't risk it.

2 Place the rinsed quinoa, water, and chicken broth in a 1½-litre (2¾-pint) saucepan and bring to the boil. Reduce to a simmer, cover, and cook until all the water is absorbed (about 15 minutes). Fluff with a fork and set aside.

3 While the quinoa is cooking, heat the oil in a nonstick pan. Sauté the onions until they begin to caramelise. Add the cumin, turmeric, cinnamon, and ginger, cooking until fragrant. Stir in the almonds and raisins until heated.

4 Add the hot quinoa to the pan. Toss to combine. Heat until the mixture is heated through. Serve garnished with fresh mint, if desired.

Per serving: *Kilocalories 274; Fat 9g (Saturated 1g); Cholesterol 1mg; Sodium 80mg; Carbohydrate 38g; Dietary Fibre 5g; Protein 9g.*

Exchanges: *2 starch, 1 fat, ½ fruit.*

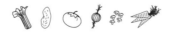

Trying out barley

Barley is a whole grain that can make a delicious side dish to serve with meats and poultry. Try the following recipe to include some barley in your diet.

Barley Pilaf

Barley that still retains the bran takes a long time to cook, and so manufacturers *pearl* the barley, which means they remove the bran. Pearl barley is the kind you usually find in supermarkets. In comparison with rice and wheat, barley has significantly less effect on blood glucose. Barley is also tasty added to soups.

Preparation time: *10 minutes*

Cooking time: *50 minutes*

Serves: *6*

175-gram piece smoked ham hock	*960 millilitres water*
2 stalks celery, cut into 5-centimetre lengths	*1 tablespoon olive oil*
2 bay leaves	*Medium onion, chopped*
½ teaspoon dried sage	*200 grams pearl barley*
Ground black pepper	

1 In a large pot, put the ham hock, celery, bay leaves, sage, pepper to taste, and water. Bring to the boil over a high heat, and then lower the heat to medium and cook, uncovered, for 20 minutes. The volume of the broth reduces by about one-quarter.

2 In a medium pot, heat the olive oil over a medium heat. Cook the onion, stirring occasionally, until soft (about 5 minutes). Add the pearl barley and cook, stirring, for 1 minute.

3 When the ham hock stock is prepared, pour the broth through a sieve into the barley. Bring to a boil.

4 Turn the heat to low, cover the pot, and cook the barley until tender and all the liquid is absorbed (about 30 minutes). If the barley is not quite done, add 1 or 2 tablespoons of water and continue to cook. If the barley is cooked but liquid remains, turn off the heat and let the barley rest in the covered pot while the grain continues to absorb the liquid.

Per serving: *Kilocalories 146; Fat 3g (Saturated 0g); Cholesterol 0mg; Sodium 20mg; Carbohydrate 22g; Dietary Fibre 6g; Protein 4g.*

Exchanges: *2 starch.*

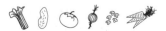

Preparing Perfect Pasta

Pasta comes in many shapes and sizes (see Figure 10-1 for a sample). Here are some guidelines to help you decide what works for your recipe:

✔ For lighter, brothy sauces and pesto choose delicate, long pasta, such as vermicelli, spaghetti, linguine, or angel hair.

✔ For meatier, chunkier sauces or pasta salads, choose shorter shapes with ridges or holes, such as cavatelli, penne, farfalle, and wagon wheels. The smaller pieces make it easier to grab pasta and sauce with every bite. And the ridges and holes in the pasta grab bits and chunks of your sauce.

✔ For heavier and creamier sauces, choose flat, ribbon-like pasta, such as fettuccine or tagliatelle.

Most pasta is made from semolina flour, not refined white flour. Pasta is a complex carbohydrate, rather than a simple carbohydrate, meaning that it gives your body more lasting energy and a more gradual release of sugar. A 70-gram (2½-ounce) serving of cooked pasta contains 92 kilocalories, less than half a gram of fat, and less than 5 milligrams of sodium; and it costs you only 1 starch exchange.

Here are a few other benefits of choosing pasta:

✔ Pasta has a relatively low glycaemic index of 44. For more about the glycaemic index and how it can help you manage your blood glucose levels, check out Chapter 2.

✔ Pasta is a quick food to prepare and makes a filling side dish that's ready in about 10 minutes.

✔ Pasta is so versatile that it goes with just about anything. You can toss it with chicken broth and fresh herbs, or fresh vegetables and a little bit of olive oil. Here are some other ideas:

• Create Chinese flavoured dishes with a splash of sesame oil, crunchy water chestnuts, pak choi, and coriander. Add thinly sliced beef for a full meal.

• Mix up a Mediterranean delight with tomatoes, garlic, and fresh basil. Throw in some pine nuts and seafood for a low-fat, tasty weeknight supper.

- Invent your own Latin lunch, by including grilled onions, chicken breast, chilli peppers, and squash.

- Introduce flavours from the Caribbean by tossing pasta with prawns, flaked coconut, jerk seasonings, and vegetable stock.

- Work in some Vietnamese inspired cuisine, by adding pasta to vegetable broth, chopped chilli peppers, coriander, and lean pork.

✔ Pasta is very filling. A 70-gram (2½-ounce) serving may not seem like much, but a little goes a long way, especially if you bulk up the fibre content of your dish with fresh vegetables. Or opt for 2 starch servings, and have 140 grams (5 ounces) of cooked pasta and enjoy as a main course.

Although most of the pasta in your local shops is made from semolina flour, you can find pasta made from a variety of different flours, including the following:

✔ **Brown rice:** This pasta is a great alternative for people who are sensitive to wheat. Check the label, but most brown rice pasta is both wheat-free and gluten-free. Some are also dairy-free and organic. Try this delicious pasta in the Buckwheat and Brown Rice Pasta recipe in this section.

✔ **Soy:** Pasta made with soy flour is usually higher in protein and lower in carbohydrate than semolina pasta, but always read the label to ensure that you're making the right choice for your needs.

✔ **Wholewheat:** If you're looking for a higher fibre pasta, wholewheat pasta is ideal, and has a more robust flavour than its semolina counterpart.

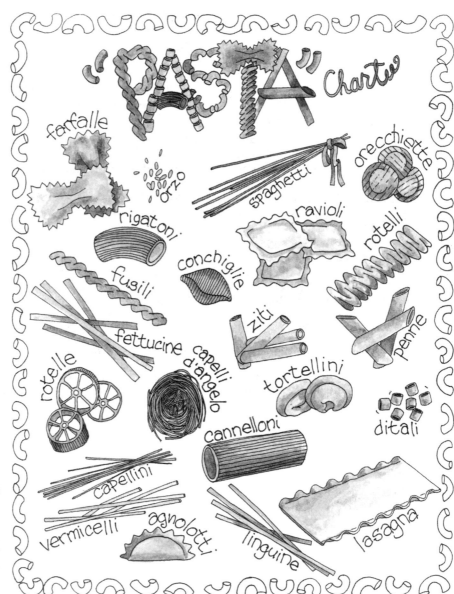

☜ Butterfly Pasta with Sun-Dried Tomatoes and Artichoke Hearts

The few ingredients that this simple recipe calls for complement each other perfectly. The dish is a certified crowd pleaser, full of colour and flavour and ideal for entertaining. The pasta is best served at room temperature, so you can make it hours in advance, freeing you for the last-minute details of throwing a party.

Preparation time: *15 minutes (plus overnight marinating time)*

Cooking time: *10 minutes*

Serves: *4*

55 grams sun-dried tomatoes, chopped

120 millilitres extra-virgin olive oil

3 garlic cloves, crushed

20 grams finely chopped basil leaves, plus extra whole leaves for garnish

425-gram jar marinated artichoke hearts, drained

225 grams uncooked butterfly pasta (farfalle)

Freshly ground black pepper (optional)

Grated Parmesan cheese (optional)

1 In a shallow bowl, combine the tomatoes, olive oil, garlic, and basil. Let it rest overnight so that the tomatoes rehydrate.

2 Transfer the tomato mixture to a large bowl and add the artichoke hearts. Lightly toss together.

3 Bring a large pot of water to the boil and cook the pasta according to the directions on the package until the pasta is *al dente,* cooked but not soft. Drain and add to the tomato artichoke mixture. Adjust seasoning with ground black pepper (if desired).

4 Serve at room temperature, garnished with whole basil leaves and Parmesan cheese on the side, if desired.

Per serving (without Parmesan): Kilocalories 550; Fat 32g (Saturated 4g); Cholesterol 0mg; Sodium 160mg; Carbohydrate 53g; Dietary Fibre 6g; Protein 13g.

Exchanges: 4 starch, 6 fat, 2 vegetable.

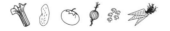

Seafood Farfalle Salad

Unsurprisingly, because Italy has many coastal cities, loads of pasta dishes include fish. The Italians even use the black ink of octopus in one special pasta dish. This recipe is much tamer, however, and is a low-kilocalorie but quite satisfying combination of seafood and pasta. Using farfalle, pasta shaped like a butterfly or a bow tie, adds eye appeal. If you have access to a specialty Italian food market, you may even find far-fallini, the smallest butterflies, or farfallone, the largest.

Preparation time: *25 minutes*

Cooking time: *20 to 25 minutes*

Serves: *4*

225 grams uncooked farfalle pasta

Nonstick cooking spray or 2 tablespoons olive oil

225 grams fresh scallops

225 grams cooked baby prawns

1½ teaspoons white wine vinegar

1 tablespoon extra-virgin olive oil

1 teaspoon freshly squeezed lemon juice

1 teaspoon dried thyme leaves

Garlic clove, crushed

2 teaspoons chopped fresh parsley

Pinch of black pepper

90 grams plum tomatoes, peeled, seeded, and diced

Small cucumber, peeled, seeded, and diced

2 tablespoons seeded and finely chopped green bell pepper

1 Bring a large pot of water to the boil. Add the farfalle and cook according to package directions. Drain, rinse under cold running water, and drain again. Set aside.

2 Meanwhile, coat a medium nonstick frying pan with cooking spray or 2 teaspoons of olive oil and place over a medium heat until hot. Add the scallops and prawns, a few at a time, and sauté, turning them as they brown, allowing 1½ to 2 minutes per side; remove them to a bowl as they finish.

3 In a large bowl, whisk together the vinegar, olive oil, lemon juice, thyme, garlic, parsley, and black pepper. Add the tomatoes, cucumber, and green pepper and mix thoroughly. Combine the pasta, scallops (and their released juices), and prawns. Toss the pasta mixture with the dressing mixture.

Per serving: *Kilocalories 350; Fat 7g (Saturated 1g); Cholesterol 182mg; Sodium 1,005mg; Carbohydrate 44g; Dietary Fibre 3g; Protein 26g.*

Exchanges: *3 starch, 3 very lean meat, 1 fat.*

☞ Buckwheat and Brown Rice Pasta

Sometimes simple food, such as this delicious combination of buckwheat and pasta, tastes the best. Kasha is buckwheat *groats,* which means it's hulled and crushed buckwheat. The flavours are mellow and nutty with just a hint of mushroom, a step beyond blandness but still a comfort food. This mixture is a good background dish, served with savoury foods such as chicken roasted with herbs or slow-cooked flank steak prepared with onion and dried fruits. This merger of whole grains and pasta is especially popular in Eastern European and Russian cooking.

Preparation time: *10 minutes*

Cooking time: *25 minutes*

Serves: *6*

2 teaspoons olive oil

Medium onion, chopped

Egg, slightly beaten

160 grams kasha (buckwheat groats)

35 grams sliced button mushrooms

480 millilitres boiling vegetable broth or water

Ground black pepper

960 millilitres water

160 grams brown rice pasta rotini/spirals

1 In a heavy medium-sized saucepan, heat the oil and sauté the onion until translucent (5 to 7 minutes).

2 Beat the egg in a small bowl. Add the buckwheat and mix together, coating each grain with the egg. Add to the onions. Cook the kasha while stirring until the grains are dry and separated.

3 Add the mushrooms, broth or water, and pepper. Cover the pan and simmer until all the liquid is absorbed (about 15 minutes).

4 In the meantime, bring the 960 millilitres of water to a boil in a large pot. Add the rice pasta rotini/spirals and cook for 6 minutes, or until tender but still firm. Drain and, if necessary, keep warm while the kasha finishes cooking.

When the kasha is fully cooked, fluff with a fork and stir in the rotini/spirals.

Per serving: Kilocalories 187; Fat 4g (Saturated 1g); Cholesterol 35mg; Sodium 20mg; Carbohydrate 31g; Dietary Fibre 3g; Protein 6g.

Exchanges: 2 starch, ½ fat.

Letting Legumes into Your Diet

Legumes (pronounced *lay*-gooms) are the protein-packed staple of a vegetarian diet, but you don't have to swear off meat to enjoy them. The legume family includes thousands of plant species, including beans, soybeans, lentils, peas, and the beloved peanut.

Finding a more perfect all-round food than legumes is tough. They're rich in protein, low in fat (what fat they do have is the good fat), high in dietary fibre, and rich in complex carbohydrates and vitamins. Besides their healthy benefits, they're also inexpensive, versatile, and easy to use. They store well when dried, and have a shelf life of a full year.

Because legumes are also high in carbohydrate, diabetics still need to take care with their portion sizes. The benefits that the fibre and protein provide, however, make them a better option than the usual carbohydrates such as bread, pasta, or rice.

Lentils cook quickly, so you don't need to soak them before cooking as you do with dried beans. If you're extra conscious, feel free to pick over the lentils, as you would with dried beans. Rinse them well to remove any dirt or other debris, and then sort through a handful at a time, looking for dirt clods, stones, and other foreign particles. Try lentils in soups, saucy Indian curries, or this terrific 'salad'.

○ Olive and Lentil Salad

This dish is considered a 'salad', but don't let that word fool you! This dish is unlike most salads – it's hearty and keeps you full and satisfied for a long time. This olive and lentil mix has a ton of fibre and protein (from the lentils) and enough heart-healthy monounsaturated fats (from the olives) that digest slowly to keep you feeling full for longer. This one-pot meal has only a moderate amount of carbohydrate, so it's kind to your blood sugar level, and it offers you a significant amount of iron, calcium, and vitamins A, C, B6, and folate (another B vitamin) .

Preparation time: 30 minutes

Cooking time: 40 minutes

Serves: 6

Salad:

190 grams dry lentils

2 bay leaves

Sprig fresh thyme

Carrot, finely chopped

Stalk celery, finely chopped

2 tablespoons chopped shallots

1 tablespoon crushed garlic

2 plum tomatoes, seeded and sliced thinly

½ yellow bell pepper, diced

225 grams unsalted green olives, roughly chopped (reserve any juice for the dressing)

2 tablespoons roughly chopped fresh oregano

Ground black pepper

115 grams goats' cheese, crumbled

Dressing:

60ml red wine vinegar

2 tablespoons green olive juice

1 tablespoon chopped shallot

3 teaspoons Dijon mustard

1 teaspoon ground black pepper

60 millilitres olive oil

1 In a large saucepan, combine the lentils, bay leaves, thyme, carrot, celery, shallots, and garlic. Cover with water. Bring to a low boil and cook until the lentils are just tender (about 40 minutes). Drain and set aside to cool.

2 After the lentils have cooled, add the tomatoes, bell pepper, olives, and oregano. Mix thoroughly. Add black pepper to taste. Gently stir in the goats' cheese.

3 In a blender, combine the vinegar, olive juice, shallot, mustard, and pepper. Remove the knob from the lid of the blender. With the blender running, slowly pour in the olive oil to emulsify the dressing. Adjust seasonings as necessary. Pour over the salad and toss gently to coat.

Per serving: Kilocalories 343; Fat 21g (Saturated 5g); Cholesterol 0mg; Sodium 1,066mg; Carbohydrate 20g; Dietary Fibre 8g; Protein 14g.

Exchanges: 1 starch, 1 very lean meat, 1 medium-fat meat, 3½ fat.

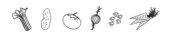

Red Wine Braised Lentils

This recipe is an easy accompaniment to any poultry or meat dish. The hearty lentils are softened during the slow-cooked method of braising in which they soak-up the delicious flavour of the red wine. Lentils are a complex carbohydrate full of fibre, as well as a good source of protein.

Preparation time: *10 minutes*

Cooking time: *1 hour and 20 minutes*

Serves: *6*

1 tablespoon butter

2 tablespoons olive oil

160 grams chopped onions

2 stalks celery, chopped

Medium carrot, chopped

Ground black pepper

½ teaspoon thyme leaves

60 grams diced prosciutto

28 grams dried porcini mushrooms, reconstituted and sliced (see the tip at the end of the recipe)

360 millilitres red wine

380 grams dried brown lentils

Bay leaf

1,200 millilitres low-sodium chicken broth

1 In a medium saucepan, heat the butter and olive oil. Sauté the onions, celery, and carrot until they begin to *sweat,* or give off a bit of liquid. Season the vegetables with black pepper to taste and cover. Cook until the vegetables are soft (approximately 10 minutes).

2 Add the thyme, prosciutto, and dried porcini mushrooms. Add the wine and reduce by one-third. Add the lentils, bay leaf, and chicken broth and simmer for about 1 hour, until the lentils are soft.

3 Remove the bay leaf. Adjust the pepper if needed. You can refrigerate this dish for up to 3 days, until ready to use.

Tip: To reconstitute the dried porcini mushrooms, place them in 60 millilitres of hot water for 30 minutes, chop them, and strain the liquid. If you want, you can use the liquid as part of the cooking liquid. Just substitute the mushroom broth for the equivalent amount of chicken broth in Step 2.

Per serving: *Kilocalories 348; Fat 10g (Saturated 3g); Cholesterol 17mg; Sodium 241mg; Carbohydrate 28g; Dietary Fibre 16g; Protein 23g.*

Exchanges: *3 starch, 3 very lean meat, 1½ fat.*

'Beans, beans, they're good for your heart.' This saying is in fact true. Beans offer a tremendous amount of fibre, more specifically soluble fibre – the type that lowers your LDL (low-density lipoprotein), or 'bad' cholesterol. (Refer to Chapter 2 for more on 'good' and 'bad' cholesterol.) Because beans are plant based, they have no cholesterol.

☞ White Bean, Spinach, and Mushroom Medley

Beans are a dietary staple in almost every culture. This recipe uses cannellini beans together with nutritious, carotenoid-rich spinach. Use canned beans and pre-washed spinach to make this nutritious powerhouse, which is as easy to make as to enjoy.

Preparation time: *10 minutes*

Cooking time: *20 minutes*

Serves: *4*

1 tablespoon olive oil

80 grams chopped onion

3 garlic cloves, peeled and sliced thinly

70 grams sliced Italian cremini (portobello) mushrooms

60 millilitres dry white wine

1 tablespoon Dijon mustard

140 grams well-washed spinach

425 grams cooked white beans (like navy, cannellini, or great northern), rinsed and drained

2 tablespoons fresh chopped oregano

Ground black pepper

1 Heat the olive oil in a frying pan over a medium-high heat. Add the onions and sauté until translucent. Add the garlic and mushrooms, and cook until just fragrant. Add the white wine and mustard. Scrape up any browned bits that are stuck to the pan.

2 Add the spinach and cover. Steam the spinach for 3 to 4 minutes, or until wilted but still bright green. Add the white beans. Continue to cook until heated through. Add the oregano and black pepper to taste.

Per serving: *Kilocalories 122; Fat 4g (Saturated 1g); Cholesterol 0mg; Sodium 385mg; Carbohydrate 13g; Dietary Fibre 5g; Protein 5g.*

Exchanges: *½ starch, 1 vegetable, ½ very lean meat, 1 fat.*

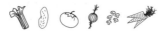

Many different kinds of canned beans are available in shops and supermarkets. They're a bit more expensive than the dried variety, but they help you create a well-balanced nutritious meal super-fast. Keep a few cans in your cupboard, for quick and satisfying meals, such as the following Black Bean Pie, which keeps you full and your blood glucose level stable.

When using canned anything, such as beans or vegetables, whenever possible, drain and rinse the food before cooking to get rid of excess sodium. But before you toss out the liquid, remember to double-check the recipe. Some recipes, such as the one for Black Bean Pie in this section, use the liquid in the recipe.

☺ *Black Bean Pie*

This recipe is a great way to get a well-balanced meal that includes most of the basic food groups. The beans, peppers, and coriander stop a craving for Mexican food dead in its tracks. Serve with a crisp green salad to round out your meal plan.

Preparation time: *45 minutes*

Cooking time: *20 minutes*

Serves: *6*

400 grams canned black beans	*½ small green bell pepper, chopped*
100 grams jasmine rice, uncooked	*1 tablespoon chopped fresh coriander*
23-centimetre frozen pie shell	*1 teaspoon cumin, ground*
Nonstick cooking spray	*1 teaspoon chilli powder*
80 grams chopped onion	*½ teaspoon cayenne pepper*
Garlic clove, crushed	*2 tablespoons cornflour*
½ small red bell pepper, chopped	*85 grams grated cheddar cheese*

1 Preheat the oven to 180°C/350°F/Gas Mark 4. Drain the black beans and reserve the juice. Set to one side.

2 Cook the jasmine rice according to the packet's directions. Set aside. While the rice is cooking, bake the pie shell until slightly browned (approximately 5 to 7 minutes), and set aside.

3 Heat a medium frying pan over a medium-high heat. Once heated, spray the pan with the cooking spray. Add the onions, garlic, and red and green peppers. Sauté until the vegetables are crisp but tender (approximately 5 to 7 minutes). Set aside.

4 In a bowl, combine the beans, rice, onion mixture, coriander, cumin, chilli powder, and cayenne pepper. In another bowl, combine the reserved black bean juice with the cornflour to make a paste. Mix the paste into the black bean mixture.

5 Spread the black bean mixture in the pie shell. Cover with the cheese. Bake for 15 to 20 minutes, until the cheese starts to brown. Allow to set for 15 minutes before serving.

Per serving: *Kilocalories 303; Fat 12g (Saturated 5g); Cholesterol 15g; Sodium 372mg; Carbohydrate 32g; Dietary Fibre 5g; Protein 10g.*

Exchanges: *2 starch, 1 high-fat meat, 1 fat.*

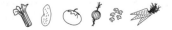

⏲ Spicy Hummus

Hummus is a classic Mediterranean and Middle Eastern dish, but this version has a spicy twist. This creamy spread (with little fat!) makes a surprisingly healthy appetiser – great served with wholewheat pitta bread wedges, baked tortilla chips, or raw vegetables. (If you're looking for other delicious dipper ideas to pair with this tasty spread, check out Chapter 7.) The main ingredients here are chickpeas, which are an excellent vegetarian source of protein, as well as dietary fibre – two great reasons why hummus makes a perfect snack. Protein and fibre are essential for good blood glucose control, so keep a bowl of hummus on hand when you're looking for something light, quick, and easy.

Preparation time: *10 minutes*

Serves: *4*

Garlic clove, crushed

2 425-gram cans chickpeas, drained and rinsed

65 grams ready-made tomato–chilli salsa

2 tablespoons fresh lime juice

1 teaspoon cumin

½ teaspoon chilli powder

1 teaspoon cayenne pepper (more or less as you prefer)

1 tablespoon olive oil

Handful of roughly chopped coriander

Ground black pepper

Garnishes (optional):

1 tablespoon light sour cream

2 tablespoons chopped avocado

1 tablespoon chopped coriander

1 tablespoon minced black olives

1 Place the garlic, chickpeas, salsa, lime juice, cumin, chilli powder, cayenne pepper, olive oil, and coriander into a food processor and blend. Add black pepper and adjust other seasonings to taste. Place in a covered bowl. Chill in the refrigerator for 2 to 3 hours to allow flavours to mingle thoroughly.

2 When ready to serve, spread the hummus in the bottom of a medium-sized serving bowl, and top with the garnishes in the following order: light sour cream, avocado, coriander, and black olives.

Per serving: *Kilocalories 170; Fat 5g (Saturated 1g); Cholesterol 0mg; Sodium 389mg; Carbohydrate 18g; Dietary Fibre 6g; Protein 7g.*

Exchanges: *1 starch, 1 very lean meat, 1 fat.*

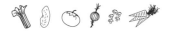

Chapter 11

Adding Veg to Your Meals

In This Chapter

▶ Converting vegetables into food exchanges

▶ Giving old favourites a fresh taste

▶ Including starchy vegetables in your diet

▶ Making 'noodles' from firm vegetables

▶ Dressing up vegetables for special occasions

*Y*our body thrives on the fantastic phytochemicals, must-have vitamins and nutrients, and fabulous fibre found in vegetables, but most people just don't eat enough of them. And yet you can eat vegetables in so many ways: in soups, in salads, puréed in sauces, on the side, or as the main event. Whether you eat them cooked or raw, using fresh or frozen products, you can improve your health today by increasing the amount of vegetables you eat.

In this chapter, we show you how to translate vegetables into food exchanges and how to use common vegetables in exciting new ways. We also help you to create some special-occasion recipes to impress your guests.

Translating Vegetable Servings into Exchanges

For people with diabetes, not all vegetables are created equal. In relation to food exchanges, vegetables fall into one of three categories:

❙ **Starchy vegetables:** These vegetables are so high in carbohydrates that in food exchange lists (see Appendix B for all the lists) they count as a starch, not a vegetable. Starchy vegetables include sweetcorn, parsnips, plantains, potatoes, pumpkin, sweet potatoes, winter squash, and legumes, including beans, lentils, lima beans, and peas.

✔ **Vegetables that count as a single vegetable exchange:** Many common vegetables do count as vegetables, including artichokes, asparagus, aubergines, bamboo shoots, bean sprouts, beets, broccoli, Brussels sprouts, cooked cabbage, carrots, chard, green pepper, kale, kohl rabi, leeks, mangetout, okra, onions, swede, sauerkraut, cooked spinach, string beans, tomatoes, turnips, and water chestnuts.

✔ **Free vegetables:** A few vegetables, typically those with a high water content, don't count at all! They contain so little fat, protein, or carbohydrates that you can consider them freebies. You can have up to two helpings of the following with little effect on your blood glucose: alfalfa sprouts, raw cabbage, celery, chicory, Chinese cabbage, courgette, cucumber, endive, spring onions, fresh spinach, hot peppers, lettuce, mushrooms, radishes, rhubarb, fresh salad greens, and watercress.

Adding a New Twist to Old Favourites (And Not-So-Favourites)

Most people have a vegetable that haunts them from their childhood. Whether you're unfortunate enough to remember Aunt Betty's Brussels sprout casserole at a family reunion when you were 9 years old, or you were forced to sit in front of a plate of lukewarm boiled carrots that you were unable to choke down, you probably have one vegetable you just don't like. Well, hopefully, we're about to change your view of vegetables.

In this section, we give you delicious recipes using traditional vegetables that you may not feel kindly towards – yet. But never fear, after trying a few, you're sure to have a whole new appreciation for these previously shunned vegetables.

Including delicious extras

The following recipes focus on adding tasty flavours such as lemon, herbs, and cheese to old stand-by vegetables such as Brussels sprouts, broccoli, and courgette. Try them the next time you want to add some zing to your veggies.

↺ Brussels Sprouts Roasted with Lemon and Capers

These Brussels sprouts are simple to prepare and surprisingly good! And luckily for you they're also full of wonderful nutrition. Just one serving gives you 25 per cent of your daily vitamin A requirement, 25 per cent of your dietary fibre goal, and more than 100 per cent of your daily vitamin C needs. These sprouts are also a great source of antioxidant carotenoids such as lutein, an important nutrient for eye health. No need to add any large amounts of salt here. Just a small touch of capers (which contain sodium) does the job.

Preparation time: *20 minutes*

Cooking time: *25 minutes*

Serves: *6*

675 grams Brussels sprouts	*3 tablespoons olive oil*
Juice from 2 lemons	*Ground black pepper*
2 tablespoons capers	

1 Preheat the oven to 200°C/400°F/Gas Mark 6. Trim the bottoms from the Brussels sprouts, cut them in half, and place in a pan of boiling water. Cook for 8 to 10 minutes, or until fork-tender.

2 Remove them from the water and drain. Toss the sprouts with the lemon juice, capers, and olive oil. Season with black pepper to taste and place in a roasting pan.

3 Roast for 10 minutes.

Per serving: *Kilocalories 114; Fat 7g (Saturated 1g); Cholesterol 0mg; Sodium 63mg; Carbohydrate 5g; Dietary Fibre 5g; Protein 3g.*

Exchanges: *2 vegetable, 1½ fat.*

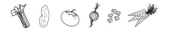

Broccoli is one of the most nutritious vegetables out there. If you still can't seem to acquire a liking for it though, look no further. Prepare the following elegant recipe for your family or guests, and surprise everyone – especially when you tell them that the rich, savoury sauce has barely any fat.

⏱ Broccoli with Creamy Lemon Sauce

Who doesn't love broccoli and cheese? And for most of us, the more cheese the better! And what's even better, you can enjoy this one guilt-free. This creamy sauce is made with mainly low-fat ingredients instead of the full-fat dairy products that usually go into rich sauces. Just ensure that you don't add any more salt. The cottage cheese and Parmesan already contribute enough for flavour.

Preparation time: *10 minutes*

Cooking time: *35 minutes*

Serves: *6*

150 grams low-fat cottage cheese

60 millilitres evaporated skimmed milk

2 tablespoons grated Parmesan cheese

1 teaspoon lemon juice

Pinch of ground turmeric

White pepper

220 grams hot cooked broccoli florets

1 In a blender, combine the cottage cheese, milk, Parmesan cheese, lemon juice, turmeric, and white pepper to taste, and purée until the mixture achieves a thin consistency (about 30 seconds).

2 Heat the sauce in a pan, stirring occasionally, until heated through, but don't boil.

3 Serve the sauce over the warm broccoli.

Per serving: *Kilocalories 45; Fat 1g (Saturated 1g); Cholesterol 3mg; Sodium 155mg; Carbohydrate 3g; Dietary Fibre 1g; Protein 6g.*

Exchanges: *1 vegetable, ½ very lean meat.*

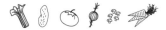

⏱ Courgette and Parmigiano-Reggiano Salad

This dish is sure to become a favourite in your household. The recipe uses simple, quality ingredients, such as Parmigiano-Reggiano (the original and best Parmesan cheese in the world), extra-virgin olive oil, and fresh lemon juice, to provide rich flavours with very little effort.

Preparation time: *15 minutes*

Serves: *4*

3 medium courgettes, peeled and sliced	4 tablespoons extra-virgin olive oil
50 grams Parmigiano-Reggiano, shaved thin	½ teaspoon ground black pepper
1 tablespoon lemon juice	2 tablespoons chopped lemon verbena

Place the courgettes in a bowl and shave the Parmigiano-Reggiano over them. Add the lemon juice, olive oil, black pepper, and verbena. Toss to incorporate the ingredients and serve.

Tip: *Lemon verbena is a potent herb, with a strong lemon flavour. You can find it in specialty food shops. Alternatively, look for it at your local nursery and grow your own. If you can't find lemon verbena, you can always pick another herb (such as tarragon or basil). The substitution changes the flavour but this dish is still fresh and delicious.*

Per serving: Kilocalories 188; Fat 17g (Saturated 4g); Cholesterol 8mg; Sodium 266mg; Carbohydrate 3g; Dietary Fibre 2g; Protein 6g.

Exchanges: 1 vegetable, 3 fat, 1 lean meat.

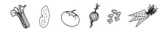

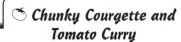
☞ Chunky Courgette and Tomato Curry

This vegetable curry is delicious, perfect as a side dish, as a dip, or on top of crisp bruschetta. The recipe's full of Indian-inspired spices and remains modestly low in kilocalories and fat. No added salt is needed as the spices already offer plenty of flavour. Be creative with spices, like the ones used here, to make unique ways of serving simple vegetables that you and your guests are sure to love.

Preparation time: *10 minutes*

Cooking time: *20 minutes*

Serves: *4*

2 tablespoons olive oil	1 teaspoon ground coriander
1 medium red onion, finely diced	2 teaspoons curry powder
2 teaspoons grated fresh ginger	250 grams canned, chopped tomatoes
4 garlic cloves, crushed	450 grams courgette, quartered lengthwise and chopped into large chunks

(continued)

1 Heat the olive oil in a large nonstick frying pan. Sauté the onion, ginger, and garlic for about 5 minutes, or until the onions are translucent. Add the coriander and curry powder. Continue cooking for 1 minute.

2 Stir in the tomatoes and courgette. Simmer for approximately 10 minutes, until the courgette is tender.

Per serving: Kilocalories 97; Fat 8g (Saturated 1g); Cholesterol 0mg; Sodium 38mg; Carbohydrate 5g; Dietary Fibre 3g; Protein 2g.

Exchanges: 2 vegetable, 1½ fat.

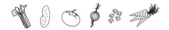

Enhancing natural flavours with dry steaming

Dry steaming refers to cooking vegetables in their own natural juices rather than adding additional moisture. In the case of carrots, they have a medium to high moisture content, so that when you heat them in a closed environment (for example, in a pot with a tight-fitting lid), they use the liquid that they give off during the cooking process to create steam and facilitate the cooking process. So the food is essentially steamed without adding any water. You get a similar effect when you microwave vegetables without adding water.

Don't microwave vegetables, or anything else, in a completely closed container. Always provide a vent of some sort for steam to escape.

☺ Dill-Scented Carrots

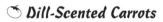

Here's a tasty twist on a vegetable favourite, which uses fresh herbs to give carrots a new and interesting flavour. Carrots are one of the best sources of antioxidants such as lutein and betacarotene, which are important for eye health. The orange fruits and vegetables are all good sources of these antioxidants, so get them in whenever you can!

Preparation time: *10 minutes*

Cooking time: *35 to 40 minutes*

Serves: *12*

2 tablespoons unsalted butter

450 grams baby carrots

1 tablespoon chopped fresh dill

Ground black pepper

1 Melt the butter in a deep frying pan or wok with a tight-fitting lid. Add the carrots. Cook over a medium to medium-low heat for approximately 35 to 40 minutes. Shake the pan occasionally during cooking, without removing the lid.

2 Remove the lid after 35 to 40 minutes and check to confirm that the carrots are tender. Allow any excess moisture to evaporate from the pan. Toss the carrots with the dill. Add black pepper to taste.

Per serving: *Kilocalories 31; Fat 2g (Saturated 1g); Cholesterol 5mg; Sodium 34mg; Carbohydrate 2g; Dietary Fibre 1g; Protein 0g.*

Exchanges: *1 vegetable, ½ fat.*

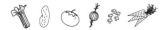

Blanching vegetables for optimum taste and nutrition

As well as being surprisingly simple, *blanching* is also a terrific technique for cooking vegetables without losing too many of the vitamins that make them so healthy for you. You immerse vegetables in boiling water, leave them in the water for a short period of time, and then *shock* them, or immerse them in ice-cold water to stop the cooking. This technique helps to prevent the vegetables from getting mushy.

Here are the detailed steps to follow for blanching vegetables.

1. **Bring water to a vigorous boil in a large saucepan.**

2. **While the water is working up to a boil, prepare the ice bath.**

   Fill a medium-sized mixing bowl one-half to three-quarters full with ice. Add water to just cover the ice.

3. **Blanch the vegetables.**

   Place the trimmed vegetables, in batches if necessary, in the boiling water. Cook the vegetables until they're crisply tender.

   You want to keep a constant boil, but adding too many veggies at a time can slow down the process.

4. **Shock the vegetables.**

   Remove the vegetables with a slotted spoon and immediately place them in the ice bath. Remove them from the ice bath after the vegetables are completely cooled, usually 1 to 2 minutes.

To check they are done, remove a single vegetable piece from the boiling water with a slotted spoon; submerge it in the ice bath until cool enough to place in your mouth. Then actually taste it to check the texture. Do this step quickly so that if the vegetables are ready, the rest of them in the boiling water don't overcook while you're testing.

5. Reheat the vegetables and season as desired.

Blanching times vary based on the vegetable and the size of the pieces, but Table 11-1 shows a few approximate times.

Table 11-1	Approximate Blanching Times for Vegetables	
Vegetable	*Size*	*Approximate Time*
Asparagus	Spears	3 to 4 minutes
Aubergine	Slices	3 minutes
Broccoli	Florets, bite sized	3 minutes
Brussels sprouts	Whole	3 to 5 minutes
Cabbage	Leaves	5 to 10 minutes
Carrots, baby	Whole	5 minutes
Carrots	Diced or strips	2 minutes
Cauliflower	Florets, bite sized	3 minutes
Corn	Cob	4 minutes
Courgette	Bite-sized chunks	3 minutes
Green beans	Whole	3 minutes
Greens like spinach	Leaves	2 minutes
Mushrooms	Whole or caps	5 minutes
Okra	Pod	3 to 5 minutes
Peas, shelled	Whole	1½ minutes
Peas	Pod	2 to 3 minutes
Summer squash	Bite-sized chunks	3 minutes
Tomatoes	Whole, for peeling	1 minute

Give blanching a try with several of the recipes in this book, including the following recipe for Haricot Vert and the Yellow Tomato Sauce later in this chapter.

⟳ *Haricot Vert*

Haricot vert (pronounced ah-ree-co *vehr*) is a fancy French word that literally means 'green beans' and refers to (surprise!) green beans, or what you may call string or runner beans. If you find true French haricot vert in the supermarket, use them in this recipe. They're a bit smaller and thinner than common string beans, but the flavour is very similar. If you can't find them, feel free to substitute fresh string beans, however. Canned beans don't work because they're already cooked beyond tender. Enjoy this elegant vegetable with any hearty entrée.

Preparation time: *10 minutes*

Cooking time: *10 minutes*

Serves: *6*

600 grams string beans

2 tablespoons butter

Ground black pepper

Cut off the ends of the beans and blanch in boiling water for 1 minute (see the instructions earlier in this section on blanching). Remove and place them in an ice water bath. Drain and reheat in a pan with the butter and pepper to taste.

Tip: *Serve these tasty veggies with the Veal Tenderloin and Chanterelle Mushrooms recipe in Chapter 14.*

Per serving: *Kilocalories 71; Fat 4g (Saturated 2g); Cholesterol 10mg; Sodium 38mg; Carbohydrate 5g; Dietary Fibre 4g; Protein 2g.*

Exchanges: *1 vegetable, 1 fat.*

Serving Up Starchy Vegetables

Potatoes and sweetcorn – two of the most commonly eaten starchy vegetables – have surprisingly high glycaemic index values (refer to Chapter 2 for more on the glycaemic index). Processed versions of these foods, such as instant mashed potatoes and cornflakes, which enter the bloodstream more quickly than foods in their natural state, rank even higher on the scale. Believe it or not, these convenience foods have an effect on your bloodstream similar to low-fat ice cream.

Potatoes and sweetcorn can have a place in your diet, but you need to eat them in smaller portions and balance their carbohydrate content with protein and fat from other foods at the same meal. But with all the great recipes in this chapter, you don't need to default to those high-starch foods regularly. Try out this excellent substitute for mashed potatoes the next time you're looking for a nutritious side dish.

☞ *Mashed Sweet Potatoes*

Here's a perfect example of a great substitution for a traditional food – a substitution that adds lots more colour on your plate and, usually, many more key nutrients from the antioxidant pigments. Instead of the usual white potatoes, this recipe uses sweet potatoes. The orange variety is rich in carotenoids such as lutein and betacarotene, cancer-fighting antioxidants and key nutrients for eye health. This recipe calls for just a bit of low-fat evaporated milk, providing a more concentrated flavour without the extra kilocalories and fat. Because sweet potatoes already have a natural sweet flavour, little added butter and salt are needed.

Preparation time: *10 minutes*

Cooking time: *35 minutes*

Serves: *6*

900 grams sweet potatoes (roughly 4 large sweet potatoes), peeled and cubed

1 tablespoon butter

Ground black pepper

80 millilitres evaporated low-fat milk

Boil the sweet potatoes in a saucepan until fork-tender, then drain. Place them in a bowl and, using an electric mixer, whip. Add the butter and pepper to taste, and the milk.

Per serving: *Kilocalories 184; Fat 3g (Saturated 2g); Cholesterol 11mg; Sodium 102mg; Carbohydrate 32g; Dietary Fibre 4g; Protein 4g.*

Exchanges: *2 starch, 1 fat.*

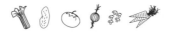

Using Vegetables in Place of Pasta

Pasta gets a lot of bad press these days, but the biggest problem is the portion size that most people typically eat. For healthy ways to include pasta and other grains in your diet, check out Chapter 10.

When you crave the rich, delicious Italian sauces but have run out of starch exchanges for the day, vegetables make a terrific substitute. Make 'noodles' from slices of aubergine, strings of cucumber, or slices of courgette. Get started with the great Aubergine Lasagne recipe below.

A *mandoline* is a handy tool to have around your kitchen. Take a look at one in Figure 11-1. A mandoline is a manual slicing device that quickly makes consistently sized cuts of foods. You can use it to make julienne strips or even thin slices of aubergine (for the Aubergine Lasagne recipe below). You can make paper-thin strips of sweet potatoes for your own baked chips or thick lemon wheels for water. Consider getting one to ease the prep work of making your own vegetable noodles. Look for a mandoline at your local kitchen or gourmet shop.

Figure 11-1:
A mandoline
makes quick
work of
slicing and
creating
julienne
cuts.

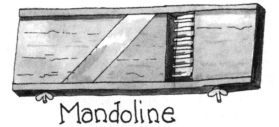

Mandoline

⊘ Aubergine Lasagne

This recipe uses slices of aubergine in place of traditional lasagne sheets. Although some time is necessary to get these 'sheets' ready to layer, the effort is definitely worthwhile. When you slice into this cheesy, layered, flavourful dish, you aren't going to miss the pasta.

Preparation time: *45 minutes*

Cooking time: *60 minutes*

Serves: *6*

Nonstick cooking spray

Large aubergine, unpeeled, halved lengthwise, and sliced ½-centimetre thick

2 tablespoons olive oil

2 garlic cloves, crushed

Small onion, finely chopped

2 225-gram cans low-sodium tomato sauce

400-gram can low-sodium diced tomatoes, drained

Pinch of crushed red chilli pepper flakes

Pinch of dried oregano

Pinch of dried basil

Pinch of dried thyme

Ground black pepper

125 grams low-fat ricotta cheese

60 grams grated low-fat mozzarella cheese

2 tablespoons grated Parmesan cheese

1 Preheat the oven to 220°C/425°F/Gas Mark 7. Cover a baking sheet with foil. Coat the foil with the cooking spray and arrange the aubergine in a single layer on the foil-lined baking sheet. Lightly coat the aubergine with 1 tablespoon of the oil. Bake for 5 minutes, turn the aubergine, bake for an additional 5 minutes, and set aside to cool.

2 Reduce the oven temperature to 180°C/350°F/Gas Mark 4. Make the tomato sauce: Place a medium saucepan over a medium-high heat. Add the remaining 1 tablespoon of olive oil, the garlic, and the onions. Sauté for about 5 minutes, until the onions are tender. Add the tomato sauce, chopped tomatoes, red pepper flakes, oregano, basil, and thyme. Lower the heat to a medium-low heat and simmer the sauce for 30 minutes. Season with pepper to taste.

3 In a 20 × 20 centimetre (8 × 8 inch) ovenproof lasagne dish, spoon enough sauce to coat the bottom and then cover with a layer of aubergine. Spread the ricotta cheese over the aubergine and then cover with sauce. Continue to layer twice more in the same manner (so that you have three layers in total), ending with the sauce. Sprinkle the mozzarella cheese over the top and the Parmesan cheese over the entire dish. Place in the oven and bake for 35 minutes, until the cheese is melted and golden.

Per serving: *Kilocalories 231; Fat 13g (Saturated 4g); Cholesterol 23mg; Sodium 191mg; Carbohydrate 17g; Dietary Fibre 6g; Protein 11g.*

Exchanges: *4 vegetable, 1 medium-fat meat, 1½ fat.*

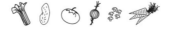

Courgette and Cucumber Linguine with Clams

After steeping in the delicious wine and clam sauce of this shellfish lover's delight, the courgette and cucumbers actually begin to taste much like linguine, without the kilo-calories and carbohydrate. You're sure to impress your guests when you serve this light appetiser at your next dinner party. Because this dish is low in kilocalories, they even have plenty of room left for the main course.

Clams are full of vitamin B12 and iron. If you're cutting back on fat by avoiding red meat, you can feel confident that you aren't missing out on these essential nutrients, which are abundant in carnivorous diets. By the way, when purchasing clams and other shell-fish, ensure that the shells are closed. The open ones are sometimes contaminated and cause severe foodborne illness.

Preparation time: *20 minutes*

Cooking time: *20 minutes*

Serves: *4*

2 tablespoons olive oil

2 tablespoons chopped garlic

2 tablespoons chopped shallots

40 grams chopped red peppers

18 to 24 Manila or littleneck clams

360 millilitres white wine

2 lemons (juice and zest)

1 tablespoon butter

Ground black pepper

1 teaspoon crushed red chilli pepper flakes

1 large seedless cucumber, cut into long, julienne strips to resemble noodles (use a mandoline or a sharp knife)

Large courgette, julienned

4 tablespoons chopped parsley

1 Heat the olive oil in a frying pan. Add the garlic, shallots, and red peppers and sauté until golden (approximately 10 minutes). Add the clams, white wine, and lemon juice and zest. Cover and bring to the boil. Continue to cook until the clams open (approximately 5 minutes).

2 When the clams open, add the butter and black pepper to taste, and the red pepper flakes. Remove the clams. Toss in the cucumber and courgette noodles and heat until they're warm and wilted (approximately 7 minutes).

3 Divide among 4 bowls and top each with the clams and the remaining juice. Garnish with the chopped parsley and lemon zest.

Per serving: *Kilocalories 171; Fat 11g (Saturated 3g); Cholesterol 28mg; Sodium 138mg; Carbohydrate 7g; Dietary Fibre 3g; Protein 11g.*

Exchanges: *2 vegetable, 1 very lean meat, 2 fat.*

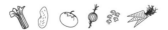

Giving Veggies the Gourmet Treatment

Vegetables are ripe for dressing up with the full gourmet treatment. They're flavourful on their own, but they also take most seasonings, spices, and cooking techniques very well. You really can't mess vegetables up unless you overcook them. Use the techniques in this chapter to experiment with your favourite recipes. Also, try a few that you haven't tried before just to broaden your vegetable horizon.

○ Pickled Vegetables

Here's a great way to have your favourite veggies, but pickled in a creative way; and you can try this with any vegetables you like. This tasty recipe satisfies your hunger pains without sending your blood glucose through the roof (don't worry, most of the sugar and salt in this recipe is discarded in the juice).

Preparation time: *30 minutes*

Cooking time: *3 minutes*

Serves: *20, or makes 1.3 kilograms of pickled vegetables*

1 tablespoon yellow mustard seed

1 teaspoon fennel seed

1 teaspoon black peppercorns

4 dried pepperoncini (sweet Italian peppers)

2 bay leaves

720 millilitres water

240 millilitres white wine vinegar

3 sprigs thyme

200 grams sugar

3 tablespoons salt

1.3 kilograms vegetables (such as carrots, cauliflower, baby red (cherry) peppers, fennel, onions, or turnips), cleaned and cut into bite-sized pieces

1 Combine the mustard seed, fennel seed, peppercorns, pepperoncini, bay leaves, water, vinegar, thyme, sugar, and salt in a large pot and bring to a boil. Add the vegetables and simmer for about 3 minutes.

2 Turn off the heat, but leave the vegetables in the pickling solution. The residual heat cooks them through.

3 Discard the pickling juice and store in the refrigerator for up to 5 days.

Tip: *Serve these pickled vegetables with sandwiches or fried fish, or just snack on them on their own.*

Per serving: *Kilocalories 28; Fat 0g (Saturated 0g); Cholesterol 0mg; Sodium 283mg; Carbohydrate 5g; Dietary Fibre 2g; Protein 1g.*

Exchanges: *1 vegetable.*

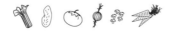

Courgette is a terrific all-around vegetable. You can eat it raw or bake it in muffins; you can stew, grill, steam, or blanch it; or you can melt cheese on it. Courgette makes excellent 'noodles' (check out the Courgette and Cucumber Linguine with Clams recipe earlier in this chapter). To get an idea of just how versatile this veggie is (and how much you can dress it up), try the following recipe.

☉ Goats' Cheese Stuffed Courgette with Yellow Tomato Sauce

This dish makes a lovely appetiser, a side entrée, or even a small meal. The distinct tastes of garlic, lemon, tomato, and savoury goats' cheese meld into one phenomenal flavour, and yet each flavour also stands strong alone and comes alive with every moment in your mouth. This vibrant dish is high in protein and quite low in carbohydrate, making it suitable for people managing their blood glucose carefully. Keep in mind, however, that goats' cheese is quite rich and high in saturated fat. So, enjoy these courgettes in moderation.

Serve with the Yellow Tomato Sauce as indicated below (note that the sauce can be served on top of any favourite vegetable).

Preparation time: *40 minutes*

Cooking time: *25 to 30 minutes*

Serves: *6*

6 medium green courgettes

450 grams goats' cheese (room temperature)

30 grams breadcrumbs

Zest of 1 lemon

4 tablespoons basil chiffonade (see the tip at the end of this recipe)

Ground black pepper

1 tablespoon olive oil

1 Preheat the oven to 180°C/350°F/Gas Mark 4. Wash the courgettes and pat dry. Cut the ends off the courgettes, and then cut each one in half to create 2 pieces of equal length. Use a paring knife or melon baller to core out the centre of the courgettes.

2 Put the goats' cheese in a bowl and add the breadcrumbs, lemon zest, and basil. Season with black pepper. Mix well and taste for seasoning. Spoon the cheese mixture into the courgette shells.

3 Drizzle the olive oil on the courgettes, season with more black pepper to taste, and place on a baking sheet. Bake until the cheese begins to bubble and the breadcrumbs start to brown (about 30 minutes).

4 Remove the courgettes from the oven, drizzle the Yellow Tomato Sauce (see the next recipe) on top of them, and return to the oven for 1 to 2 minutes.

Tip: *Chiffonade literally means 'made of rags', which pretty well describes what the final product looks like. Leafy lettuce or herbs are rolled together tightly and then thinly sliced widthwise to form long, stringy strips.*

Yellow Tomato Sauce

4 ripened yellow tomatoes (substitute red tomatoes if yellow ones aren't available)

4 garlic cloves crushed

2 tablespoons olive oil

Ground black pepper

1 De-seed the tomatoes, blanch the flesh in salted water for 10 seconds, and then shock in an ice water bath. Allow the tomatoes to chill for a few minutes, and then remove from the water and peel the skin. Cut the tomatoes in half and squeeze out the pulp and seeds.

2 Place the tomatoes in a blender, add the garlic, and blend. With the blender on high, drizzle in the olive oil until the sauce achieves a smooth, even consistency (approximately 3 to 5 minutes). Season with black pepper to taste.

Per serving: *Kilocalories 411; Fat 30g (Saturated 17g); Cholesterol 60mg; Sodium 361mg; Carbohydrate 13g; Dietary Fibre 4g; Protein 21g.*

Exchanges: *2 vegetable, 2 high-fat meat, 1½ fat.*

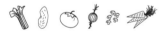

No doubt many of you love Chinese food, but sometimes find that your favourite dishes are loaded with sweeteners and other starches. This situation limits the frequency with which you can enjoy this food. The next time you get a craving for stir-fry, try out this flavourful dish, which doesn't have any added sugars.

⌒ *Asian Vegetable Stir-Fry*

With this stir-fry, act creatively and use any vegetables you like. The health benefits here don't get any better! All these vegetables in combination are rich in countless vitamin and minerals, notably vitamins A, C, B6, folate (another B vitamin), calcium, and potassium. This stir-fry is prepared with minimal oil, and so remains quite low in total fat and kilocalories. The dish is also rich in fibre, which makes it great for weight management, heart health, and especially blood glucose control. If you like, round out the stir-fry with some tofu or chicken to get a bit of lean protein, and serve over a bed of brown rice for some more fibre as well.

Preparation time: *40 minutes*

Cooking time: *20 minutes*

Serves: *4*

55 grams dehydrated wild mushrooms	*140 grams baby pak choi, sliced in half*
60 millilitres boiling water	*Red pepper, seeded and cut into juliennes*
1 tablespoon light soy sauce	*½ carrot, thinly sliced on the diagonal*
2 garlic cloves, crushed	*70 grams broccoli florets*
1½ teaspoons grated fresh ginger root	*60 grams mangetout, trimmed*
2 tablespoons olive oil	

1 Place the mushrooms in a heatproof bowl and cover them with the boiling water. Allow them to reconstitute for 30 minutes. Remove the mushrooms from the water. Chop them and put to one side. Strain the liquid through a coffee filter to remove the grit. Combine the mushroom liquid, soy sauce, garlic, and ginger root. Set aside.

2 Heat the oil in a wok or nonstick pan. Stir-fry the mushrooms, pak choi, red pepper, carrots, and broccoli for 3 minutes. Add the soy sauce mixture and mangetout. Reduce the heat and continue cooking until the veggies are crisply tender and the sauce thickens.

Per serving: *Kilocalories 137; Fat 7g (Saturated 1g); Cholesterol 0mg; Sodium 176mg; Carbohydrate 13g; Dietary Fibre 4g; Protein 4g.*

Exchanges: *3 vegetable, 1½ fat.*

Moderation is the key when enjoying any fried food, and you may even have received advice to avoid it altogether. In general, this advice is good because many fried foods are heavily battered with starchy concoctions that no one needs to eat. But on occasion, you can enjoy fried foods that are lightly *dredged,* or lightly coated, in flour, as in this Vegetable Fritto Misto.

✎ *Vegetable Fritto Misto*

This dish calls for significant amounts of milk and white flour, but not to worry. Because they're used only to coat the vegetables, neither ingredient provides a significant amount of kilocalories or carbohydrates. The flour and milk help to create a thick, crispy coating on the veggies when they're sautéed. Though rapeseed or olive oil are wonderful sources of monounsaturated, heart-healthy fat, they're still very dense in kilocalories, so go thriftily here! When the vegetables are finished, drain them well on paper towels to get rid of some of the excess oil. You may also want to pair these veggies with a light entrée, such as fish or chicken, both low-kilocalorie, lean sources of protein.

Preparation time: *30 minutes*

Cooking time: *35 minutes*

Serves: *4*

4 tablespoons olive or rapeseed oil	*480 millilitres low-fat milk*
85 grams artichoke hearts	*250 grams flour*
½ head cauliflower, chopped into florets	*Ground black pepper*
10 pitted green olives	*Lemon wedges (optional)*
Large portobello mushroom, chopped into chunks	

1 Heat the oil in a deep saucepan until it starts smoking. While you're waiting for the oil to heat, place the artichoke hearts, cauliflower, olives, and mushrooms in the milk in a shallow bowl and soak. Place the soaked veggies in a resealable plastic bag with the flour. Shake to coat them with flour. Put the floured vegetables into a strainer and shake off the excess flour.

2 Carefully place the vegetables in batches into the hot oil. Fry for 3 to 5 minutes, or until golden brown.

3 Remove the vegetables from the oil onto paper towels and season lightly with pepper. Place them in a bowl and serve with a wedge or two of lemon, if desired.

Tip: *To ensure that your food absorbs the least amount of oil possible, make sure that the oil is very hot before you begin frying it. This step ensures that your food gets a quick, crispy outer coating without getting saturated in oil.*

Per serving: *Kilocalories 192; Fat 10g (Saturated 1g); Cholesterol 1mg; Sodium 180mg; Carbohydrate 19g; Dietary Fibre 3g; Protein 5g.*

Exchanges: *3 vegetable, 2 fat, ½ starch.*

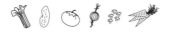

Chapter 12

Boning Up on Fish Cookery

Seafood is a great source of protein, especially for people with diabetes, and also contains lower saturated fat, cholesterol, and carbohydrates than any other protein source. Much seafood has a mild flavour that takes on the taste of its accompanying ingredients and preparation methods, and so you can have an almost endless variety of flavours and dishes. In addition, seafood cooks quickly, and so is ready when you are.

In this chapter, we convince you (in case you need convincing) that seafood is an excellent food choice to include in your diet. We give you plenty of recipes and fun new ways to prepare all kinds of fish dishes, as well as tips for preparing shellfish.

Identifying Good Reasons to Serve Seafood

Like meat and poultry, seafood supplies high-quality protein, balancing the fats and carbohydrates in the meal and providing kilocalories that have little effect on blood glucose. But the benefits of eating fish extend further, as the following list shows:

▶ Eating fish means that you also consume iodine, selenium, phosphorus, potassium, iron, and calcium, because the oceans are a rich reservoir of these minerals.

✔ Eating seafood regularly may help improve kidney function in people with severe diabetes.

✔ Eating seafood provides a good source of B vitamins, especially niacin, and fat-soluble vitamin A. In addition, fatty fish is one of the few food sources of vitamin D.

✔ Eating fish provides you with omega-3 fatty acids (one of the most important of all the nutrients in fish). These polyunsaturated fatty acids are especially high in cold-water fish, because these oils stay liquid at room temperature and help to insulate these fish against the cold. The omega-3 fatty acids appear to lower the undesirable form of cholesterol, LDL cholesterol, and to raise the desirable form, HDL cholesterol. These fats also have an anti-inflammatory effect. The fish with the highest percentage of these healthy oils are salmon, sardines, tuna, and mackerel.

To reduce exposure to possible deep-sea pollutants such as dioxins and mercury, women who are or may become pregnant at some time are recommended to eat only one or two portions of oily fish each week. Everyone else can eat up to four portions a week.

Preparing Fish in Healthy Ways

You don't need to deep-fry your catch of the day, or order deep-fried fish when you eat out, in order to get fish that tastes good. Not only is this type of fish loaded with fat, but also the type of fat is usually unhealthy. When fats heat to high temperatures, such as in deep-frying, toxic by-products are formed. Far better to eat seafood prepared using methods such as poaching, baking, or grilling – all delicious and healthy ways of cooking fish. The following sections cover a variety of methods that you can use to cook fish the healthy way.

Baking your way to fish bliss

Baking is one of the first techniques that most people discover when they start to cook. Technically speaking, *baking* means to cook something by surrounding it with dry heat. In most cases, you bake in an oven, a closed environment where you control the temperature.

Baking doesn't mean boring. Try out this flavourful baked cod to see how baking can be both easy and delicious.

Horseradish-Crusted Cod with Lentils

This recipe shows that you can develop a great-tasting meal for a person with diabetes. The cod is a lean source of protein and prepared simply by baking, a great low-fat cooking technique. The fillets are topped with a touch of horseradish, which lends a ton of flavour but very little added fat and kilocalories. The lentils are full of fibre and complex carbohydrate, making them a perfect choice. They are combined with crème fraîche, a heavy cream with a nutty flavour. This ingredient is included in such a modest amount, however, that it contributes very little fat and kilocalories. The lentils, however, are left creamy and decadent.

Preparation time: *20 minutes*

Cooking time: *30 minutes*

Serves: *4*

450 grams Puy lentils (or substitute the lentils of your choice)

2 sprigs fresh parsley

4 tablespoons crème fraîche (or substitute 3 tablespoons heavy cream and 1 tablespoon sour cream)

4 tablespoons chopped fresh parsley

Ground black pepper

4 teaspoons horseradish sauce

4 175-gram cod fillets

4 tablespoons panko breadcrumbs (substitute crushed cornflakes if you can't find these Japanese breadcrumbs in the Asian section of your supermarket)

1 teaspoon olive oil

1 Preheat the oven to 190°C/375°F/Gas Mark 5. Place the lentils in a large saucepan with enough cold water to cover them, plus 5 extra centimetres (2 inches). Add the whole sprigs of the parsley and bring to a boil. Simmer for 25 minutes, or until tender. Discard the parsley sprigs. Drain the lentils and toss with the crème fraîche and chopped parsley. Season to taste. Set aside and keep warm.

2 Spread the horseradish sauce over each fish fillet and then press in the breadcrumbs to coat. Grease a nonstick baking sheet with the olive oil. Place the fish fillets on the baking sheet and bake for 14 to 17 minutes, until the fish is just cooked and the breadcrumbs are golden.

3 Place one-quarter of the lentils on each of four plates. Top each with one piece of baked fish.

Per serving: *Kilocalories 590; Fat 9g (Saturated 4g); Cholesterol 81mg; Sodium 281mg; Carbohydrate 47g; Dietary Fibre 26g; Protein 58g.*

Exchanges: *4 starch, 6 very lean meat, 1 fat.*

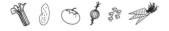

Poaching to perfection

Poaching is a method of cooking that gently cooks the food in a small amount of liquid, just below the boiling point. In the case of seafood, this liquid is often highly flavoured with herbs, wine, stock, and other seasonings. Give poaching a shot with this terrific salmon recipe.

Poached Salmon with Steamed Asparagus and Tapenade Salsa

This recipe poaches the salmon, which is the lightest method of cooking, requiring only water. The dish contains a wonderful source of omega-3 fatty acids as well as other beneficial heart-healthy fats. Combined with asparagus, the vitamin A content of this dish is off the chart; so eat up for eye health! Asparagus also lends a significant source of fibre, some good protein, and lots of folate – an important B vitamin that helps to lower your risk of heart disease, stroke, and even some forms of dementia, by helping to protect against hardening and furring up of your arteries. For women of childbearing age, folate is essential for the prevention of birth defects and has even healthier outcomes in people with diabetes. For everyone else, adequate folate intakes can also lower blood levels of an amino acid called homocysteine, high levels of which are linked to heart disease.

By the way, if you don't have the time or energy to prepare your own fish stock, you can find pre-prepared versions in most supermarkets and specialty food stores. Just remember though that homemade always tastes better and is healthier for you too!

Preparation time: *45 minutes*

Cooking time: *15 minutes*

Serves: *4*

Fish stock (see the following recipe)	*4 175-gram salmon fillets*
225 grams green asparagus	*Tapenade Salsa (see the accompanying recipe)*
225 grams white asparagus (if not available, use an additional 225 grams green asparagus)	

1 Prepare the fish stock.

2 While the stock is cooking, prepare the asparagus. Add the asparagus to lightly boiling water and cook until tender. Immediately remove the asparagus from the boiling water and shock it in an ice-water bath. (Check out Chapter 11 for tips on blanching and shocking vegetables.)

3 Bring the prepared fish stock to a gentle simmer over a medium heat. Add the salmon fillets to the simmering fish stock and cook for 5 minutes. Remove from the broth and keep warm.

4 Prepare the Tapenade Salsa (see the accompanying recipe).

5 Just before serving, reheat the asparagus in the simmering fish stock (approximately 5 minutes).

6 Serve each salmon fillet with the asparagus tips and top with the Tapenade Salsa.

Fish Stock

450 grams fish bones

480 millilitres water

Small onion, diced

225 grams leeks, sliced and well rinsed

Pinch of ground cloves

60 millilitres dry white wine

Juice of 1 lemon

1 In a large sauté pan, add the fish bones to half the cold water and bring to a simmer.

2 Add the onion, leeks, clove, and white wine and return to a simmer; add the remaining water and the lemon juice. Continue to cook the bones for an additional 30 minutes.

3 Strain the broth through a fine mesh strainer. Reserve the broth; discard the bones and other solids.

Tip: *You can purchase fish bones at fish markets or at specialty food stores that sell fresh fish. Alternatively, you can find concentrated fish stock bases in most supermarkets, which you just dilute.*

Tapenade Salsa

55 grams anchovies

130 grams pitted black olives

2 garlic cloves

240 millilitres olive oil

2 tablespoons balsamic vinegar

1 In a food processor, combine the anchovies, olives, and garlic until the mixture becomes a paste (about 45 seconds).

2 In a separate bowl, combine the olive oil and vinegar.

3 Combine the two mixtures and stir.

Per serving: *Kilocalories 838; Fat 71g (Saturated 10g); Cholesterol 109mg; Sodium 1,226mg; Carbohydrate 6g; Dietary Fibre 1g; Protein 43g.*

Exchanges: *1 vegetable, 5 lean meat, 13 fat.*

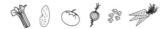

Pan roasting seafood sensations

In the strictest culinary terms *pan roasting* is a two-step process that first sears and seals a thicker piece of meat or chicken in a pan on the hob and then finishes that piece in the oven, in the same pan with which you started. So when we're talking about seafood, the term *pan roasting* is probably not exactly accurate: Because seafood cooks so fast, no need usually exists to finish it in the oven. But you can make a terrific sauce in the same pan in which you seared your fish.

Whatever you call it, pan-roasted food is good for you, as these next three recipes prove. Use a quality sauté pan that heats evenly. And make sure that you heat it up well before placing your fish in, to ensure an even, quick crust.

Plaice Franchaise

If you're new to the world of seafood, this recipe is the plaice to start! (Sorry about that.) Seriously, plaice is a mild-flavoured white fish that really takes on the flavours of the food with which it's cooked. This dish is simple to make, because you cook the whole thing in a single pan, but it's very impressive for guests. Sear the fish and then create the rich sauce – all without changing pans or washing a single dish. What can be simpler?

Preparation time: *10 minutes*

Cooking time: *15 minutes*

Serves: *2*

Nonstick cooking spray	*60 grams wholewheat flour*
2 175-gram pieces plaice (or other flat white fish)	*60 millilitres white cooking wine*
	1 tablespoon lemon juice
Egg	*120 millilitres low-salt chicken broth*

1 Coat a medium frying pan with the cooking spray and place over a medium heat.

2 Rinse and dry the plaice. In a small bowl, lightly beat the egg. Place the flour on a flat plate. Lightly coat both sides of the fish with the flour, coat the fish with the egg, and place directly in the hot pan.

3 When the fish is golden brown on the first side (approximately 4 minutes), flip it over to brown the other side.

4 When the fish is golden brown (after roughly 2 to 3 minutes), reduce the heat to low. Add the wine and let it reduce to half the amount. Add the lemon juice and broth and let the liquid reduce as it cooks the fish.

5 When the liquid has reduced to approximately one-quarter and appears to have slightly thickened, remove from the heat and serve.

Tip: Serve with fresh vegetables, salad, wholewheat couscous, or brown rice for extra fibre.

Per serving: Kilocalories 291; Fat 5g (Saturated 2g); Cholesterol 190mg; Sodium 156mg; Carbohydrate 19g; Dietary Fibre 4g; Protein 40g.

Exchanges: 1 starch, 5 very lean meat, ½ medium-fat meat.

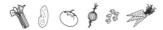

Pan-Roasted Salmon Fillet with Lemon–Dill Butter Sauce

This recipe makes an excellent pan-roasted dish. The sauce is fantastic, the butter adds the right creaminess, the lemon juice provides the perfect acidity, and the pungent dill ties them together. Look for baby leeks because they're more tender and subtly flavoured for a great addition to the salad. If you need instructions for the right way to wash and slice leeks, take a look at Chapter 8.

Preparation time: 25 minutes

Cooking time: 15 minutes

Serves: 2

½ cucumber

Bunch of salad rocket leaves

6 baby leeks, trimmed, cleaned, and blanched (or substitute 1 large leek, sliced)

Ground black pepper

3 tablespoons olive oil

2 175-gram salmon fillets, 2.5 centimetres (1 inch) thick

1 tablespoon lemon juice

3 tablespoons unsalted butter

3 sprigs dill, chopped

1 Prepare the cucumber salad first. Chop the cucumber into half moons and place in a bowl with the rocket and blanched baby leeks. Season with black pepper to taste and 1 tablespoon of the olive oil.

2 To cook the fish, heat a sauté pan with the remaining 2 tablespoons of olive oil. Season the fish with black pepper and, when the pan is hot, add the fillets. Cook for 3½ minutes on each side (medium-rare to medium). Keep warm.

3 To make the sauce, wipe clean the same sauté pan and add the lemon juice. Allow the juice to reduce in half, and then add the butter. Swirl the butter vigorously into the lemon juice and season with black pepper to taste before adding the chopped dill.

4 To serve, place the salad in the centre of the plate, put the fish on top, and drizzle over the sauce.

Per serving: Kilocalories 589; Fat 23g (Saturated 14g); Cholesterol 143mg; Sodium 86mg; Carbohydrate 8g; Dietary Fibre 2g; Protein 39g.

Exchanges: 2 vegetable, 5 lean meat, 9 fat.

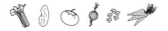

A *fumet* (pronounced foo-*may*) is a heavily concentrated stock. In the next recipe, this stock is made from prawn shells. You can make a fumet by boiling fish heads, bones, shellfish shells, or whole fish with wine, aromatic herbs, and vegetables, and then reducing it to concentrate the flavour.

Use a fumet to season sauces and soups or to braise or poach fish or vegetables. The subtle flavour imparts the delicate essence of seafood with a slight acidity (thanks to the wine), but doesn't overpower the main event.

If you'd rather not make your own fumet, look for fish stock or fish stock base (an even more concentrated product that's reconstituted with water before using) at your local fishmonger or supermarket.

Pan-Roasted Cod with Prawn and Butternut Squash

If you're keeping in mind blood sugar control and heart-health, fish is always a great choice – and this recipe makes use of two. The cod and prawns come together well with the squash ragout.

Butternut squash – which is full of antioxidant carotenoids – makes a wonderful addition to soups, stews, and casseroles, and has a lovely buttery flavour. Although often available all year round, you can substitute courgettes instead for a lighter, more summery flavour. This dish is rich in lean protein, low in carbs and saturated fat, and full of vitamins A and C.

Preparation time: *1 hour*

Cooking time: *40 minutes*

Serves: *4*

Prawn Fumet:

20 tiger prawn shells (from the prawns used in the ragout)

Shallot, chopped

Bay leaf

Thyme sprig

120 millilitres Chardonnay

Ragout:

20 tiger prawns, peeled and de-veined

250 grams 5-millimetre cubes of peeled butternut squash, blanched (see Chapter 11 for blanching instructions)

180 grams peeled, cubed tomato

120 millilitres Prawn Fumet

2 tablespoons butter

2 teaspoons fresh lemon juice

2 tablespoons parsley (whole leaves)

Cod:

4 175-gram cod fillets

Ground black pepper

2 teaspoons flour

2 tablespoons olive oil

1 Preheat the oven to 180°C/350°F/Gas Mark 4. Place the prawn shells, shallot, bay leaf, thyme, Chardonnay, and enough water to cover the ingredients in a small saucepan.

Slowly bring to a boil and simmer for 15 to 20 minutes to extract some flavour from the shells. After the flavour is extracted, strain the liquid. Discard the shells and other solids and reserve the liquid.

2 Make the ragout: Place the prawns, butternut squash, tomato, Prawn Fumet, butter, lemon juice, and parsley in a medium saucepan. Simmer until the prawns are done, for approximately 5 to 7 minutes, and hold until ready to serve. Adjust seasoning as needed.

3 Lightly season the cod fillets with black pepper to taste and dust one side with flour.

4 Heat the olive oil in a sauté pan and place the cod fillets flour side down in the oil. Sauté to a golden brown, for approximately 4 minutes, and then turn and transfer to the oven for 4 to 6 minutes.

5 When the cod is finished baking in the oven, place each fillet in a bowl and pour the ragout on top.

Per serving: Kilocalories 292; Fat 14g (Saturated 5g); Cholesterol 134mg; Sodium 276mg; Carbohydrate 5g; Dietary Fibre 2g; Protein 34g.

Exchanges: ½ starch, 7 very lean meat, 3 fat.

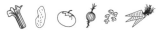

Grilling your seafood bounty

You may find that many recipes call for grilling – known in some parts of the world as broiling. Basically, you grill food by cooking it using a heat source from above, usually called (you guessed it) a grill (or broiler). Typically, food is heated for relatively short periods of time at a high heat, which usually creates a crispy coating. In most cases, grilling is a low-fat cooking technique that requires little additional fat *and* allows the natural fats present in the food to drip away. All in all, a pretty healthy combination!

Grilled Salmon with Herb Sauce and Cucumber

As if a pile of reasons to include salmon in your diet didn't already exist, here's one more: Salmon is a wonderful source of selenium, which is another of those disease-fighting antioxidants. Add that to the long list of this seafood's many health benefits!

This salmon recipe is grilled and paired with a sauce flavoured with a variety of herbs. Although most creamy sauces are usually quite high in fat and kilocalories, this one remains extremely light. The recipe takes advantage of low-fat yoghurt instead of its full-fat counterpart. You can make simple substitutions like this with most dairy products, thus doing away with a lot of fat and kilocalories with a barely noticeable change in taste.

Preparation time: *20 minutes*

Cooking time: *10 minutes*

Serves: *4*

4 tablespoons finely chopped fresh chives	280 grams plain low-fat yoghurt
2½ tablespoons extra-virgin olive oil	Juice of 1 lemon
60 grams finely chopped fresh parsley	Medium cucumber, unpeeled, thinly sliced
30 grams finely chopped fresh coriander leaves	4 175-gram fresh salmon fillets
	Ground black pepper

1 Place an oven-safe grilling pan in a hot oven to heat through. Meanwhile, preheat the grill (on a low setting if possible).

2 Place the chives in a blender with 1 tablespoon of the oil. Blend for approximately 1 minute, until well combined. Place the chive mixture in a small bowl. Add half of the chopped parsley and all the coriander, yoghurt, and lemon juice. Set aside.

3 Mix the cucumber slices with the remaining chopped parsley.

4 Prepare 4 dinner plates by spreading the herb sauce in each one. Arrange the cucumber slices over the sauce. Put aside.

5 Brush the salmon fillets with 1 tablespoon of the olive oil. Sprinkle with black pepper to taste.

6 Remove the grill pan from the oven, using oven gloves. Brush the pan with the remaining olive oil. Place the salmon fillets in the heated, oiled pan.

7 Place the pan under the grill, about 12 centimetres (5 inches) from the heating element.

8 Cook for 5 to 7 minutes, until the top of the salmon acquires a golden to light brown colour. Flip the fish to the other side. Allow the fillets to remain under the grill for an additional 2 to 3 minutes.

9 Place one salmon fillet in the centre of each dinner plate, over the cucumber slices and sauce.

Per serving: Kilocalories 351; Fat 16g (Saturated 3g); Cholesterol 101mg; Sodium 146mg; Carbohydrate 8g; Dietary Fibre 1g; Protein 42g.

Exchanges: ½ milk, 5 lean meat, 2 fat, 1 vegetable.

Getting your barbecue on

Barbecuing is similar to grilling, but the heat comes from a different direction. In a barbecue, the heat source is under the food, whereas in grilling, the heat source is above the food.

Tuna is an excellent fish for the barbecue, because the flesh is firm, not flaky like white fish, and it stands up nicely to spices and flavourings. And because tuna's usually served quite rare, it takes very little time to cook. Try barbecued tuna in the following recipe.

In recent years, concern has grown regarding the methyl mercury content of some fish. Water pollution may increase the level of this metal to toxic amounts in certain areas. Pregnant and nursing women should avoid eating swordfish, shark, and marlin, because these fish have the greatest mercury levels compared with other species. These women are also advised to limit their consumption of canned tuna to two cans per week. In addition, all women who are already pregnant, or likely to experience pregnancy at some point in the future, are advised to limit their intake of oily fish to two portions per week. Everyone else can have up to four portions weekly.

Barbecued Tuna with Asian Coleslaw

If you're in the mood for something light yet delicious and satisfying, this dish is just perfect, being full of protein yet low in total kilocalories and fat. The slaw provides a good source of vegetables, and the dressing helps to round out the dish with few added kilocalories.

Fresh tuna is best when prepared very rare in the middle – nearly raw. For this reason, only purchase ultra-fresh, sushi-grade tuna from the fishmonger, which is less likely to cause food poisoning. Pregnant and nursing women should always avoid all raw fish, including rare tuna. Otherwise, it's still a good idea to consume at least two servings of fish per week, for their heart-health benefits, as long as you limit your intake of oily fish as described previously.

Preparation time: *30 minutes, plus 2 hours for marinating*

Cooking time: *6 to 10 minutes*

Serves: *4*

4 fresh tuna steaks, about 900 grams in total (ensure that they're sushi grade)

Marinade:

60 millilitres light soy sauce

60 millilitres mirin (sweet rice wine)

1 tablespoon toasted sesame oil

2 tablespoons rice wine vinegar

2 tablespoons minced fresh ginger root

Spring onion, finely chopped

4 garlic cloves, crushed

Dressing:

160 millilitres rice wine vinegar

½ tablespoon granulated Splenda (or to taste)

1 teaspoon honey

1 teaspoon light soy sauce

3 tablespoons chopped coriander leaves

1 teaspoon finely grated ginger root

1 tablespoon toasted sesame seeds

Coleslaw:

Small head Chinese cabbage, shredded

Medium carrot, shredded

Large spring onion, chopped

½ small red pepper, julienned

½ small yellow pepper, julienned

100 grams julienned daikon (Japanese) radish

1 Make the marinade by combining the soy sauce, mirin, sesame oil, vinegar, ginger, spring onion, and garlic in a resealable plastic bag. Place the tuna steaks in the bag. Gently coat the steaks in the marinade. Place in the refrigerator for 2 hours, turning occasionally.

2 About a half hour before the tuna finishes marinating, prepare the coleslaw: First mix the dressing ingredients (vinegar, Splenda, honey, soy sauce, coriander, ginger root, and sesame seeds) in a large bowl. In another large bowl, mix the coleslaw ingredients (Chinese cabbage, carrot, onion, red and yellow peppers, and Japanese radish). Toss the cabbage mixture with most of the dressing. Reserve a small amount of dressing for later.

3 Allow to stand for 20 minutes at room temperature. If you prefer to refrigerate the coleslaw, extend the standing time to 1 hour (and start preparing it about 40 minutes after you start marinating the tuna). Preheat the grill.

4 Grill the tuna for 2 to 3 minutes per side, about 12 centimetres (5 inches) from the heating element. The tuna's perfectly done when the outside is grey-brown; however, the inside remains red. Don't overcook the steaks, as they quickly dry out and lose flavour.

5 Slice the tuna thinly and serve with the coleslaw. Drizzle the reserved dressing on top.

Per serving of tuna: Kilocalories 258; Fat 3g (Saturated 1g); Cholesterol 99mg; Sodium 232mg; Carbohydrate 2g; Dietary Fibre 0g; Protein 51g.

Exchanges (tuna): 1 fat, 6 very lean meat.

Per serving of coleslaw and dressing: Kilocalories 57; Fat 1g (Saturated 0g); Cholesterol 0mg; Sodium 73mg; Carbohydrate 7g; Dietary Fibre 3g; Protein 3g.

Exchanges (coleslaw and dressing): 2 vegetable.

Barbecue Cedar-Planked Salmon

This sumptuous feast of salmon uses a plank of cedar wood on which the fish is barbecued. You can prepare it in the oven or on an outdoor grill. As the plank roasts on the fire, the salmon retains the aroma and begins to acquire the earthy cedar flavour of the wooden plank. Note: You can find cedar planks in most timber yards – specifically look for *untreated* cedar shingles – or in kitchen supply stores or in some gourmet shops. If you can't find any, you can still cook the salmon without – it just won't taste quite as deliciously woody, although you can add hickory-wood chips to the coals for additional flavour.

Try to get wild salmon if you can – it contains more beneficial omega-3 fatty acids and far less saturated fat than its farmed counterpart. Salmon is a gift of nature and a gift to your health as well. Enjoy this oily fish and reap its medicinal benefits.

Special tool: *1 cedar plank, 1 to 2 inches larger than salmon fillet all the way around, soaked in water for at least 2 hours*

Preparation time: *30 minutes, plus optional marinating time of 1 to 2 hours*

Cooking time: *20 minutes*

Serves: *6*

1 teaspoon sea salt	5 tablespoons olive oil
70 grams brown sugar	6 garlic cloves, finely chopped
Zest from 1 orange	20g chiffonade basil (roll the basil together tightly and then thinly slice widthwise to form long, stringy strips)
Salmon fillet (900g), pin bones removed (ask the person at the seafood counter to do this for you)	
	Large onion, peeled and thinly sliced

1 To cook in an oven: Preheat the oven to 230°C/450°F/Gas Mark 8.

2 Mix up the dry marinade. In a small bowl mix the salt, brown sugar, and orange zest and spread it generously on both sides of the salmon fillet. (You can marinate the fish 1 to 2 hours in advance, if you prefer. Refrigerate the fish while it's marinating if you marinate it in advance.)

3 Brush one side of the cedar plank with 3 tablespoons of the olive oil and place it in the oven for 15 to 20 minutes.

4 Spread the garlic on the olive-oil-coated side of the plank and then place the salmon fillet on top. Sprinkle the salmon fillet with the basil. Cover the fish generously with the sliced onions and then drizzle it with the remaining 2 tablespoons olive oil.

5 Place the planked fish in the preheated oven. Cook the salmon for approximately 10 to 15 minutes, or until the fish is medium-rare. The cooking time will vary with the thickness of your fish. Allow approximately 10 minutes per inch of thickness.

If you prefer to cook the salmon on a barbecue, follow these instructions: Preheat the barbecue to a medium-high heat. Place the oiled plank directly on the barbecue. Let the plank smoke a bit before adding the fish. If the plank catches fire, spritz it with water. Close the lid of the grill and cook the salmon for approximately 10 to 15 minutes, or until the fish is medium-rare. The cooking time will vary with the thickness of your fish. Allow approximately 10 minutes per inch of thickness.

Per serving: Kilocalories 373; Fat 17g (Saturated 2g); Cholesterol 86mg; Sodium 400mg; Carbohydrate 20g; Dietary Fibre 1g; Protein 33g.

Exchanges: 1 other carbohydrate, 5 lean meat, 3 fat.

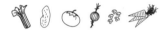

Surveying Superior Shellfish

Shellfish includes seafood such as prawns, lobsters, oysters, clams, mussels, and scallops, which all have a shell instead of fins and gills. The term also includes some seafood with a not-so-obvious shell, such as octopus and squid.

Shellfish are sold according to their size and weight. For tips on how to pick the right shellfish for your recipe, see Chapter 7.

The texture of these tasty titbits ranges from exceptionally tender, in the case of lobster and some prawns, to a bit chewy, in the case of octopus and squid. No surprise, therefore, that the tenderness of these delicate creatures depends, in part, on how well you cook them.

Avoid overcooking shellfish: Doing so causes the texture to become rubbery and unpleasant.

Mussels with Pastis

Mussels are a wonderful source of lean protein, as is true of most fish. Pastis (pronounced pas-*tees*) is a French aniseed-flavoured liqueur. Enjoy these shellfish on top of a small bed of pasta or along with any steamed vegetables of your choice.

Note that you don't need any additional salt in this dish: The sodium content is already mildly high, mainly due to the naturally high sodium levels of saltwater shellfish. Just ensure that you limit or avoid any added salt for the remainder of the meal.

Choose mussels that are closed, with their shells intact. Discard any with open, chipped, or broken shells. Soak your raw mussels for about 20 minutes in cool, clean water before cooking. They take in water and expel excess salt and sand. Clean the soaked mussels by scrubbing them with a stiff brush. Remove any beard (the hair-like thread that mussels use to attach to rocks) by pulling the beard towards the mussel's hinge. Rinse again in cool, clean water before using them.

Preparation time: *20 minutes*

Cooking time: *15 minutes*

Serves: *6*

2 tablespoons olive oil	*1 kilogram mussels, raw, scrubbed, and de-bearded*
½ white onion, diced	
1 tablespoon chopped garlic	*6 tablespoons pastis*
1 tablespoon chopped anchovy	*Splash of white wine*
2 tablespoons chopped parsley	*60 millilitres tomato sauce*

1 Heat the olive oil in a sauté pan. Add the onion and sauté until tender. Add the garlic, anchovy, parsley, and mussels. Continue to cook until the mussels start to open, after about 2 to 3 minutes.

2 Add the pastis. (If you're cooking on a gas hob, remove the sauté pan from the burner before adding the pastis. Because it contains quite a bit of alcohol, the pastis can easily catch fire, so you don't want it near an open flame. Return your pan to the burner after you've added the pastis). Add the white wine and tomato sauce. Cover and simmer for another 2 to 3 minutes, until most of the shells are open.

If most, but not all, the shells are open, you can cover the dish and cook for another minute or two. But if they don't open after these additional minutes, discard any unopened mussels. Eating closed mussels isn't safe because they can contain harmful bacteria. And don't waste your time continuing to cook them, hoping that they may open. You just end up overcooking the good ones. Cut your losses with a few that don't open, and savour the ones that do!

3 Scoop the mussels, along with their tomato broth, into a large serving dish.

Tip: *Serve alone, with crusty bread, or on top of pasta. Add a green salad for a great meal in minutes.*

Tip: *If you can't find pastis in your local spirits shop, substitute Sambuca, Ouzo, or Pernod instead. You get a similar aniseed or licorice flavour.*

Per serving: Kilocalories 261; Fat 10g (Saturated 2g); Cholesterol 66mg; Sodium 949mg; Carbohydrate 11g; Dietary Fibre 1g; Protein 28g.

Exchanges: ½ other carbohydrate, 4 very lean meat, 1 fat.

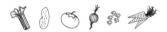

Ceviche (pronounced se-vee-*chee*) is an amazing food. Born out of the necessity of using acid to retard food spoilage, ceviche is a delicious and healthy cooking technique. In a nutshell, raw seafood, usually whitefish or prawns, is placed in an acid – usually lime juice – which in essence 'cooks' the fish. Feel free to add chillies, onions, and tomatoes to your ceviche for a full-flavoured experience.

Use only very fresh sushi-grade seafood in ceviche because this method of cooking never reaches temperatures high enough to kill bacteria.

Seared Diver Scallops with Bacon and Shallots

If you're looking to show off some cooking skills, this scallop dish is sure to impress. Just a small amount of bacon as a condiment helps to achieve a lovely, rich flavour – without breaking the day's saturated fat and cholesterol limit. Scallops are a great source of protein while remaining low in total and saturated fat, so they're a healthier alternative to red meats. Serve this dish on top of a bed of wholewheat couscous to complete the meal.

Diver scallops are sea scallops that are harvested by, well, divers. They are a bit more expensive than standard sea scallops because people harvest them rather than boats dragging chains along the ocean floor, but typically diver scallops are less gritty and have a better texture. Plus, they're more environmentally friendly because divers generally take only the larger mature scallops, leaving the smaller young scallops to grow for future scallop eaters.

Preparation time: *30 minutes*

Cooking time: *30 minutes*

Serves: *2*

4 slices bacon, cut into 1-centimetre (½-inch) strips

Shallot, peeled and thinly sliced

120 millilitres low-sodium chicken stock

2 tablespoons butter

1 tablespoon chopped fresh chives

Ground black pepper

6 diver scallops (you can substitute 450 grams of sea scallops)

2 tablespoons olive oil

12 asparagus stalks, cleaned, trimmed, and blanched (see Chapter 11 for blanching instructions)

60 millilitres Balsamic Syrup (see the following recipe)

1 Add the bacon to a small sauté pan and cook for 2 minutes. Add the shallots and continue cooking for an additional 3 minutes. Add the chicken stock and butter and bring to a simmer until the stock has reduced in volume by half and the shallots are tender (approximately 20 minutes). Add the chives and season to taste with black pepper. Set aside.

2 Preheat a medium sauté pan over a high heat. Season the scallops evenly on both sides with black pepper. Add the oil to the hot pan and sauté the scallops for approximately 2 minutes per side. Remove the scallops from the pan and place 3 scallops in the centre of each plate. Reheat the asparagus in the pan that you used to cook the scallops. Put the bacon and shallot reduction (from Step 1) around the scallops. Arrange the asparagus around the scallops. Drizzle the Balsamic Syrup over the scallops and asparagus.

Per serving: *Kilocalories 652; Fat 34g (Saturated 11g); Cholesterol 154mg; Sodium 590mg; Carbohydrate 27g; Dietary Fibre 2g; Protein 52g.*

Exchanges: *6 lean meat, ½ high-fat meat, 6 fat, 2 vegetable, 1 other carbohydrate.*

Balsamic Syrup

240 millilitres balsamic vinegar   *1½ teaspoons granulated Splenda*

Combine the balsamic vinegar and Splenda in a medium saucepan. Cook over a medium-high heat until the sauce thickens and reduces to around 60 millilitres (one-quarter of original volume), which takes approximately 30 minutes.

Per serving (2 tablespoons): Kilocalories 80; Fat 0g (Saturated 0g); Cholesterol 0mg; Sodium 31mg; Carbohydrate 19g; Dietary Fibre 0g; Protein 0g.

Exchanges: 1 other carbohydrate.

Langoustine Ceviche

With this simple-to-prepare ceviche dish, you and your guests are in for a treat. Langoustines (also known as Dublin Bay prawns or scampi) are a sweet type of prawn with an almost lobster-like flavour and texture. They are extremely succulent and cook quickly, so langoustines are a natural choice for this no-heat cooking method. The acidic nature of the lime juice actually cooks the fish – without any heat, pots, or pans. Leave to marinate for an hour, and the dish is ready to serve. Ceviche makes for a great first course, especially in the hot summer months, because it contains almost no fat and is quite light and refreshing. Enjoy!

Preparation time: 10 minutes, plus marinating time of 1 hour

Serves: 4

450 grams fresh scampi tails, roughly chopped

Mango, diced into small pieces

Shallot, finely chopped

20 grams chopped fresh coriander leaves

60 millilitres fresh lime juice (about 4 limes)

Pinch of chilli flakes

Ground black pepper

Place the fresh scampi tails in a bowl and mix together with the mango, shallot, coriander, lime juice, and chilli flakes. Season with black pepper to taste and place in the refrigerator for 1 hour. The ceviche looks particularly attractive served in a martini glass on a bed of shredded lettuce.

Per serving: Kilocalories 131; Fat 1g (Saturated 0g); Cholesterol 168mg; Sodium 240mg; Carbohydrate 12g; Dietary Fibre 1g; Protein 19g.

Exchanges: 1 fruit, 3 very lean meat.

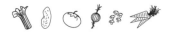

Chapter 13

Flocking to Poultry

*W*hen you first find out that you have diabetes, you may assume that you're going to be restricted to a diet of little more than grilled chicken breasts and steamed vegetables. Well, even a cursory glance through all the delicious recipes in this chapter (and the rest of the book) dispels that assumption.

In this chapter, we show you how to use poultry safely in your diet. We give you tips to keep the most popular piece of chicken – the breast – tasty, moist, and downright exciting. We also give you recipes and ideas for using other parts of the bird, such as the legs and thighs. And finally, we cover some great things to do with turkey.

Including Poultry in Your Diet

In the food exchange lists for diabetes (see Appendix B) poultry fits into the categories of very lean meat (0 to 1 gram of fat per 30 grams), lean meat (3 grams of fat per 30 grams), and medium-fat meat (5 grams of fat per 30 grams):

✔ **Very lean-meat poultry:** Examples include white-meat chicken or turkey without the skin.

✔ **Lean-meat poultry:** Examples include dark-meat chicken or turkey without the skin, white-meat chicken with the skin, domestic duck or goose well drained of fat and without skin.

✔ **Medium-fat meat poultry:** Examples include dark-meat chicken with the skin, minced turkey or chicken, fried chicken with the skin.

Nutritionists define a portion of meat as 100 grams (3½ ounces), which is typically half a chicken breast or a chicken drumstick and thigh. Most people eat more than this amount. When eating a whole breast, choose one that is smaller rather than larger. To reduce the fat content, eat the meat but don't eat the skin.

Maintaining good hygiene practices in your kitchen is important when working with poultry, no matter how much poultry you're cooking. Keep the following hints in mind to minimise bacterial contamination from poultry:

✔ Don't rinse poultry, as was often previously advised, because any bacteria present are killed during proper cooking. In fact, rinsing may spread bacteria from the chicken to your kitchen sink!

✔ Don't place raw poultry near, over, or in any foods that you don't intend to cook before they're eaten. Proper cooking kills most bacteria found in poultry, but never let the liquid in raw poultry drip onto salads, sauces, condiments, and so on. Place raw meat in the bottom of the fridge.

✔ Do keep a separate colour cutting board that you only use for raw poultry. You can significantly reduce the chances that you cut lettuce on the same board you use to slice raw chicken if they're different colours.

✔ Do clean your knife immediately after cutting raw poultry: Wash it thoroughly in hot, soapy water.

✔ Do sanitise thoroughly any surfaces that come into contact with any raw poultry or its juices. Use detergent or an antibacterial cleaner that's specifically made for this purpose.

✔ Do always cook poultry to the appropriate food-safe temperature, as listed in Table 13-1.

Table 13-1	Safe Cooking Temperatures for Poultry
Product	*Temperature*
Minced turkey, chicken	165°C/320°F/Gas Mark 3
Poultry breasts	170°C/325°F/Gas Mark 3
Chicken, whole	180°C/350°F/Gas Mark 4
Duck and goose	180°C/350°F/Gas Mark 4
Poultry thighs, wings	180°C/350°F/Gas Mark 4
Turkey, whole	180°C/350°F/Gas Mark 4

Making the Breast of Chicken

The breast is the leanest part of a chicken, with the lowest total and saturated fat content, which makes it the healthiest option for your heart.

Chicken Breasts with Lemon and Garlic

This dish takes full advantage of a chicken breast's delicious, white, lean meat. Just remember to remove the skin after the chicken is cooked.

Preparation time: *20 minutes*

Cooking time: *25 minutes*

Serves: *6*

2 tablespoons extra-virgin olive oil

30 garlic cloves

4 tablespoons butter

6 small chicken breasts, bone in, with skin

Juice and zest of 2 lemons

240 millilitres dry white wine

720 millilitres chicken stock or water

A few thyme sprigs

(continued)

1 In a small sauté pan, heat 1 tablespoon of the olive oil and add the garlic. Cook over a medium-low heat, allowing it to brown but not burn. Shake the pan occasionally or stir the garlic with a spoon to keep it from burning. Add a little water if the garlic starts to brown too much. Cook the garlic until it's soft (about 15 to 20 minutes).

2 When the garlic is soft, heat the remaining olive oil and 2 tablespoons of butter over a medium heat, in a large cast-iron/enameled casserole with a tight-fitting lid. Slowly brown the chicken, skin side down, until the skin is golden and crisp. Turn the breasts over and reduce the heat to medium-low.

3 After you turn over the breasts, add the garlic and olive oil sauce to the chicken pan. Add half the lemon juice and zest, and all the white wine, chicken stock, and thyme. Bring the sauce to a simmer and cover. Continue cooking for approximately 5 to 7 minutes, or until the breasts are cooked through and tender, but not dried out. Check the chicken and sauce occasionally, stirring as needed. If the pan begins to dry, add a little water to maintain about a 1-centimetre (½-inch) depth of liquid.

4 When the chicken is cooked and its juices run clear, remove from the pan to a warm serving platter. Keep warm. Increase the heat in the pan until the sauce begins to boil, and then turn off the heat and add the remaining 2 tablespoons of butter. Adjust the seasonings with pepper, and the remaining lemon juice/zest, if desired. Pour the sauce over the chicken.

5 Garnish with the remaining lemon zest. Remove the chicken skin before eating.

Per serving: *Kilocalories 288; Fat 17g (Saturated 7g); Cholesterol 91mg; Sodium 135mg; Carbohydrate 6g; Dietary Fibre 1g; Protein 26g.*

Exchanges: *4 very lean meat, 3 fat.*

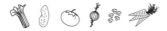

Chicken Scampi

This dish is an excellent example of what we mean when we say that you can enjoy good food that's good for you – it's both delicious and low fat. The total fat and saturated fat content are low simply because you're using skinless chicken breast – the leanest part of the chicken. The recipe calls for some butter, but just enough to enrich the flavour without significantly raising the fat content. The chicken is full of wonderful flavour from fresh herbs, lemon juice, wine, and a sprinkle of Parmesan cheese. The longer you marinate the chicken, the more flavour it has when done.

Preparation time: *6 to 7 hours (mostly marinating time)*

Cooking time: *20 to 30 minutes*

Serves: *4*

Pinch of pepper	1 tablespoon olive oil
2 garlic cloves, crushed	60 millilitres chicken stock
2 tablespoons roughly chopped fresh oregano	1 tablespoon butter
4 tablespoons roughly chopped fresh parsley	100 grams plum tomatoes, diced
3 tablespoons lemon juice	Ground black pepper to taste
60 millilitres white wine	3 tablespoons grated Parmesan cheese
5 120-gram skinless, boneless chicken breast halves, cut into 2½-centimetre (1-inch) strips	

1 Combine the pepper, half the garlic, oregano, parsley, lemon juice, and half of the wine in a resealable plastic bag. Add the chicken. Mix gently to coat the chicken with the marinade. Marinate in the refrigerator for several hours (overnight is best).

2 When ready to cook the chicken, preheat the grill, on a low setting. Remove the chicken from the marinade (save the remaining marinade) and place in a shallow pan. Grill 20 centimetres (8 inches) from the heat, turning once, until the chicken is no longer pink inside (about 15 minutes).

3 While the chicken is grilling, heat the olive oil in a sauté pan. Sauté the remaining garlic, until fragrant but not browned. Add the remaining white wine to the sauté pan and scrape to remove any bits on the pan. Add the remaining marinade and chicken stock, and bring to a boil. Reduce the sauce by half, and stir in the butter and tomatoes. Season with black pepper, pour the sauce over the chicken, and top with Parmesan cheese.

Per serving: *Kilocalories 241; Fat 11g (Saturated 4g); Cholesterol 89mg; Sodium 196mg; Carbohydrate 2g; Dietary Fibre 1g; Protein 31g.*

Exchanges: *4 very lean meat, ½ medium-fat meat, 2 fat.*

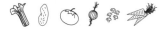

Many supermarkets and some butchers sell hot, delicious-smelling rotisserie-roasted chickens. They're a great choice for a quick shortcut to a homemade meal. Pick one up to shave time off your prep work for this next recipe, featuring oven-roasted chicken breast.

Barbecue Chicken with Potato and Oven-Dried Tomatoes

You may be surprised, but this dish is a nutritional powerhouse! The oven-dried tomatoes and barbecue sauce (find the sauce recipe in Chapter 15) contribute lots of vitamin C, lycopene, and betacarotene, important antioxidants that also play a key role in eye health. Enjoy this dish and all its benefits – with little fat and few carbohydrates, but lots of great flavour.

Preparation time: *15 minutes*

Cooking time: *35 minutes for chicken, 2½ hours for tomatoes*

Serves: *2*

2 tablespoons unsalted butter

Shallot, diced

Garlic clove, chopped

Tomato, chopped

1 tablespoon diced peppers

Potato, cut into cubes

Oven-roasted chicken breast, skinless, shredded

60 millilitres Barbecue Sauce (such as Wolfe's, Chapter 15)

2 tablespoons chicken stock (or broth)

Ground black pepper

1 tablespoon chopped parsley

1 In a large, hot sauté pan, melt the butter. Add the shallot, garlic, tomato, and peppers and sauté for 4 minutes.

2 Add the potato and cook for 15 minutes.

3 Fold in the shredded chicken, potato, barbecue sauce, and chicken stock. Season with black pepper to taste.

4 Cook for approximately 4 minutes.

5 Garnish with the oven-dried tomatoes (see the following recipe) and parsley.

Oven-Dried Tomatoes

2 to 3 plum tomatoes, sliced into quarters

Ground black pepper

1 Preheat the oven to 120°C/250°F/Gas Mark ½.

2 Place the tomato quarters skin side down on a nonstick baking sheet (or one that is lined with greaseproof paper). Season the tomatoes with the pepper and bake for 2½ hours.

Per serving: Kilocalories 418; Fat 17g (Saturated 8g); Cholesterol 121mg; Sodium 418mg; Carbohydrate 28g; Dietary Fibre 3g; Protein 36g.

Exchanges: 1 starch, 1 other carb, 1 vegetable, 4 very lean meat, 3 fat.

A *paillard* (pronounced *pie*-yarhd) is a fancy French word that means a cutlet, or a slice of meat that's pounded to a thin, even thickness (or thinness depending on your viewpoint). Some people call it a medallion (when it's small) or a scaloppine. This process has two benefits:

✔ The meat cooks evenly, because no thicker or thinner sections exist.

✔ The meat cooks fairly quickly because it's thin.

Try this handy technique for yourself – take a look at Figure 13-1 and the following recipe.

Figure 13-1:
Pound chicken into paillards with a mallet or the bottom of a heavy pan.

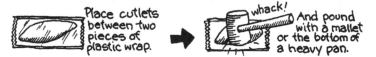

Chicken Cutlets Pounded to an Even Thickness

Paillard of Chicken Breast with Fennel and Parmigiano-Reggiano

Although you can enjoy this wonderful meal at any time of the year, it's perfect for summer: The dish is light, has fresh ingredients, and is easily cooked on the barbecue. The fennel and Parmigiano-Reggiano cheese offer two very opposing flavours but come together with the chive and sun-dried tomato vinaigrette. The ingredients create deep layers of flavour, requiring no added salt.

Notice that the skin is removed before cooking the chicken. Searing the breasts in a hot pan locks the juices inside the chicken's crisp coat, stopping the breast from drying out.

Preparation time: 30 minutes

Cooking time: 30 minutes

Serves: 4

Bunch of fresh chives	*550 grams cherry tomatoes*
5 tablespoons extra-virgin olive oil	*Ground black pepper*
Bulb Florence fennel	*4 boneless skinless chicken breasts, pounded flat*
80 grams baby rocket leaves	
115 grams Parmigiano-Reggiano, sliced paper thin	*90 grams sun-dried tomatoes in olive oil, puréed*
	2 lemons, halved

1 Chop the chives and, using a blender, blend with 3 tablespoons of olive oil.

2 Slice the fennel into paper-thin slices.

3 Arrange four dinner plates with baby rocket on one side and layer fennel slices with Parmigiano-Reggiano slices on top. Halve the cherry tomatoes and place on either side of the salad.

4 Lightly sprinkle ground black pepper on both sides of the chicken breasts.

5 Warm the remaining 2 tablespoons of olive oil in a large saucepan. When the pan is very hot, place in the 4 chicken breasts. Cook the breasts for 2 to 3 minutes until they gain a golden colour. Flip the breasts over and do the same to the other side. Don't overcook or the breasts become dry.

6 Place 1 chicken breast paillard on each plate next to the salad. Season with black pepper. With a spoon, dribble the chive sauce and the puréed tomato sauce over and around the chicken breast paillards to create a colourful design.

7 Dress the salad plate with a drizzle of olive oil and half a lemon.

Tip: *Fennel is a terrific herb. The bulb (sometimes called the head) has a thick, cabbage-like texture and the rich flavour and aroma of aniseed. Save the feathery tops, which resemble dill, for a fun and unusual garnish.*

Per serving (with 2 tablespoons chive and sun-dried tomato vinaigrette): Kilocalories 589; Fat 33g (Saturated 9g); Cholesterol 116mg; Sodium 404mg; Carbohydrate 17g; Dietary Fibre 7g; Protein 51g.

Exchanges: 4 vegetable, 4 very lean meat, 1 medium-fat meat, 5 fat.

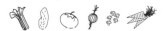

Marinating chicken for hours or even overnight is a great way to maximise flavour and add moisture to chicken breasts. Make up your own marinades to suit your mood. Here are some ideas to get you started:

  ✔ Balsamic vinegar, olive oil, and oregano

  ✔ Light soy sauce, lime juice, crushed garlic, and crushed ginger

  ✔ Low-fat salad dressing or vinaigrette

Include an acid of some sort in your marinade to help break down some connective tissue in the meat, making it more tender and helping it to absorb the marinade flavour more completely. Good acid choices include citrus juice and vinegar. The marinade in the following recipe features lemon juice.

Roast Free-Range Chicken Breast Stuffed with Porcini Mushrooms, Caramelised Leeks, and Pancetta

This dish is fantastic – yet surprisingly simple. Although you want to keep the skin on while cooking the chicken, remember to remove it after you sit down to eat: The skin is full of artery-clogging saturated fat. But after you taste the pancetta, you aren't going to miss the skin. Pancetta is essentially Italian bacon, although it has a higher fat content and slightly saltier flavour than traditional bacon. For this reason, use pancetta in moderation, more as a condiment than a main ingredient in dishes. Just a small amount imparts a delicious, smoky flavour.

To create the delightful sauce, you need to rehydrate dried mushrooms. Rehydrating is easy, but remember: Always strain the liquid used to rehydrate mushrooms before adding it to any recipe. Gently pour it through a coffee filter paper to remove any dirt or grit.

Preparation time: *30 minutes*

Cooking time: *50 minutes*

Serves: *4*

28 grams dried porcini mushrooms

480 millilitres warm water

3 sun-dried tomatoes

115 grams lean pancetta (approximately 8 thin slices), diced

2 tablespoons butter

Medium leek, tough greens removed, rinsed well, chopped small

4 chicken breasts, skin on, boned and tendons removed

Ground black pepper

1 teaspoon finely chopped fresh thyme

125 grams watercress, washed

1 tablespoon extra-virgin olive oil

1 tablespoon balsamic vinegar

480 millilitres low-sodium chicken stock

1 Place the oven rack in the lower part of the oven. Preheat the oven to 200°C/400°F/Gas Mark 6. Set aside a large roasting pan.

2 Place the porcini mushrooms in 240 millilitres (9 fluid ounces) of warm water. Allow to rest for 15 minutes. Repeat the process in a separate bowl of water with the sun-dried tomatoes. Strain the porcini from the water and reserve the water. Cut the mushrooms into fine juliennes. Strain the sun-dried tomatoes from the water and discard it. Cut the tomatoes into fine juliennes.

3 Sauté the pancetta in a pan until the fat is rendered out, but not browned (3 to 4 minutes).

4 Heat the butter in a small sauté pan over a medium heat. When hot, add the leeks and cook until lightly browned (about 4½ minutes). Add the mushrooms, tomatoes, and pancetta to the sauté pan.

5 To assemble the chicken breasts, pull the skin back and season both sides with black pepper. Sprinkle with thyme on both sides. Spread just under a quarter of the mushroom mixture over each chicken breast. Cover with skin. Place in the reserved roasting pan. Top the chicken breasts with the small amount of remaining stuffing mixture.

6 Place in the oven and roast until browned (approximately 25 to 30 minutes). Transfer the chicken to a warm platter.

7 Toss the watercress with the olive oil and vinegar.

8 Deglaze the pan. Combine the porcini mushroom water and chicken stock in the pan used for the chicken. Simmer until reduced to 80 millilitres (3 fluid ounces), after about 6 to 8 minutes.

9 Serve the chicken breasts over the watercress and pour the sauce on top.

Per serving: Kilocalories 527; Fat 30g (Saturated 10g); Cholesterol 145mg; Sodium 346mg; Carbohydrate 11g; Dietary Fibre 4g; Protein 50g.

Exchanges: 4 lean meat, 1 high-fat meat, 4 fat, 1 vegetable.

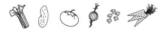

Divvying Up Different Bits of the Bird

Although chicken breasts are a heart-healthy option, trying something else makes a nice change. If you're looking to maximise your enjoyment of poultry and try some different pieces of chicken, this section is for you.

Loving chicken legs

Chicken legs are fun to eat whatever your age, because they come with their own handle! They cook fairly quickly because they have a large bone running right through the centre. If you think that chicken legs are just for kids, give this sophisticated recipe a try. The recipe also features a variety of mushrooms, some of which are shown in Figure 13-2.

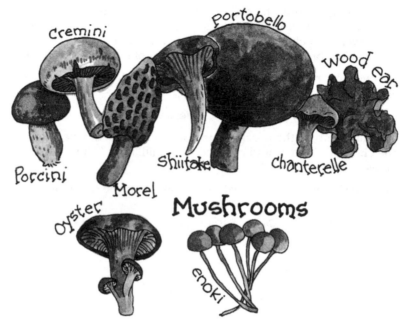

Figure 13-2:
Mushrooms
come in
many
shapes and
sizes.

Braised Chicken Legs with Mushrooms

This recipe is a great one-pot dish. With the good, however, comes the chicken skin. Feel free to keep the skin on the chicken while cooking. Just remember to take it off before your first bite. Eat the good stuff and leave the saturated fat behind.

Preparation time: *45 minutes*

Cooking time: *1 hour and 15 minutes*

Serves: *3 to 4*

28 grams dried porcini mushrooms

240 millilitres warm water

1 tablespoon olive oil

6 chicken legs

80 grams chopped onion

10 garlic cloves

2 medium carrots, chopped

Medium red potato, chopped

100 grams assorted mushrooms (button, portobello, shiitake)

240 millilitres dry red wine

120 millilitres low-sodium chicken stock

1 tablespoon chopped parsley

Ground black pepper

1 Soak the porcini mushrooms in 240 millilitres (8 fluid ounces) of warm water for about 10 minutes before use.

2 Heat a heavy-bottomed roasting pan large enough to hold all 6 chicken legs and vegetables over a medium-high heat. Add the oil and sear the legs for 7 to 10 minutes, browning the chicken on all sides.

3 Preheat the oven to 190°C/375°F/Gas Mark 5. Remove the legs from the pan and add the onion and garlic. Cook for 2 minutes over a medium heat. Add the carrots and potato and cook for 2 minutes more. Add the mushrooms. Return the chicken legs to the pan and add the red wine. Bring to a simmer for 2 minutes and then add the chicken stock.

4 Cover with aluminum foil, place in the oven, and cook for 2 hours. Remove from the oven, add the parsley, and season well with black pepper. Serve with good crusty bread and a glass of dry red wine.

Per serving (2 legs): Kilocalories 590; Fat 22g (Saturated 5g); Cholesterol 179mg; Sodium 322mg; Carbohydrate 24g; Dietary Fibre 8g; Protein 63g.

Exchanges: 7 lean meat, 1 fat, 3 vegetable, ½ starch.

Tasting flavoursome thighs

Chicken thighs are full of flavour. If you've sworn off dark meat in favour of boneless, skinless chicken breast, this next recipe may change your mind.

Look in the frozen food section of your grocery store for individually quick-frozen, boneless, skinless chicken thighs to make this (and any other chicken) dish quickly and easily.

Coriander and Lime Chicken Thighs

Eliminating the skin from the chicken thighs reduces the fat content of this dish by more than a half. The wonderful sauce in which the chicken is marinated and cooked offers so much good flavour that you don't even miss the skin! Grill or serve them at your next barbecue.

Yoghurt is a great ingredient to use as a marinade when baking chicken. As the thighs cook, the yoghurt hardens and creates a nice thick crust, similar to fried chicken but without all the added fat.

Preparation time: *6 to 8 hours (mostly marinating time)*

Cooking time: *1 hour*

Serves: *6 (2 thighs each)*

350 millilitres plain low-fat yoghurt	*2 teaspoons pepper, coarse grind*
Bunch of coriander, roughly chopped	*12 boneless, skinless chicken thighs, about 1.8 kilograms*
Juice from 2 limes	
7 garlic cloves	*Nonstick cooking spray*

1 Combine the yoghurt, coriander, lime juice, garlic, and pepper in a food processor. Pulse to combine in order to make the marinade.

2 Place the chicken in an extra large resealable plastic bag. Pour the marinade over the chicken and seal the bag. Gently work the marinade over the chicken to coat thoroughly. Place in the refrigerator and allow to marinate for 6 to 8 hours.

3 When ready to cook the chicken, preheat the oven to 180°C/350°F/Gas Mark 4. Spray a roasting pan with the nonstick cooking spray and arrange the marinated chicken in the pan. Reserve the marinade. Cook the chicken for 1 hour, basting with marinade as necessary for the first half of the cooking time.

4 Cook the chicken until the internal temperature reaches 180°C/350°F, measured with a meat thermometer.

Per serving (2 chicken thighs): *Kilocalories 263; Fat 12g (Saturated 4g); Cholesterol 102mg; Sodium 51mg; Carbohydrate 7g; Dietary Fibre 0g; Protein 30g.*

Exchanges: *4 lean meat, ½ milk.*

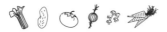

Talking Turkey to Liven Up Your Meals

A standard 100 grams (3½ ounce) serving of white meat turkey, without the skin, has less than a gram of saturated fat, which is lower than the same size serving of chicken breast. Turkey is also a good source of B vitamins and many minerals, including iron, potassium, selenium, and zinc, especially in the dark meat.

When you buy a whole turkey, try to buy a larger bird because you tend to get more meat for your money. With a small bird, in the 2.7 to 6.8 kilogram (6 to 15 pound) range, much of what you get is bones, so you're disappointed with the meagre meat that results from all your hard work. If you have more leftovers than you can (or want to) eat in a couple of days, freeze the extra with a touch of chicken broth or gravy to help keep it moist.

'Rotisserie'-Roasted Turkey Breast

Rotisserie chicken, which is available in just about every supermarket, is a great convenience food, and a relatively healthy one as well. Here's a low-sodium version of this perennial favourite that uses turkey instead. Roast the turkey up out of its own fat (on a rack or on foil balls) for a true 'rotisserie' experience at home.

Preparation time: *20 minutes*

Cooking time: *2 hours and 15 minutes*

Serves: *Varies based on weight of turkey, 175 grams serving size*

1 tablespoon olive oil	*4 tablespoons lemon pepper*
Turkey breast, 2.7 to 3 kilograms with skin	*1 tablespoon ground sage*

1 Preheat the oven to 200°C/400°F/Gas Mark 6. Rub the olive oil into the turkey breast. Place the turkey breast in a roasting pan with a rack. (If you don't have a rack, roll up 6 balls of foil and place them under the turkey in the roasting pan to support the turkey breast.) To get a rotisserie-like final product, you need to make sure that the turkey doesn't sit in any fat as it cooks. Set aside.

2 In a small bowl, combine the lemon pepper and ground sage. Sprinkle the combined seasonings evenly over the oiled turkey breast. Place the roasting pan in the oven. Cook for 45 minutes at 200°C/400°F/Gas Mark 6. Then reduce the oven temperature to 150°C/300°F/Gas Mark 2 to finish cooking (approximately 1½ hours, depending on the size of your bird). Cook the turkey until it reaches an internal temperature of 165°C/325°F measured with a meat thermometer.

Tip: Use this easy dry rub on any poultry you like: It's great with chicken, Cornish game hens, capons, and game birds.

Per serving (with skin): *Kilocalories 329; Fat 14g (Saturated 4g); Cholesterol 125mg; Sodium 589mg; Carbohydrate 1g; Dietary Fibre 0g; Protein 48g.*

Exchanges: *6 lean meat.*

Turkey Loaf with Portobello Sauce

Meat loaf is an old-fashioned food that's increasingly finding a place on the menus of trendy gourmet restaurants. This recipe is a dressed-up version that uses minced turkey and is topped with fancy portobello mushrooms, those meaty giants you find in the vegetable section of most supermarkets. Have this meat loaf for dinner and then in a sandwich the next day for lunch.

Preparation time: *25 minutes*

Cooking time: *60 minutes*

Serves: *4*

The meat loaf:

Nonstick cooking spray

Medium onion, finely chopped

Stalk celery, finely chopped

450 grams lean minced turkey

4 tablespoons chopped parsley

1 tablespoon fine breadcrumbs

60 millilitres skimmed milk

Egg white, lightly beaten

Garlic clove, crushed

1 teaspoon dried thyme leaves

Pinch of nutmeg

Pinch of pepper

The sauce:

2 teaspoons olive oil based margarine

Large portobello mushroom, cleaned and cut into small pieces

240 millilitres low-sodium chicken broth

Pinch of ground nutmeg

Pinch of ground black pepper

1 Preheat the oven to 180°C/350°F/Gas Mark 4.

2 For the meat loaf, coat a large frying pan with cooking spray and place over a medium heat until hot. Add the onion and celery. Sauté, stirring often, until translucent (about 5 minutes).

3 Meanwhile, in a large bowl, combine the turkey, parsley, breadcrumbs, milk, egg white, garlic, thyme, nutmeg, and pepper. Add the onion and celery and mix well.

4 Form into a loaf and place in an oiled loaf tin. Bake for 50 minutes or until the internal temperature is 165°C/320°F/Gas Mark 3 measured with a meat thermometer.

5 For the sauce, melt the margarine in a saucepan placed over a medium heat. Add the mushrooms and sauté, stirring, until tender.

6 Remove from the heat. Add the chicken broth, nutmeg, and pepper. Return to heat. Cook until fragrant and slightly thickened (approximately 5 minutes).

7 When the meat loaf is cooked, turn out, slice, and place portions on warmed dinner plates.

8 Ladle mushroom sauce over the sliced turkey loaf.

Tip: Minced turkey is a great substitute for minced beef. Choose minced turkey without skin, for the greatest savings in the saturated fat department. You can use minced turkey anywhere in place of beef, such as pasta sauce, burgers, or casseroles.

Per serving: Kilocalories 203; Fat 4g (Saturated 1g); Cholesterol 76mg; Sodium 181mg; Carbohydrate 9g; Dietary Fibre 2g; Protein 31g.

Exchanges: ½ starch, 4 very lean meat, 1 vegetable.

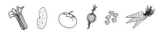

Chapter 14

Creating Balanced Meals with Meats

*L*ean meat is an ideal food for people with diabetes because it's a rich source of protein and contains only minimal carbohydrate. As a result, lean meat doesn't raise your blood glucose levels significantly. Every time you eat, you need to include some protein to balance the fat and carbohydrate in your diet, because meals that contain protein, as well as fat and starch, help stabilise blood glucose and give you a more consistent supply of energy.

Your body uses protein to build and repair tissues. Meat is an excellent source of protein because it contains all nine essential amino acids that you can't make in your body and must therefore obtain from your diet. Meat is also a source of B vitamins and many minerals needed for good health. In particular, meat is a good source of vitamin B12 – essential for normal functioning of the nervous system – and iron for transporting oxygen to the cells.

In this chapter, we show you three great techniques for cooking meats: searing, braising, and roasting. We also give you great recipes for each technique and other tips along the way.

Always cook meats to a safe temperature for the appropriate degree of 'done-ness' using a meat thermometer to assess the temperature of the centre of the meat. Push the meat thermometer into the thickest section of the meat, making sure it isn't touching any bones. Leave the thermometer in the meat through the cooking process. See Table 14-1 to find out what temperature the meat of your choice needs to reach.

Table 14-1	Safe Internal Cooking Temperatures for Meats
Product	*Meat Thermometer Temperature*
Ground veal, beef, lamb, pork	70°C/160°F
Beef, medium rare	55 to 60°C/130 to 140°F
Beef, medium	60 to 65°C/140 to 150°F
Beef, well done	70°C/160°F and above
Veal, medium rare	55 to 60°C/130 to 140°F
Veal, medium	60 to 65°C/140 to 150°F
Veal, well done	70°C/160°F and above
Lamb, medium rare	60 to 65°C/140 to 150°F
Lamb, medium	70°C/160°F
Lamb, well done	75°C/170°F and above
Pork (fresh)	65 to 70°C/150 to 160°F
Ham (fully cooked)	70°C/160°F
Ham, precooked (to reheat)	60°C/140°F

Searing for Sealing Meats

A cooking technique called searing is particularly helpful for keeping meat as low fat and delicious as possible. *Searing* subjects meat to extremely high heat on the hob for a short period of time. Usually you sear one side and then the other. This technique produces a beautifully caramelised skin on the meat and essentially seals in its juices. Searing also helps to retain the moisture content of the meat and therefore much of the flavour.

Searing is a great way to avoid the use of rich sauces and salt.

Thai Rare Beef with Red Onion and Kaffir Lime

Try this dish the next time you have a craving for some Thai food. Purchase a lean beef cut, such as the top sirloin used here. Beef is a wonderful source of protein, but ensure that you trim away all excess fat from the meat. And don't add any extra salt: The Thai fish sauce and light soy sauce already contain plenty! In fact, ordinarily, we wouldn't suggest a dish with this much sodium, but every now and then, splurge a little – just don't make it a habit! To round out the meal, serve on a bed of brown rice or quinoa (a grain high in protein and fibre.) Check out Chapter 10 for great grain recipes.

Preparation time: *1 hour and 20 minutes*

Cooking time: *20 minutes*

Serves: *4*

450 grams beef top sirloin (fat removed)	*1 tablespoon Nam pla (Thai fish sauce)*
120 millilitres light soy sauce	*2 tablespoons olive oil*
Handful of chopped coriander stems	*Large red onion, thinly sliced*
240 millilitres freshly squeezed lime juice	*2 spring onions, diagonally sliced*
60 grams palm sugar (if not available, use granulated)	*Handful coriander leaves*
	3 kaffir lime leaves, chiffonade (optional)

1 In a bowl, marinate the beef with the soy sauce and the coriander stems for 1 to 3 hours – the longer you leave it, the more tender and flavoursome it becomes.

2 In a small pot, place the lime juice, sugar, and fish sauce. Heat over a medium-low to low heat, stirring frequently, until the sugar melts. Set aside and chill.

3 Heat a sauté pan over a high heat, for at least 5 minutes. Remove the sirloin from the marinade and discard the marinade. Add the olive oil and sear the top sirloin on both sides (approximately 3 to 4 minutes on each side). Remove from the pan and thinly slice.

4 In a large bowl, add the red onion, spring onions, coriander leaves, and, if desired, the kaffir lime leaves. (See Chapter 9 for info on how to make a herb chiffonade.) Place the sliced beef on top and pour the chilled sauce over all.

Per serving: Kilocalories 304; Fat 12g (Saturated 3g); Cholesterol 64mg; Sodium 707mg; Carbohydrate 26g; Dietary Fibre 1g; Protein 23g.

Exchanges: 1 other carbohydrate, 3 lean meat, 1½ fat.

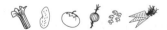

Veal tenderloin is a healthy option compared with many other cuts of meat. Veal is naturally low in fat, so cook it quickly at high temperatures to keep in as many of the natural juices as possible. Searing veal is a great option.

Veal Tenderloin with Chanterelle Mushrooms in a Muscat Veal Reduction Sauce

A *medallion* is a small, coin-shaped piece of meat. Medallions are very thin, and so once you sear them, you don't need to finish them in the oven. With just a short searing time, you create perfectly tender slices of veal. Serve this terrific recipe with pasta and the Haricot Vert from Chapter 11.

Preparation time: *15 minutes*

Cooking time: *15 minutes*

Serves: *4*

1½ teaspoons cracked black pepper (plus more to taste)

4 veal tenderloin medallions, approximately 165 grams each (silver skin removed), pounded thin (check out Chapter 13 for details on pounding meat into paillards)

70 grams plain flour

2 tablespoons extra-virgin olive oil

115 grams wild mushrooms (chanterelle if available)

60 millilitres Muscat wine

185 millilitres veal reduction sauce (reduced veal stock, also known as demi-glace)

1 Press ½ teaspoon black pepper into each veal medallion and coat in the flour.

2 Heat a medium sauté pan over a high heat. Add olive oil; sear the medallions on both sides (about 4 minutes on each side). Remove the medallions and set aside.

3 Add the mushrooms, Muscat, remaining 1 teaspoon pepper, and veal sauce to the same sauté pan, and cook for 2 minutes over a high heat. Adjust seasoning to taste. Pour the mixture over the veal slices.

Tip: *If you can't find veal reduction sauce in your supermarket or online, use beef stock.*

Per serving: *Kilocalories 424; Fat 24g (Saturated 8g); Cholesterol 111mg; Sodium 471mg; Carbohydrate 17g; Dietary Fibre 1g; Protein 32g.*

Exchanges: *5 lean meat, 1½ fat, ½ starch.*

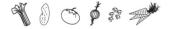

If you sear a thicker piece of meat, such as a chop or even a roast, quickly sear the outside and then *finish* the meat in the oven. Searing seals in the natural juices, and roasting finishes the cooking process to desired perfection. Check out Table 14-1, earlier in this chapter, for tips on choosing the right temperature for your meat.

Pan-Roasted Veal Chops with Sweetcorn and Gouda Ragout

This dish is bursting with flavour without providing a prohibitive amount of kilocalories. Even without much salt, you don't miss a thing – the dish remains full of other herbs and ingredients that offer intense flavours and great taste.

A *ragout* (pronounced ra-*goo*) is a thick, flavourful stew-like concoction that usually features meat and sometimes vegetables. In this recipe, pan-roasted sweetcorn is paired with creamy Gouda cheese, and the result is great with the delicate veal chops.

Preparation time: *1 hour and 15 minutes*

Cooking time: *45 minutes*

Serves: *4*

Steak seasoning:
Pinch of salt
1 tablespoon cracked black pepper
3 garlic cloves, crushed
1 tablespoon chopped fresh sage

Sweetcorn ragout:
350 grams sweetcorn kernels, fresh or frozen
Garlic clove, chopped

240 millilitres milk
Spring onion, chopped
½ teaspoon ground black pepper
30 grams grated Gouda cheese

Veal chops:
4 veal chops, 200 grams each
2 tablespoons steak seasoning (see Step 1)
2 tablespoons olive oil

1 To prepare the steak seasoning, preheat the oven to 120°C/250°F/Gas Mark ½. Place the salt, pepper, garlic, and sage into a food processor and process for 15 seconds. Transfer to an oven-safe dish and place in the oven for 30 minutes. After the garlic dries out, transfer back to the food processor and process for a further 15 seconds. Set the seasoning aside. Increase the oven temperature to 200°C/400°F/Gas Mark 6.

2 To make the ragout: Heat a cast-iron pan over a high heat for at least 5 to 6 minutes. Add the sweetcorn and continue to cook until charred (approximately 8 to 10 minutes). Add the garlic, milk, spring onion, and pepper. Cook for 2 minutes and reserve.

3 Heat a large oven-proof sauté pan over a high heat. Season the veal chops with the prepared steak seasoning. Add the olive oil to the heated pan. Sear the chops in the olive oil until golden brown on both sides (approximately 4 minutes per side). Transfer to the hot oven and roast until desired 'doneness'. Check out Table 14-1 to find the right temperature for you and test your chops with a meat thermometer.

4 When ready to serve, place the sweetcorn ragout on plates and sprinkle the Gouda cheese over the corn. Place the veal chops on top of the sweetcorn and serve.

Per serving: Kilocalories 351; Fat 18g (Saturated 5g); Cholesterol 104mg; Sodium 464mg; Carbohydrate 16g; Dietary Fibre 3g; Protein 30g.

Exchanges: 1 starch, 4 lean meat, 2 fat.

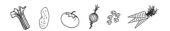

Understanding the Basics of Braising

Braising is a terrific cooking method for meats, vegetables, and anything else you want to make tender and tasty. Basically, *braising* involves cooking a cut of meat in a small amount of liquid. The meat gently cooks and steams, or *braises,* at the same time. Braising is particularly effective for less expensive cuts of meat, because you cook it slowly and break down the tougher muscle over time.

Braising is also a great cooking method because it requires very little added fat, like butter or oil. You can braise foods in the oven or in a pot on the hob. Try this latter technique out with the following great recipe.

Beer-Braised Pork and Crisp-Herb Cabbage with Apple–Tarragon Dipping Sauce

This diabetes-friendly dish contains pork, so it must have a high fat content, right? Not necessarily. Pork is gaining a good reputation as another white meat alternative to chicken. The amount of fat in pork depends on the cut of the meat, however. The rump and rib roast, for example, are much higher in fat and cholesterol than the pork tenderloin, boneless sirloin chops, or boneless loin roasts. This dish uses the lean tenderloin of pork, which remains beautifully moist during the slow-cook method of braising.

Preparation time: *1 hour and 45 minutes*

Cooking time: *1 hour*

Serves: *6*

¼ teaspoon ground black pepper	1 tablespoon melted butter
4 tablespoons low-sodium soy sauce	525 millilitres pale ale
2 tablespoons minced shallots	2½ tablespoons olive oil
1 tablespoon chopped garlic	450 grams pork tenderloin sliced into 12 medallions
1 tablespoon Dijon mustard	Red pepper, julienned

1 Combine the pepper, soy sauce, shallots, garlic, mustard, butter, and ale. Marinate the pork in this mixture in a resealable plastic bag in the refrigerator for 30 to 60 minutes before cooking.

2 Heat the oil in a medium-hot large sauté pan. Add the pork medallions, reserving the marinade, and cook until golden brown (about 3 to 4 minutes on each side).

3 Reduce the heat to medium-low and add the reserved marinade and the red pepper. Simmer gently, uncovered, for 25 to 30 minutes until the sauce volume reduces in half.

4 To serve, place the cabbage (see the next recipe) on a warm plate. Place 2 pork medallions next to the mound of cabbage. Pour the dipping sauce (see the accompanying recipe) into a ramekin and place it next to the pork and cabbage.

Crisp-Herb Cabbage

Head of cabbage, thinly shredded

Medium red onion, julienned

2 garlic cloves, crushed

30 grams chopped parsley

15 grams chopped fresh basil

1½ teaspoons chopped fresh thyme

120 millilitres rice vinegar (seasoned)

60 millilitres white vinegar

½ tablespoon crushed red chilli pepper flakes

2 level teaspoons granulated sweetener

½ teaspoon allspice

½ teaspoon ground coriander

Juice from 2 lemons

1 Combine the cabbage, onion, garlic, parsley, basil, and thyme in a large mixing bowl.

2 Combine the rice vinegar and white vinegar in a small bowl. Add to the cabbage mixture.

3 Add the red pepper flakes, sweetener, allspice, coriander, and lemon juice to the bowl and mix ingredients well.

4 Let stand at room temperature 45 minutes while getting the other ingredients together.

Apple–Tarragon Dipping Sauce

240 millilitres water

120 millilitres rice vinegar

Juice of 1 lemon

2 peeled and diced Granny Smith apples

Garlic clove, crushed

Bay leaf

Pinch of ground cinnamon

Pinch of ground allspice

½ teaspoon crushed red pepper flakes

1 tablespoon chopped tarragon

Combine all the dipping sauce ingredients in a medium saucepan and bring to a boil. Simmer for 20 to 25 minutes, until the apples are tender. Remove the bay leaf. Purée in a food processor until smooth (approximately 3 to 4 minutes).

Per serving (pork, cabbage, and dipping sauce): Kilocalories 284; Fat 12g (Saturated 3g); Cholesterol 47mg; Sodium 946mg; Carbohydrate 23g; Dietary Fibre 6g; Protein 19g.

Exchanges: ½ fruit, 4 vegetable, 2 lean meat, 2 fat.

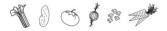

Recommending Roasting

Roasting is a simple technique that requires little effort. Season the meat with herbs and spices and cook in the oven until it reaches a desired degree of 'doneness'. You just need to ensure that the meat doesn't dry out, which is a distinct possibility with this dry-heat method of cooking. Here are some suggestions:

- Slow-roast meat at a low temperature, 180°C/350°F/Gas Mark 4 and below.
- Wrap meat in foil for most of the cooking time and remove only for the last half hour of cooking – to allow the meat to brown.
- Cook roasts with the bone still attached, when possible, as the meat cooks faster and has more flavour that way.

Putting roast pork on your table

Try the recipes in this section the next time that you have a taste for pork – a great source of lean meat if you select the right cut.

Roast Pork Loin with White Beans all'Uccelletto

This is fine dining and comfort food at its best, and leaves you satisfied in several ways. The pork loin remains tender all the way through, with noticeable hints of rosemary and thyme, and is delicious, yet with little trace of fat. The White Beans all'Uccelletto are a wonderful complement to the meat (as well as a great source of protein and fibre). This recipe is pure guilt-free dining, so enjoy!

Uccelletto is the general Italian term for small game birds. So to cook something *all'uccelletto* means to cook it like you would a small game bird. No need to pluck feathers, truss your beans, or even stuff them. The term just means that you season the beans as you would (or rather as the Italians would) for small game birds, specifically with tomatoes, garlic, and sage. You can definitely add other spices, but these three are almost always present. This dish is old school Italian comfort food, so enjoy.

Preparation time: *1 hour*

Cooking time: *1 to 2 hours*

Serves: *6*

1.3 to 1.8 kilogram pork loin, bone in

Bunch of sage (approximately 7 or 8 picked leaves)

Bunch of rosemary (leaves picked)

1 teaspoon crushed red chilli pepper flakes

Ground black pepper

1 To prepare the pork loin, cut down the back of the loin along the rib bones to separate the meat from the bones. Do not completely remove the bones. Place the sage leaves, rosemary leaves, chilli flakes, and pepper to taste between the loin and the bones. Bring the bones and the loin back together and tie the roast with butcher's twine. Season the outside of the roast with pepper and set aside until ready to roast. You can do this process up to 2 days before roasting, and doing it at least one day ahead is best so that the herbs can really flavour the meat.

2 Insert a meat thermometer in the joint and place the roast in a roasting pan. Roast at 230°C/450°F/Gas Mark 8 for 10 minutes, and then reduce the heat to 180°C/350°F/Gas Mark 4. Continue to cook, for approximately 40 to 45 minutes, until the internal temperature of the roast (as measured by a meat thermometer) reaches 70°C/160°F. Remove from the oven, cover loosely with foil, and let it rest for approximately 15 to 20 minutes before slicing.

3 To serve, place the warm beans (see the accompanying recipe) on a platter. Remove the butcher's twine from the pork roast. Slice the roast into 6 equal chops and place the chops next to the beans.

White Beans all'Uccelletto

2 tablespoons extra-virgin olive oil

Onion, chopped

3 garlic cloves, crushed

2 rosemary sprigs

6 to 8 sage leaves

1 kilogram cooked cannellini beans (approximately 450 grams dry beans) and their liquid

115 grams prosciutto, diced

2 tablespoons tomato purée

Pinch of salt

Pour the olive oil into a medium saucepan. Over a low heat cook the onion, garlic, rosemary, and sage until the onions are soft and translucent. Add the beans and some of the juice (roughly 3 to 4 tablespoons), reserving the rest in case you want the beans moist later. Add the prosciutto and the tomato purée. Combine thoroughly to achieve a dark orange colour. Season with salt to taste and simmer for up to 2 hours to fully flavour the beans.

Per serving: Kilocalories 575; Fat 18g (Saturated 6g); Cholesterol 108mg; Sodium 349mg; Carbohydrate 36g; Dietary Fibre 12g; Protein 55g.

Exchanges: 2 starch, 2 very lean meat, 5 lean meat, 1 fat.

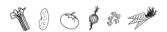

Loin of Pork Glazed with Roasted Vegetable Salsa

Loin of pork is preferred for oven roasting because slicing it for serving is so easy. However, loin of pork can easily become dry. This recipe specifies loin of pork with the bone left in, which yields moister, more flavourful meat and gives you more flexibility in timing.

Preparation time: 15 minutes

Cooking time: 1½ to 2 hours

Serves: 6 or more

2 garlic cloves, crushed	2 tablespoons olive oil, plus more as needed
2 teaspoons chopped fresh sage leaves or 1 teaspoon dried sage	80 millilitres Roasted Vegetable Salsa (see the following recipe)
Ground black pepper	80 millilitres Dijon-style mustard
1 kilogram potatoes, peeled and cut into 2.5-centimetre (1-inch) cubes	1.3 to 1.8 kilogram pork loin roast, bone-in

1 Preheat the oven to 230°C/450°F/Gas Mark 8.

2 In a small bowl, mix together the garlic, sage, and pepper to taste.

3 Arrange the potatoes in a roasting pan that is also large enough to hold the pork. Toss the potatoes with 1 teaspoon of the garlic–sage mixture and the olive oil. Place the pan in the heated oven while you prepare the pork.

4 In a bowl, combine the Roasted Vegetable Salsa (see the next recipe) and mustard. Spread the mixture over the pork.

5 Take the potatoes out of the oven, place the pork loin on top of the potatoes or along-side them, and put the pan back in the oven. Roast undisturbed for 30 minutes.

6 Remove the roasting pan from the oven. Stir the potatoes, using a spatula to scrape them off the bottom of the pan if necessary. Lower the heat to 180°C/350°F/Gas Mark 4 and continue to cook, stirring the potatoes every 15 minutes or so.

7 After 1¼ hours total cooking time, check the pork for doneness by inserting an instant-read thermometer into several places in the meat. When the thermometer reads 70°C/160°F, remove the roasting pan from the oven. Transfer the pork to a platter and let it rest for 15 minutes before carving. During the resting time, the temperature continues to rise, to ensure that there is no trace of rosiness in the centre of the meat.

8 Return the potatoes to the oven to keep warm, lowering the heat to 160°C/325°F/Gas Mark 3.

9 Carve the meat and serve the potatoes. Enjoy with a green vegetable such as sautéed courgettes. Savour the pork the next day in a sandwich, along with sautéed onions and more salsa.

Roasted Vegetable Salsa

Preparation time: *30 minutes, plus 2 hours for salsa to stand*

Cooking time: *20 minutes*

Makes: *600 millilitres*

450 grams ripe tomatoes	*120 millilitres tomato purée*
2 medium red or green peppers	*2 tablespoons chopped fresh coriander leaves*
2 red onions, sliced	
4 garlic cloves, crushed	*2 teaspoons fresh thyme leaves*
2 teaspoons extra-virgin olive oil	*2 teaspoons cider vinegar*

1 Place the tomatoes and peppers under a grill or on a barbecue until they are charred and blackened on all sides. Remove from the grill or barbecue and transfer to a large bowl. Loosely cover and set aside.

2 Heat the oven to 220°C/425°F/Gas Mark 7.

3 Drizzle the onions and garlic with the olive oil. Toss them together to coat and then spread them in one layer on a baking sheet. Roast them, stirring occasionally, until the onions are soft and brown (about 15 minutes). Remove and cool at room temperature.

4 Peel the charred tomatoes and remove the cores, catching any juice in a bowl, and add the peeled, cored tomatoes to the juice. Set aside. Peel the peppers, remove the seeds and stems, and cut into thin slices. Place the peppers in a medium-size bowl.

5 Place the roasted onion and garlic in a food processor fitted with a metal blade and process until moderately finely chopped. Add to the bowl with the peppers and stir. Put the grilled tomatoes in the processor and process coarsely. Add the chopped tomatoes, tomato purée, coriander, and thyme to the bowl.

6 Season the tomato salsa with black pepper, and stir in the vinegar. Cover and refrigerate for a couple of hours to allow the flavours to develop. Taste again before using and adjust the seasoning if necessary.

Per serving: Kilocalories 435; Fat 18g (Saturated 5g); Cholesterol 99mg; Sodium 341mg; Carbohydrate 26g; Dietary Fibre 3g; Protein 39g.

Exchanges: 4½ lean meat, 1½ starch, 1 fat.

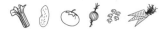

Looking at roast lamb dishes

Try roasting lamb with the following recipes. Leave the bones on the chops in the first recipe for quicker cooking and a beautiful presentation.

Roast Lamb Sirloin with Herbes de Provence, Spinach, and Onion Ragout with Lamb au Jus

Herbes de Provence is simply a mix of herbs commonly used in southern French cooking. They happen to go wonderfully well with this lamb dish. Lamb is typically one of those meats with more fat, so do your best to choose a leaner cut, such as the sirloin. Choose cuts with the least amount of white marbling (or fat) within the meat and, as with all meat dishes, remember to trim excess fat whenever possible!

The ragout contributes a wonderful flavour to the lamb and spinach, and the only ingredient is onion! Use your blender creatively – you can make many wonderful, flavourful sauces and spreads even when using just a single fruit or vegetable.

Preparation time: *45 minutes*

Cooking time: *1 hour*

Serves: *4*

4 175-gram lamb sirloin chops	*480 millilitres water*
2 tablespoons Dijon mustard	*Bunch of spinach*
2 tablespoons herbes de Provence	*120 millilitres port*
Ground black pepper	*3 garlic cloves, chopped*
2 tablespoons olive oil	*2 tablespoons butter*
3 onions, sliced	

1 Preheat the oven to 200°C/400°F/Gas Mark 6.

2 Place the lamb sirloin chops in a roasting pan. Spread the Dijon mustard evenly over the lamb chops. Sprinkle on herbes de Provence and season with black pepper. Drizzle lightly with 1 tablespoon of the olive oil and roast for 15 minutes. Reduce the heat to 150°C/300°F/Gas Mark 2. Continue roasting until the chops are medium rare (light pink inside) or a meat thermometer inserted in the centre of a chop reaches 65°C/150°F.

3 While the chops are cooking, combine the onions and water in a large sauté pan or saucepan. Cover and simmer until the onions become soft. Remove the onions from the pan and process them in a food processor until they're smooth.

4 In the same sauté pan, heat the remaining olive oil. Add the spinach. Cover and cook the spinach for about 3 to 4 minutes. Fold the onion purée into the spinach, season lightly with salt and pepper, and set aside; make sure that you keep it warm.

5 Remove the chops from the roasting pan to another dish and cover them with foil to keep them warm.

6 Place the baking pan on the stove. On a low heat, deglaze the pan with the port, garlic, and butter. Reduce the mixture by a quarter.

7 To serve, place the spinach mixture in the middle of each plate. Place one lamb chop on top of the spinach and pour the port sauce over it.

Per serving: Kilocalories 281; Fat 14g (Saturated 6g); Cholesterol 84mg; Sodium 160mg; Carbohydrate 6g; Dietary Fibre 6g; Protein 26g.

Exchanges: 1 vegetable, 3 lean meat, 1½ fat.

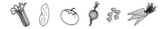

Roast Leg of Lamb Scented with Coriander

The delectable natural juices of this meat make a simple sauce that's hard to beat. Enjoy this leg of lamb, as the French would say, *au jus*.

Preparation time: *10 minutes, plus 1 hour standing time for the lamb*

Cooking time: *About 1½ hours*

Serves: *6 or more*

2 tablespoons coriander seeds

Large garlic clove, crushed

1 teaspoon freshly ground black pepper

2.2- to 3.2-kilogram leg of lamb, with as much surface fat removed as possible and preferably at room temperature

1 Preheat the oven to 220°C/425°F/Gas Mark 7.

2 Put the coriander seeds in a plastic bag and crush with a rolling pin.

3 In a small bowl, mix the crushed coriander with the garlic and pepper.

4 Using a thin-bladed knife, cut several small slits in the lamb. Press the spice mix into these cuts and rub the remaining spices all over the outer surface of the meat. Set aside in the refrigerator for an hour or more to blend the flavours.

5 Spray a large nonstick roasting pan with cooking spray. Put the pan on the stove and place the lamb in the pan. Cook the lamb over a medium-high heat, turning to sear and brown all sides.

6 Move the lamb in the pan to the oven, roast the lamb for 30 minutes, and then lower the heat to 180°C/350°F/Gas Mark 4. Cook for another half hour and check the internal temperature of the lamb with a meat thermometer. Continue to check every 10 minutes until the desired temperature is reached. (An internal temperature of 60 to 65°C/140 to 150°F indicates medium-rare, and 70°C/160°F indicates medium. Checking in several places for 'doneness' is also a good idea. Total cooking time is less than 1½ hours.)

7 Before carving, let the lamb roast rest for a few minutes. Serve with the pan juices.

Per serving: Kilocalories 354; Fat 14g (Saturated 5g); Cholesterol 162mg; Sodium 16mg; Carbohydrate 0g; Dietary Fibre 1g; Protein 52g.

Exchanges: 6 lean meat.

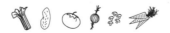

Chapter 15

Nibbling on Snacks

*H*ow many times do you hear, 'It's all about portion control'? Well, in this case, the conventional wisdom is true. Your blood glucose level benefits from a steady stream of food – little and often – and so portion control and snacking are your new best friends. Consider a snack before or after a workout to give you an energy boost. Plan on having a light bite between lunch and dinner. Just keep track of everything and make sure that your eating plan is well rounded.

Any food that's part of your healthy daily regimen is a good candidate for a snack, as long as you eat the right portion size. Here's a list of good snack options for people with diabetes:

✔ 1 piece of cheese and 4 wholewheat crackers

✔ 1 rice cake

✔ 2 crispbreads

✔ 6 smoked almonds

✔ 8 dried apricot halves

✔ Handful of roasted soy nuts

✔ Small carton of cottage cheese

✔ 170 grams (6 ounces) vegetable juice (for example, tomato with a dash of Worcester sauce)

Watch out for snacks from vending machines and pre-packaged foods such as mini pork pies, muffins, oat cakes, and pastries. Although convenient, these foods are often loaded with sugar, salt, and fat. Read labels carefully before making your food choices. For more on reading food nutrition labels, check out Chapter 5.

In this chapter, we show you how to stock up on handy snacks, supplement snacks with dips and sauces, and whip up light and easy mini meals.

Keeping Healthy Snacks at the Ready

Do you grab whatever you can find for a quick snack when you're incredibly hungry? Reaching for a bag of crisps, chocolate bar, or fizzy drink is easy if they're handy. Instead of keeping these convenient, high-fat, high-sodium, high-sugar foods handy, stock your fridge, freezer, and larder with healthy snacks that are satisfying yet keep you on a healthy eating plan. For example, you can make snack-size servings of cut-up fresh vegetables, and keep them ready and waiting in the fridge for instant crudités.

For a special liquid treat, keep some single-serving tubes of sugar-free drink mixes handy. Just add the contents to your water bottle for an instant treat.

Mixing it up with whole grains

Stock your larder today with healthy wholegrain snacks such as raisins and peanuts. In the following recipe we include whole grains, nuts, and dried fruit for a good all-around snack option. Feel free to substitute your favourite fruits and nuts as you experiment with this tasty treat.

⏱ Wholegrain Almonds and Cranberries

You can give good old peanuts and raisins an update with delicious, wholegrain cereals and readily-available dried fruits. If you can't find dried cranberries, use golden raisins, diced dried apricots, or any other fruit that appeals to you. This recipe is a great any-time snack to keep ready and waiting in resealable plastic bags in your larder.

Nuts and dried fruit also make a healthy treat, as long as portions are well controlled. Good amounts of protein and some fibre make nuts a glucose-controlling snack, and almonds and walnuts are an excellent source of heart-healthy monounsaturated fats. They do, however, pack a lot of energy – over 500 kilocalories per 100 grams (3½ ounces), so go easy if you're watching your weight. As dried fruit is a concentrated source of sugar, which if eaten excessively can send blood sugars to the moon, enjoy this tasty treat and its nutritional benefits in moderation, as always.

Preparation time: *5 minutes*

Serves: *6*

100 grams bite-sized honey and nut shredded wheat

70 grams toasted unsalted almonds

60 grams dried cranberries

1 Combine all ingredients in a resealable plastic bag. Shake to mix thoroughly.

2 Store in your larder for up to one week.

Per serving: Kilocalories 165; Fat 6g (Saturated 1g); Cholesterol 0mg; Sodium 24mg; Carbohydrate 19g; Dietary Fibre 3g; Protein, 4g.

Exchanges: ½ starch, ½ fruit, 1 fat.

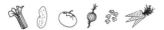

Filling your freezer with treats

Some people just can't stay away from snacks after dinner, especially sweet ones. Instead of a bowl of ice cream, a chocolate mousse, or a slice of cheese-cake, consider stocking your freezer with the following healthy quick-grab snacks.

✔ **Flavoured ice cubes:** Fill ice cube trays with your favourite sugar-free drinks, such as any flavoured water or lemonade. Freeze and then transfer the individual ice cubes to a resealable plastic bag. Try adding a few lemonade ice cubes to your next glass of apple juice. Experiment with flavours you like.

✔ **Grapes:** Clean the grapes and remove them from their stems. Place individual grapes on a clean baking sheet in the freezer. When the grapes are frozen, transfer them to a resealable plastic bag. Grab a few when your sweet tooth attacks.

✔ **Sugar-free frozen lollies:** Look for lollies made with a high percentage of juice or that include low-kilocalorie, sugar-free sweeteners.

✔ **Yoghurt tubes:** Squeezable yoghurt tubes make a terrific quick snack. Toss a few in the freezer for an extra creamy frozen treat.

Squeezable yoghurt can have added sugar, and so read labels carefully to make sure that you know what you're eating, and confirm that it fits with your eating goals.

If you love frozen desserts, consider opting for a low-sugar, pre-portioned frozen concoction, such as these Orange Cream Ices.

☞ *Orange Cream Ices*

When you feel a sugar craving coming on after dinner, think twice about that dish of ice cream. Instead, finish off a great meal with one of these low-sugar orange cream treats. They're cool, refreshing, and just sweet enough to quench a sugar craving.

Special tools: *8 frozen lolly moulds, 8 lolly sticks*

Preparation time: *4 hours (mostly freezing time)*

Serves: *8*

450 grams canned mandarin oranges in light syrup, undrained

225 grams low-fat vanilla yoghurt

2 tablespoons granulated sweetener

8 frozen lolly moulds

8 wooden lolly sticks

1 Place the oranges and yoghurt in a blender and add the sweetener. Blend to desired consistency, for approximately 2 minutes.

2 Pour the mixture into a measuring cup with a spout. Pour the mixture into freezer moulds. Freeze until firm – overnight is best.

Per serving: *Kilocalories 60; Fat 0g; Cholesterol 1mg; Sodium 22mg; Carbohydrate 14g; Dietary Fibre 0g; Protein 2g.*

Exchanges: *½ fruit, ½ milk.*

Why should you choose wholegrain snacks?

If you have a choice between 6 salted crackers and 4 wholewheat crackers, and you're really hungry, which do you choose? At first glance, the answer may seem obvious. Choose the salted ones because you get 6 crackers (compared to just 4 wholewheat crackers). But believe it or not, 4 wholewheat crackers are able to keep you fuller for longer. The whole grain is the key. Your body works harder and longer to digest the wholewheat crackers. With salted crackers, the flour manufacturer has done much of the work for you by refining the flour and removing most of the fibre and nutrients. By making your body work for its nutrition, you help it work more efficiently, in turn helping you to stabilise your blood glucose levels. Choosing the wholewheat option also reduces your sodium intake. For more about adding grains to your diet, check out Chapter 10.

Choosing kid-friendly snacks

Many children have diabetes and, often, their parents and other caregivers need to find out about the condition from scratch. Turn to Chapter 22 for more tips on helping kids cope with diabetes. Also, check out *Diabetes For Dummies,* 2nd edition, by Dr Sarah Jarvis and Dr Alan Rubin (Wiley), for more great kid-friendly tips.

Here's a list of snacks designed with diabetic kids in mind. If you can show kids how to snack well early in life, they're better equipped to deal with diabetes as they grow older.

✔ An apple with a small dollop of peanut butter

✔ Celery sticks dipped in low-fat dressing

✔ Cottage cheese

✔ Lean cooked meat, such as ham

✔ Low-fat cheese

✔ Low-fat yoghurt

✔ Snack-sized bag of light microwave popcorn

✔ Sugar-free jelly

✔ Unsalted, roasted peanuts

✔ Wholewheat pretzels

Adding Dips and Sauces to Snacks

Condiments are typically used to flavour or complement other foods. But some condiments are so delicious that you may want to eat them all by themselves. *Condiment* is a bit of an understatement for the tasty recipes in this section – try using them as terrific spreads for sandwiches or lettuce wraps, or as sauces to top grilled chicken or firm fish.

Dips are a creative way to get lots of vegetables. Unfortunately, most dips tend to have a very high kilocalorie and fat content. What is considered a light snack can quickly turn into a full meal's worth of kilocalories and fat. So skip the fat and keep the flavour with the following excellent vegetable dip. (Check out Chapter 7 for more dips to try.)

🍅 Roasted Veggie Dip

This dip is an excellent appetiser, food topper, condiment, or omelette filling – you name it, this dip can work. The roasting of the vegetables brings out their natural sugars, and the spices give a kick. Snack on this no-fat dip with wholewheat crackers or check out our list of approved dippers in Chapter 7.

Preparation time: *20 minutes*

Cooking time: *35 minutes*

Serves: *6*

½ aubergine, peeled, thick sliced

Courgette, thick sliced

Yellow squash, thick sliced

½ red onion, thick sliced

4 garlic cloves, roughly chopped

Nonstick cooking spray

½ teaspoon cayenne pepper

1 teaspoon chilli powder

Ground black pepper

1 Preheat the oven to 200°C/400°F/Gas Mark 6. Spray the aubergine, courgette, squash, onion, and garlic with the cooking spray, coating well.

2 In a small bowl, combine the cayenne pepper and chilli powder. Add a quarter of the seasoning to the vegetables. Toss well to combine. Add another quarter of the seasoning and toss well. Repeat until the vegetables are evenly coated and all the seasoning is added. Adding the seasonings in stages helps to combine the seasonings evenly.

3 Spray a baking pan with the cooking spray. Add the vegetables in a single layer. Cook the vegetables in the oven, until browned, stirring occasionally, for roughly 35 minutes.

4 Place the roasted vegetables in the bowl of a food processor. Process to desired consistency. Season with salt and pepper as necessary.

Per serving: *Kilocalories 32; Fat 0g (Saturated 0g); Cholesterol 0mg; Sodium 200mg; Carbohydrate 4g; Dietary Fibre 3g; Protein 2g.*

Exchanges: *1½ vegetable.*

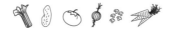

☙ Wolfe's Barbecue Sauce

You may have checked the nutrition labels of some of your favourite sauces before and noticed the really high sugar content. This sauce makes a great substitution by using sugar-free syrup instead of the usual version, which, you may have guessed, is entirely sugar. This recipe is a good reminder to make substitutions whenever you can and save your blood glucose without sacrificing your favourite foods. This sauce is great for dipping grilled chicken and vegetables, slathering on a hunk of firm fish, or topping a pitta for an impromptu barbecue chicken pizza. But definitely try it with the Barbecue Chicken with Potato and Oven-dried Tomatoes recipe in Chapter 13.

Preparation time: *10 minutes*

Cooking time: *15 minutes*

Serves: *8*

350 millilitres tomato ketchup

235 millilitres light (sugar-free) pancake syrup

1½ tablespoons low-sodium soy sauce

1½ tablespoons Worcestershire sauce

¾ tablespoon sesame oil

1 teaspoon minced ginger

1 teaspoon chilli powder

1 teaspoon onion powder

1 teaspoon fresh chopped garlic

1 teaspoon pepper

½ teaspoon salt

Place all ingredients in a non-metallic saucepan on a low heat. Warm the sauce for 10 minutes, stirring occasionally. For thicker sauce, continue to cook for 2 to 3 more minutes. Remove from the heat and cool.

Per serving: *Kilocalories 131; Fat 3g (Saturated 1g); Cholesterol 0mg; Sodium 872mg; Carbohydrate 25g; Dietary Fibre 1g; Protein 1g.*

Exchanges: *1 other carbohydrate, ½ fat.*

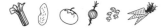

Preparing Mini Meals

Eating small portions of well-balanced meals is a great way to fit a nutritious and filling snack into your day. Maybe you ate a light brunch and are waiting for a late dinner. Maybe you had a really early breakfast and can't fit a full lunch in until late in the day. Or maybe you just find that maintaining even blood sugar levels is easier by eating five or six small meals each day. Whatever the reason, mini meals can help you eat right.

Choosing chicken

For someone with diabetes, chicken is a great basis for a mini meal because it provides protein that has minimal effect on blood glucose levels. Try the following two recipes to enjoy a taste of chicken.

Greek-Style Chicken Wraps

These wraps are quick and easy to make, and relatively low in fat because the recipe uses skinless chicken breasts. Experiment with different herbs, such as basil, and cheeses, such as feta, to find your preferred flavour combinations. The marinated chicken is also great tossed with salad greens or chopped into a quick casserole, as well as for making these wraps.

Preparation time: *20 minutes*

Cooking time: *25 minutes*

Serves: *2*

Nonstick cooking spray

2 115-gram boneless, skinless chicken breasts, pounded thin

1 tablespoon lemon juice

1 teaspoon oregano, crushed and dried

2 thin slices mild, white onion

2 25-centimetre wholewheat tortillas

60 grams low-fat plain yoghurt

30 grams peeled, seeded, and chopped cucumber

40 grams crumbled feta cheese

1 teaspoon chopped fresh mint

1 Preheat the oven to 180°C/350°F/Gas Mark 4. Coat a 20 × 20-centimetre (8 × 8-inch) baking dish with nonstick cooking spray. Brush the chicken breast on both sides with lemon juice and oregano. Place the chicken breast and onion in the baking dish. Bake for approximately 25 minutes.

2 When the chicken is done, transfer to a cutting board and cut into 1-centimetre (½-inch) strips.

3 Spread out the tortillas on a flat surface. Spread equal parts of yoghurt on top of the tortillas. Top with equal parts chicken, onion, cucumber, cheese, and mint.

4 Roll up the wraps and serve warm.

Per serving: Kilocalories 372; Fat 11g (Saturated 4g); Cholesterol 81mg; Sodium 767mg; Carbohydrate 29g; Dietary Fibre 7g; Protein 33g.

Exchanges: 2 starch, 4 lean meat, 1 medium-fat meat, 2 fat.

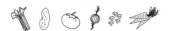

Quick Chicken Tostadas

Mexican food is often thought of as pretty high in fat and cholesterol, but that isn't always the case. In fact, common ingredients in Mexican cooking, such as beans, chicken, olives, and tomatoes, are very healthy. Not so good, on the other hand, are fried tortillas, extra cheese, and high-fat sour cream. If you have a craving for nachos or quesadillas, traditionally very high in kilocalories and saturated fat, try these light tostadas instead. They're full of flavour and incorporate traditional Mexican ingredients but have half the kilocalories and fat. When preparing tacos or other Mexican-style dishes at home, go sparingly with the toppings (cheese, sour cream, and guacamole), which contribute the most significant amounts of kilocalories and fat.

Preparation time: *20 minutes*

Cooking time: *10 minutes*

Serves: *6*

6 wholewheat flour tortillas

Nonstick cooking spray

350 grams cooked chicken (see the tip at the end of the recipe)

200 grams salsa

Pinch of cayenne pepper

Pinch of chilli powder

150 grams diced red pepper

Ground black pepper

115 grams grated cheddar cheese

1 tablespoon chopped coriander or spring onions (optional)

6 tablespoons low-fat sour cream (optional)

2 tablespoons chopped black olives (optional)

3 tablespoons prepared guacamole (optional)

1 Preheat the oven to 200°C/400°F/Gas Mark 6. Spray each tortilla lightly with cooking spray. Place prepared tortillas on a baking sheet and place in the oven. Toast the tortillas until crisp (approximately 2 to 3 minutes). Remove from the oven and set aside. Reduce the oven temperature to 190°C/375°F/Gas Mark 5.

2 Mix the chicken, salsa, cayenne pepper, chilli powder, red pepper, and ground black pepper to taste together in a mixing bowl. Top each tostada with ⅙ of the chicken mixture.

3 For each tostada, top the chicken mixture with ⅙ of the cheddar cheese. Return the tostadas to the oven. Cook until the chicken is heated through and the cheese is melted (approximately 5 to 7 minutes).

4 If desired, top each tostada with ½ teaspoon coriander or spring onions, 1 tablespoon sour cream, 1 teaspoon black olives, and ½ tablespoon guacamole.

Tip: *For this recipe, you can purchase roasted chicken breast, or you can cook the chicken breast yourself by poaching it, which means cooking in water just below the boiling point until cooked through (no longer pink inside).*

Per serving: *Kilocalories 316; Fat 13g (Saturated 5g); Cholesterol 68mg; Sodium 335mg; Carbohydrate 29g; Dietary Fibre 2g; Protein 29g.*

Exchanges: *1½ starch, 2 high-fat meat, 2 lean meat, 1 vegetable.*

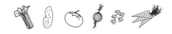

Selecting seafood

Seafood, tuna in particular, is a great item for someone with diabetes to choose as a mini meal because, like chicken, tuna is mostly protein and doesn't raise your blood glucose rapidly. The following dish is easy to reduce to a snack-size portion: Eat only one skewer full of tasty goodness, and you cut the kilocalories (and the other nutritional analyses) in half. Enjoy!

Tuna Dijon Brochettes

Fresh tuna has a beautiful ruby red colour, a firm texture, and a meaty flavour. Remember that tuna isn't just for salad anymore, but goes well with spicy sauces and spices, such as Dijon mustard. With sweet pineapple and mild vegetables, you get a full flavour experience.

Special tools: *2 metal skewers, 20 centimetres (8 inches) long*

Preparation time: *25 minutes*

Cooking time: *6 to 8 minutes*

Serves: *1 serving*

225 grams tuna, fresh, cut into 6 equal chunks

1 tablespoon Dijon mustard

4 mushrooms

4 squares red pepper, 2 × 2 centimetres (1 × 1 inch) each

4 slices courgette, ½ centimetre thick

4 chunks fresh, peeled pineapple, 2 × 2 centimetres (1 × 1 inch) each

4 medium cherry tomatoes

Ground black pepper

Nonstick cooking spray

1 Preheat the grill. In a bowl, coat the tuna chunks with the mustard.

2 Skewer the tuna, mushrooms, pepper, courgette, pineapple, and cherry tomatoes, alternating each item twice, beginning and ending with a tuna chunk.

3 Sprinkle each skewer with ground black pepper to taste. Coat a baking sheet with the cooking spray and place the skewers on the baking sheet. Grill for 6 to 8 minutes.

Per serving: *Kilocalories 351; Fat 4g (Saturated 1g); Cholesterol 98mg; Sodium 430mg; Carbohydrate 18g; Dietary Fibre 5g; Protein 56g.*

Exchanges: *2 vegetable, 7 very lean meat, ½ fruit.*

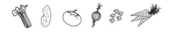

Stocking up with snacks at work

Getting through the day and avoiding food pitfalls is challenging for anyone, particularly when you have diabetes. The best defence against shared snacks of buns, cakes, muffins, pastries, and doughnuts is to be well prepared. Keep a healthy snack drawer at work for snacking emergencies, and you're sure to save yourself some kilocalories and blood glucose spikes and dips. And remember: A well-stocked snack drawer is a lifesaver when you don't have time to eat regular meals (although these occasions are very rare, right?).

Here are some ideas for a healthy snack drawer:

- Cartons of nutritional supplement drinks
- Fat-free, sugar-free puddings
- Individual servings of nuts
- Individual servings of sugar-free drink mixes
- Individual tins of low-sodium vegetable juice
- Light popcorn in snack-sized microwaveable bags
- Low-fat, low-sodium canned soups
- Low-sugar protein bars
- No-added-sugar juice cartons or bottles

When possible, choose individual serving sizes because they're proportioned and take the brainwork out of grabbing a quick snack when you're starving. Plus, keeping track of how much you eat is much easier when the nutritional information is on each snack.

Picking pasta

Indulge your cravings for Italian food with this version of the traditional potato pasta, gnocchi. If you love Italian food, but can't work in the right starch exchanges, take a look at the Aubergine Lasagne and Courgette and Cucumber Linguine with Clams recipes, both found in Chapter 11. With these recipes you get all the Italian flavour without any traditional pasta and the costly starch exchanges.

☉ *Spinach–Ricotta Gnocchi*

Here's a great twist on the traditional gnocchi, or potato pasta. Some of the white flour base to this usually high-carbohydrate food is creatively substituted with ricotta cheese, a significant source of protein. The result is that the gnocchi has far less of an effect on your blood glucose, meaning that you can eat what you may have once considered sinful! Enjoy this dish with your favourite red Italian pasta sauce.

Special tools: *Cheesecloth, pastry or icing bag, potato ricer or mouli*

Preparation time: *1 hour plus overnight straining of ricotta*

Cooking time: *4 to 5 minutes*

Serves: *4*

225 grams low-fat ricotta cheese	*Egg, beaten*
115 grams fresh spinach	*Pinch of ground nutmeg*
Floury potato	*Pinch of salt*
100 grams grated Parmesan cheese	*2 tablespoons plus 275 grams flour*

1 Place the ricotta in a strainer lined with cheesecloth and allow to sit overnight in the refrigerator to remove excess liquid.

2 Steam the spinach until wilted, and then strain and place on a baking sheet lined with parchment paper. Place the spinach in the refrigerator to cool. When cooled, squeeze out all the excess water from the spinach. Chop the spinach as fine as you can on a cutting board. This may take some time, but the finer the better.

3 Peel the potato and boil it for around 25 minutes, until soft. Drain well, allow to cool a little, then pass the flesh through a potato ricer or mouli into a bowl.

4 To make the gnocchi, place the chopped spinach, ricotta, Parmesan cheese, egg and nutmeg, and a pinch of salt into a large mixing bowl. Mix until the spinach is evenly distributed, then add the mashed potato and 2 tablespoons of flour to bind the mixture. Bring a small pan of water to a boil and drop in a spoon-sized piece of gnocchi to test the consistency and flavour. If the gnocchi is too wet and falls apart, add another egg and some flour. The key to this gnocchi is to add the minimum amount of binder so that the gnocchi is as light as possible.

5 Place a large saucepan on the stove with plenty of salted water to boil the gnocchi. Bring the water to a boil and turn down until you're ready to cook the gnocchi.

6 Place the remaining flour on a long baking tray. Shake the flour evenly around in the tray. Place the gnocchi mixture into a pastry or icing bag with a large straight tip about 12 millimetres (½ inch) in diameter. Pipe the gnocchi mixture in a long line directly into the flour, as if you're making a long snakelike piece. You can make a couple of lines like this in the flour. Alternatively, shape the mixture by rolling and stretching it between your hands before laying it onto the flour.

7 With a knife, cut the snake like pieces into 2½-centimetre (1-inch) pieces. With your hands, gently cover the gnocchi lightly with flour, shake off any excess flour, and place directly into boiling salt water. Cook the gnocchi for at least 5 minutes or until the pieces float for 2 minutes. Remove from the water.

Tip: You can serve these pieces immediately or save them for later use. If you plan to save this dish for later, place the cooked gnocchi on a lightly oiled baking sheet, and allow to cool. When cooled, you can place the gnocchi in an airtight container in the refrigerator until ready to use. You can reheat the gnocchi in boiling water for 4 to 5 minutes.

Per serving: Kilocalories 282; Fat 12g (Saturated 7g); Cholesterol 86mg; Sodium 628mg; Carbohydrate 23g; Dietary Fibre 1g; Protein 19g.

Exchanges: 2 starch, 1 medium-fat meat, 1 lean meat.

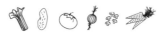

Chapter 16

Drooling over Mouth-Watering Desserts

'Sugar' is not necessarily a dirty word, even for someone with diabetes. But the truth is that the amount of sugar consumed in the UK is way too high. Manufacturers sneak sugar into all kinds of products – including pre-packaged 'ready-meals', ketchup, and, of course, baked goods – under the names *high-fructose corn syrup* and *malt syrup*. Even though diabetes is a condition that involves impaired metabolism of carbohydrates, you can still enjoy desserts that contain starches and sugar. Just select ingredients wisely and eat reasonably modest portions.

And if you crave sweet things that contain lots of table sugar (such as biscuits, jam doughnuts, pies, and boiled sweets) remember that you can retrain your taste buds to get used to less sweetness if you slowly cut back – just as you can retrain yourself to get used to less salt. Bear in mind that pure white table sugar – known as sucrose – contains no vitamins or minerals at all.

This chapter shows you how to create appealing desserts that feature nutritious ingredients and helps you to satisfy your cravings for sweet foods, including chocolate. In addition, we give you a variety of different desserts to impress your guests when you host a dinner party.

Finding a New Take on Fruit

Desserts for people with diabetes are often sugar-free gelatin concoctions or plain fruit. Although nothing is wrong with that, if you're bored with the standard take on fruit, here are several recipes that help you improve and update that old stand-by, providing desserts that you're proud to serve to anyone.

Baking with berries

Berries are nature's little juice boxes. They give a burst of juice, flavour, and fibre, all in a tiny bite. Adding them to muffins, pancakes, and cakes can add important antioxidants, fibre, and flavour, improving the taste and balance of just about any recipe. So add a few berries to your next treat.

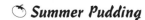 **Summer Pudding**

Summer pudding is a delicious, traditional treat that you can now enjoy all year round. Most supermarkets sell frozen berry mixtures that you can readily use when fresh berries aren't in season. Bear this pudding in mind when you have lots of wholegrain bread that needs using up. And although the original recipe calls for sugar, we make one very important substitution in this version that makes it more suitable for someone with diabetes: To maintain some of that sweetness everyone knows and loves, use a granulated sweetener (sucralose) in place of sugar.

Preparation time: *30 minutes*

Chilling time: *8 hours*

Serves: *6*

900 grams mixed fresh or frozen summer berries (raspberries, blackberries, blueberries, blackcurrants, redcurrants, strawberries)

6 to 8 tablespoons of granulated sweetener

8 to 10 thin slices of brown bread, crusts removed

1 Place the fruit and sweetener in a pan and heat gently for 3 minutes, stirring, until the sweetener dissolves and the juices start to run. Taste to check the sweetness level.

2 Cut some of the bread into wedge shapes to fit into the bottom of a 1.1-litre (2-pint) pudding basin. Use the bread to line the bowl neatly, with no spaces between the slices.

3 Fill the bread-lined basin with the fruit and most of the juice, and then cover completely with a layer of bread. If any fruit is left over, set aside to serve alongside the pudding. Spoon the remaining juice over the top layer of bread, ensuring that all the bread is coloured with juice.

4 Cover the pudding with a loose piece of cling film. Place a plate that fits inside the basin on top of the bread pudding. Put a weight (for example, a can of beans) on the plate to press it down onto the pudding, and leave in the fridge overnight so that the pudding compresses and the juices soak into the bread.

5 To serve, run a knife between the bowl and pudding and carefully invert onto a serving plate. Spoon over any remaining fruit.

Tip: *Use day old bread, which is drier and absorbs the juices more easily.*

Per serving: *Kilocalories 116; Fat 1g (Saturated 0g); Cholesterol 0mg; Sodium 185mg; Carbohydrate 25g; Dietary Fibre 5g; Protein 4g.*

Exchanges: *1 starch, 1 fruit.*

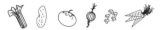

Creating luscious fruit desserts with different flavourings

Even if you don't have time to prepare a full-blown fruit recipe, you can still concoct wonderful desserts and mouth-watering nibbles that simply combine luscious fruit with a few added ingredients. You can use all sorts of herbs, spices, and nuts to enhance the flavour of fruit. Here are some examples:

- Combine low-fat vanilla yoghurt with fresh fruit and semi-freeze to create a parfait.

- Create fruit kebabs from your fresh favourites and marinate them in lemon juice, nutmeg, and crushed mint.

- Grill pineapple slices and lightly coat them with lemon juice, a dash of honey, and cinnamon.

- Peel a banana, freeze it, and then purée in a food processor, along with almonds or peanut butter, and you have a fruit version of ice cream.

- Purée ripe melon with low-fat vanilla yoghurt, a dash of nutmeg and cinnamon, and a squirt of lemon for a refreshing fruit soup.

◌ Spiced Infusion with Tropical Fruits

This recipe gives you a way to enjoy a treat without all the sugar that comes with most desserts! But remember that this dish still contains carbs, and like everything else, enjoying it in moderation is key.

Preparation time: *5 minutes*

Cooking time: *30 minutes, mostly steeping time*

Serves: *2*

4 tablespoons granulated sweetener	Zest of 1 lemon
600 millilitres water	Cinnamon stick
8 star anise	15 whole black peppercorns
2 vanilla pods	1 teaspoon coriander seed
2 tablespoons grated ginger root	230 grams fresh tropical fruits, such as mango, pineapple, star fruit, or passion fruit

1 Combine all the ingredients, except the fruit, in a large saucepan and bring to a boil. Turn off the heat, cover, and allow to steep for ½ hour. Strain spices and herbs and allow to cool completely.

2 Serve on top of the fruit.

Per serving (sauce with 115g fruit): *Kilocalories 55; Fat 1g (Saturated 0g); Cholesterol 0mg; Sodium 18mg; Carbohydrate 15g; Dietary Fibre 7g; Protein 2g.*

Exchanges: *1½ fruit.*

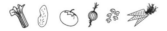

Ginger and lemon brighten the sweet flavours of the cantaloupe melon and papaya in the following recipe. Choose a cantaloupe that's heavy for its size, has a lightly sweet melon fragrance, and is firm but gives slightly when pressed. Avoid cantaloupes with mushy spots or discolourations.

The papaya is a large pear-shaped tropical fruit that contains a bed of large peppery seeds in the centre. If you're looking for a ripe papaya to use immediately or refrigerate, choose richly coloured papayas, with splotches of bright yellow, green, and some orange. Green papayas ripen in a few days if placed in a brown paper bag and left at room temperature.

☞ *Cantaloupe–Papaya Salad with Ginger Syrup*

This fruity dessert is sure to please your taste buds. The recipe is easy and uses a simple syrup made from water and sweetener in place of sugar. Enjoy the natural fruit flavours of these antioxidant-packed fruits with a little something extra drizzled lightly on top.

Preparation time: *20 minutes*

Cooking time: *10 minutes*

Serves: *6*

Syrup:	*1 tablespoon lemon zest*
4 tablespoons granulated sweetener	**Fruit salad:**
120 millilitres water	*Cantaloupe*
Thumb-sized piece of fresh ginger root, peeled	*2 papayas*
	4 mint sprigs

1 Bring the sweetener and water to a boil in a small saucepan over a medium heat. Add the ginger and reduce the heat, allowing the liquid to simmer.

2 Stir until the sweetener dissolves and the ginger infuses the syrup (about 2 minutes). Remove the pan from heat and take out the ginger. Allow the syrup to cool at room temperature. Add the lemon zest.

3 Scoop out the meat of the fruits with a melon baller and then toss with the syrup and mint when you're ready to serve.

Per serving: *Kilocalories 78; Fat 0g (Saturated 0g); Cholesterol 0mg; Sodium 20mg; Carbohydrate 16g; Dietary Fibre 3g; Protein 1g.*

Exchanges: *1 fruit.*

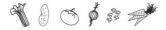

☙ *Pears Baked in Red Wine alla Piemontese*

This recipe is a classic way of preparing pears in Piemonte, Italy's most north-western region. Bake the pears until the skins turn brown and crinkly – *strafugna* as they say in the Piemontese dialect. Substitute a natural-tasting artificial sweetener for sugar in this recipe, to still give the pears great flavour. Keep in mind, however, that because fruit and wine have natural sugars, you can't completely discount the carbohydrate content of this dish, which (per serving) is equivalent to almost 3 starch servings. Enjoy this delightful dessert after a meal low in starch and only on special occasions!

Preparation time: *15 minutes*

Cooking time: *1½ hours, plus cooling time*

Serves: *4*

300 millilitres dry red wine	*Juice of 2 lemons*
7 cloves	*8 tablespoons granulated sweetener*
Cinnamon stick	*4 large dessert pears, unpeeled*

1 Preheat the oven to 150°C/300°F/Gas Mark 2.

2 Pour the wine into a 23 × 23-centimetre (9 × 9-inch) baking pan. Add the cloves, cinnamon, lemon juice, and sweetener and stir until the sweetener dissolves. Add the pears to the pan. Place them in the oven and bake for 1½ hours, brushing the pears with wine from the pan every 10 minutes.

3 Remove the pears from the oven, allow to cool at room temperature, and serve.

Per serving: Kilocalories 151; Fat 1g (Saturated 0g); Cholesterol 0mg; Sodium 13mg; Carbohydrate 28g; Dietary Fibre 5g; Protein 1g.

Exchanges: 2 fruit, ½ other carbohydrate.

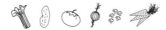

Juicing Your Way to Tasty and Healthy Treats

Fruit juice lacks the fibre of whole fruit, and without all that fibre to slow down its absorption, all the natural sugars can really raise your blood sugar. But with a little diligence you can use fruit juice to flavour your desserts and still maintain acceptable blood sugar levels.

⌚ Cranberry–Raspberry Granita

This refreshing treat makes for a sweet dessert – except that it doesn't have any added sugar. Raspberries and cranberries are some of the best sources of antioxidants, and you don't even have to wait for summer to take advantage of these nutritional power-houses. Most berries are available in frozen food sections of supermarkets and have all the great nutrition of their fresh versions.

Preparation time: *6 hours and 30 minutes, mostly unattended*

Serves: *6*

480 millilitres 100 per cent cranberry–raspberry juice blend

200 grams raspberries (fresh or previously frozen, thawed, and drained)

8 tablespoons granulated sweetener

1 In a blender, combine the juice and raspberries. Mix well. Pour the mixture through a fine-mesh sieve placed over a mixing bowl. Press the mixture gently through the sieve, as necessary, to extract as much juice as possible. Discard the mixture in the sieve or reserve for another use.

2 Add the sweetener to the strained juice mixture and stir to mix well. Cover and freeze. Stir thoroughly with a fork about every 30 minutes, for 6 hours or so, or until the granita is frozen in a crumbly, grainy texture.

Per serving: *Kilocalories 71; Fat 0g (Saturated 0g); Cholesterol 0mg; Sodium 2mg; Carbohydrate 18g; Dietary Fibre 0g; Protein 0g.*

Exchanges: *1 fruit.*

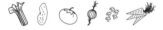

Citrus fruits make a great juice choice for adding to desserts. Their strong flavours mean a little goes a long way. And many are tart rather than sweet, so they naturally have few sugars. For tips on how to juice your own citrus, see Chapter 7.

☾ Lemon Soufflé Tart

Tarts always make a great dessert with their sweet, fruity filling and savoury, crisp crust. The only problem is all the butter needed to produce that perfect pastry shell. Pie and tart crusts, prepared traditionally with butter, are extremely high in kilocalories and fat. Unfortunately, margarine is worse, because this butter alternative is potentially high in artery-clogging trans fats. The good news is that 'lite' butters are becoming more mainstream and available in most supermarkets. Many are designed for use in place of butter, as spreads and even in cooking and baking. They're lower in total kilo-calories, cholesterol free, and most importantly, contain no trans fat. Check that the ingredients don't contain 'partially hydrogenated oils' to ensure that you buy a product with no trans fats. Also choose a brand that you can use in both cooking and baking. This soufflé tart is a great opportunity to try a trans-fat-free butter spread.

Special tool: A bain-marie. Sounds posh, but a bain-marie is just one cooking vessel inside another. Simmering water in the larger vessel supplies indirect heat to the food being cooked in the smaller one.

Preparation time: *30 minutes*

Cooking time: *1 hour*

Serves: *8*

Crust:

100 grams plain flour

100 grams wholemeal pastry flour

1 tablespoon granulated sweetener

Pinch of salt

100 grams trans-fat-free butter spread, chilled, cut into pieces

2 tablespoons cold water

Filling:

10 tablespoons sweetener

4 large eggs, yolk and whites separated

Juice of 2 fresh lemons

Zest from 1 lemon, finely chopped

1 tablespoon cornstarch

1 Make the crust: Combine the plain and wholemeal flours, the 1 tablespoon of sweetener, and the salt in the bowl of a food processor. Add the butter spread. Process using quick pulses to create a coarse mixture. Add 1 tablespoon of the water and process for 5 seconds. Add the remaining 1 tablespoon water and process for another few seconds. The dough starts to form a mass. Add a few more drops of water, if necessary, to create a ball of dough.

2 Place the dough ball between 2 large pieces of cling film. Roll the dough (still inside the cling film) into a disc, roughly 15 centimetres (6 inches) in diameter. Refrigerate the wrapped disc for an hour.

3 Preheat the oven to 190°C/375°F/Gas Mark 5. Roll the chilled dough to a 2½-millimetre (⅒-inch) thickness. Remove the top layer of cling film. Place the tart pan face down on the dough. Holding the bottom layer of cling film and the tart pan, flip the tarts over, so that the pan is resting on its bottom, the dough is in the pan, and the plastic wrap is on top. Remove the cling film. Press the dough into the fluted edge of the tart pan, allowing it to overhang slightly. Trim off any excess edges.

4 Bake the crust until it begins to brown slightly (about 5 minutes). Remove the crust from the oven and allow to cool while you make the filling.

5 Make the filling: Beat 5 tablespoons of granulated sweetener and egg yolks with an electric mixer on a medium-low heat for approximately 5 minutes, until the yolks turn a creamy pale yellow. Add the lemon juice, lemon zest, and cornstarch. Beat until smooth and fully combined. Place the egg yolk mixture in the top of a bain-marie, over simmering water. Stir constantly until the mixture thickens (approximately 7 to 8 minutes). Remove from the heat and stir for another 2 minutes to help the mixture cool.

6 With a clean whisk in a clean bowl, whip the egg whites until frothy. Gradually beat in the remaining 5 tablespoons of sweetener. Continue to beat until the egg whites form stiff peaks. Gently but thoroughly fold the egg whites into the warm egg yolk mixture. Spread the filling evenly over the baked crust.

7 Bake the tart in the centre of the oven until the filling is puffy and lightly browned (approximately 27 to 30 minutes). Remove from the oven and allow the tart to cool slightly. The filling sinks a bit as it cools. Cut into wedges and serve.

Per serving: Kilocalories 218; Fat 12g (Saturated 3g); Cholesterol 106mg; Sodium 195mg; Carbohydrate 20g; Dietary Fibre 2g; Protein 6g.

Exchanges: 1 starch, 2 fat, ½ medium-fat meat.

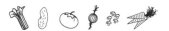

Choosing Chocolate for Dessert

Can you imagine life without chocolate? Fortunately, you don't have to speculate or experience the situation. You can mix up your own tasty chocolate concoctions if you substitute your favourite no-kilocalorie sweetener for the regular sugar.

Whenever possible, choose the highest-quality cocoa powder you can afford. The flavour is much better, and because you're only having a small portion anyway, you definitely want the best-tasting bite you can get!

Mixing up some meringues

Meringue, essentially egg whites flavoured and whipped to foamy peaks, is an extremely versatile food. You can create little clouds to hold fresh fruit, top a fruit pie, or even use to cover sponge and ice cream to create a baked Alaska. Meringue is naturally low in fat and takes on the flavour of any extracts, such as almond, mint, or chocolate; so experiment and enjoy!

☞ Chocolate Meringue Bits with Strawberries and Cream

These little meringues are a great way to satisfy chocolate cravings without all the kilocalories and fat. They are flavoured with cocoa powder and sweetener and the texture of these 'lite bites' is outstanding. Top with fresh strawberries for a dash of fibre and vitamin C.

Preparation time: *30 minutes, plus standing time of 8 hours or overnight*

Cooking time: *1 hour and 30 minutes*

Makes: *40 4-centimetre (1½-inch) meringues*

4 egg whites	*30 grams cocoa powder*
Pinch of cream of tartar	*60 grams reduced-fat tub-style whipped topping*
1 teaspoon vanilla extract	
10 tablespoons sweetener	*40 strawberries*

1 Preheat the oven to 110°C/230°F/Gas Mark ¼. Line 2 baking sheets with parchment paper.

2 Beat the egg whites, cream of tartar, and vanilla at high speed with an electric mixer until frothy. Add the sweetener, 1 tablespoon at a time, beating until stiff peaks form (roughly 5 to 7 minutes). Gently fold in the cocoa powder until completely incorporated.

3 Spoon heaped tablespoons of the mixture onto the baking sheets. Bake for 1½ hours; turn the oven off. Let the meringues stand in the closed oven for 8 hours or overnight. Store in an airtight container.

4 Just before serving, top each meringue with 1 scant teaspoon of whipped topping and a strawberry.

Per serving: Kilocalories 13; Fat 0g (Saturated 0g); Cholesterol 0mg; Sodium 6mg; Carbohydrate 1g; Dietary Fibre 1g; Protein 1g.

Exchanges: Free food.

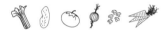

Enjoying a coffee break

Coffee is one of the most available beverages in our society these days. You can hardly stroll through most towns without smelling the aroma of your local coffee roaster. And fortunately, most coffee shops offer delicious decaffeinated versions of these aromatic beverages. Steam up a little skimmed milk to go with the coffee, and you're ready to relax for a few minutes.

For a decadent but diabetes-friendly coffee break, make your own decaf, non-fat coffee drink (sweetened with sugar-free sweeteners, of course) and pair it with our delicious, crunchy biscotti.

Chocolate–Almond Biscotti

Biscotti are a great treat, and now you can enjoy them homemade, and without all the kilocalories and sugar. This rendition of the Italian 'biscuit' is easy to make and takes no time. This recipe is also half the kilocalories and carbohydrates of the usual crusty biscuit.

Preparation time: *1 hour*

Cooking time: *45 minutes*

Serves: *20*

Nonstick cooking spray

50 grams almonds, toasted and roughly chopped

60 grams plain flour

40 grams wholemeal flour

20 grams unsweetened cocoa powder

2 teaspoons instant coffee granules

½ teaspoon baking soda

Pinch of salt

8 tablespoons granulated sweetener

Egg

Egg white

1 teaspoon vanilla extract

1 teaspoon almond extract

1 Preheat the oven to 180°C/350°F/Gas Mark 4. Line a large baking sheet with aluminum foil and spray the foil with nonstick cooking spray.

2 In a food processor, combine half the almonds with the plain flour, wholemeal flour, cocoa powder, coffee granules, baking soda, and salt. Process until the nuts are finely ground (approximately 2 minutes). Transfer the mixture to a large mixing bowl.

3 In the food processor, combine the sweetener, egg, egg white, vanilla extract, and almond extract. Mix until the mixture is slightly thickened (roughly 2 minutes). Add the egg mixture to the flour mixture in the mixing bowl. Stir in the remaining almonds.

4 Use half the mixture to form a log approximately 13 to 18 centimetres (5 to 7 inches) long on one-half of the foil-lined baking sheet. Repeat with the remaining mixture on the other half of the baking sheet. Bake until firm (approximately 15 minutes). Cool for approximately 10 minutes. Reduce the oven temperature to 150°C/300°F/Gas Mark 2.

5 Place the logs on a cutting board. Using a serrated bread knife, cut each log into approximately 10 diagonal slices. Return the slices to the baking sheets. Bake until the cut sides feel dry to the touch (approximately 20 minutes). Cool completely and store in an airtight container.

Per serving (1 biscotti): Kilocalories 60; Fat 2g (Saturated 0g); Cholesterol 11mg; Sodium 30mg; Carbohydrate 11g; Dietary Fibre 1g; Protein 2g.

Exchanges: 1 starch.

Part III
Eating Away from Home

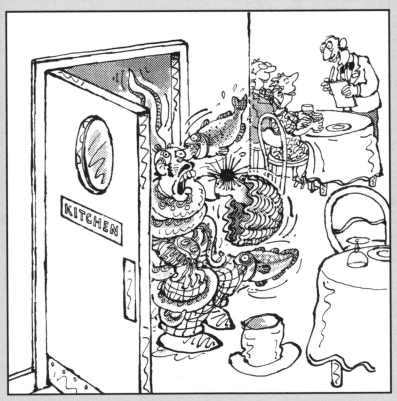

'...and we go to a lot of trouble to make
sure you get the freshest seafood
in the city.'

In this part . . .

You may believe that – because you have diabetes – you can no longer enjoy the creative cuisines and the wonderful atmospheres and service of great restaurants. This part puts that misinformation to rest with a resounding *bon appétit*, French for 'You are about to be treated to a great restaurant meal.'

This part shows you the right way to eat away from home by giving you tips for great restaurant dining experiences and showing you how to choose the best possible fast food when you're on the go. We also give you the low-down on preparing great-tasting, healthy picnic food and packed lunches.

Chapter 17

Eating Out as a Nourishing Experience

In This Chapter
- ▶ Preparing to eat out
- ▶ Arriving at a restaurant and checking the menu
- ▶ Managing meals in different kinds of restaurants
- ▶ Finding ways to enjoy your food

*P*eople eat many of their meals in restaurants these days, and so integrating restaurant eating into a nutritional plan is essential for someone with diabetes. The restaurant business is booming, and creative chefs have the same celebrity status as famous sports stars. And they deserve it. They use fresh ingredients to produce some of the most delicious and unique tastes imaginable. Unfortunately, nutrition isn't always uppermost in their minds. Interest in good nutrition is increasing among chefs, but you're still on your own most of the time when selecting healthy foods. This chapter helps you ensure that your restaurant eating fits well into your nutritional plan.

Your situation may resemble the plight of the customer who calls the waiter over and complains, 'I can't find any steak in this steak pie.' The waiter replies, 'Well, there's no horse in the horseradish either.' The point is that you're ultimately responsible for ensuring that you know what's in the food you order and for making healthy choices. And if you find a fly in your soup, thank the waiter for the extra protein but ask him to serve it separately!

Preparing for Restaurant Dining

Many restaurants believe that people need lots of food before they think they're getting value for money. However, you don't want to go to the other extreme of a trendy restaurant that offers tiny, bite-sized portions arranged artfully on a plate. Instead, you want a compromise – reasonable portions of good, healthy, quality food that's flavoursome, well-cooked, and at reasonable prices. If you find such a restaurant, cherish it and visit as often as you can.

No particular kind of food is more or less healthy than any other, with the exception of fast food which is often full of unhealthy fats, sugars, and salt. You may think that vegetarian food is healthier than animal sources, but a dish of pasta in a creamy sauce is no healthier than a piece of fatty steak. Often, restaurants have several menu items that fit into your nutrition plan.

When you don't know the ingredients in the food or whether the menu items are healthy or not, how do you assess a restaurant? Here are a few suggestions:

✔ Call ahead and find out whether you can substitute items on the menu. Non-franchise and non-fast-food restaurants are much more likely to let you substitute menu items. (In contrast, fast-food restaurants make the food entirely uniform to serve large numbers of people at lower prices, and this uniformity makes it easier to know the exact ingredients and methods of preparation.) You need to ask only a few questions to know whether a restaurant is accommodating. Ask whether the staff can

  • Bake, grill, and poach instead of frying or sautéing

  • Reduce the amount of butter, salt, and sugar in a dish

  • Serve gravies, salad dressings, and sauces on the side

  • Substitute skimmed milk for whole milk

✔ Check on the restaurant's Web site before deciding to visit a particular establishment. Many restaurants now publish their menus on the Internet, so you can make sure that it serves food you can eat.

✔ Consider choosing a restaurant that you can walk to and from. The exercise you get offsets the extra kilocalories you may consume.

✔ Consider what you've already eaten that day when choosing a restaurant. For example, if you've already eaten your daily limit of carbohydrate, selecting a restaurant where pasta or rice is the major ingredient isn't a good idea. People often choose a restaurant days in advance, so if you know ahead where you're dining, you can modify your eating accordingly, earlier in the day, especially if the restaurant specialises in foods you usually eat in small quantities.

✔ Don't go to the restaurant if the catch of the day is fish fingers.

✔ Don't visit a restaurant that you know serves huge portions of everything, unless you plan to share your meal or take part of your meal home.

✔ Drink water or have a vegetable snack before you go to the restaurant so that hunger doesn't drive you to make bad choices.

✔ Select an older restaurant, with the advantage of experienced and well-trained waiting staff who know what the kitchen staff are willing to do for you, based on previous occurrences.

You have to evaluate the food you order, so question the waiting staff carefully. Even if the balance of energy sources is right, you may receive too much food and need to take some home or leave some on your plate.

Mrs Wilson, who has type 2 diabetes, decides to go to a well-known café before she goes to the theatre. She knows that they serve huge portions but also that she can order a mini-version of many of the items. At the restaurant, she orders a cheese and ham baguette – made with french bread, ham, Swiss cheese, pickle, and mayonnaise. She expects to get half or less of the usual entrée but what arrives is the entire baguette without the usual side salad and coleslaw. She can't take half of it home because she's going directly to the theatre. She feels bad leaving part of such a delicious meal, and so she ends up eating most of it. Her blood glucose level later that night reflects the huge excess in kilocalories that she has consumed.

You can see from the information in this section that you can do plenty to prepare for dining out, even before you reach the restaurant. Your preparation may make the whole experience much more satisfying and less frustrating.

Beginning the Dining Experience

As you sit down to enjoy your meal, you can take many steps to make the experience of eating out as pleasurable as possible. A few simple considerations at this point allow you to enjoy the meal free of the concern that you're wrecking your nutritional programme. Here are some steps that you can take:

- Ask the waiting staff to show you straight to your table, to avoid sitting in the bar with cocktails or getting too hungry or even hypoglycaemic.

- Ask the waiting staff not to bring bread, or ask them to take any existing bread off the table; that goes for crisps and crackers as well.

- Ask to be served raw vegetables without a dip – what the restaurant menu calls *crudités* – so that you can munch on something before you order.

- Check your blood glucose before you order so that you know how much carbohydrate is appropriate at that time.

- Wait to administer your short-acting insulin until you're sure of the food delivery time.

Mr Phillips, a 63-year-old man with type 2 diabetes, is trying to understand, with the help of his dietitian, why his blood glucose rose unusually high after a meal at a local Mexican restaurant. 'I know the portions are large, so I ordered a bean tortilla, and I didn't even eat the whole thing. I left half of it on my plate. I ate very little of the rice as well.' The dietitian asks him if he arrived early at the restaurant. 'Oh yes, I forgot. We had to wait in the bar, and I had a virgin margarita.' 'That,' says the dietitian, 'explains your high blood glucose. The margarita is all carbohydrate.'

Ordering from the Menu

The standard menu and the specials of the day or season encourage you to order a big meal. When you order meat, fish, or poultry, you often get at least twice as much as the serving in the diabetic exchange lists. When you consider how frequently people eat out in the United Kingdom, you can see why the population is getting fatter.

Your strategy for ordering from a menu needs to include the following:

- ✔ Consider a meal of soup and salad. This combination is delicious, filling, and low in kilocalories and carbohydrate.

- ✔ Consider using a starter as your main course.

- ✔ Feel free to get a complete description, including portion size, of a starter or main course from the waiting staff so that you aren't surprised when the food arrives. Pay particular attention to how the food is cooked – in fat or butter, for example.

- ✔ Let the waiting staff know that you need to eat soon. If your food is delayed because the kitchen is slow or busy, ask politely for some vegetable snacks to be brought to the table.

- ✔ Order any wine you decide to have by the glass. Diners almost always finish a bottle of wine, and unless eight of you share the bottle, you end up drinking too much.

- ✔ Order clear soup rather than cream soups.

- ✔ Plan to leave some food or take home half your order, because the portions are almost always too large. You can also order one dish to share with another person.

- ✔ Request salad dressings and sauces on the side if possible. This approach ensures that you're in control of the amount you consume.

- ✔ Watch out for vegetarian dishes. They're often high in carbohydrates and made with a lot of dairy products that contain saturated fats.

- ✔ You're probably wise to choose fish more often than meat, both to avoid fat and to take advantage of the cholesterol-lowering properties of fish. Remember, however, that fried fish is often as fat-laden as a steak. Women who are pregnant need to limit their intake of oily fish, and of deep sea fish, however. See Chapter 12 for more on this.

The description of a main course usually offers clues that tell you whether that dish is a good option for you. The following words, in particular, indicate that the preparation keeps fat to a minimum:

- ✔ Baked
- ✔ Barbecued

- ✔ Blackened
- ✔ Cooked in its own juice
- ✔ Grilled
- ✔ Poached

On the other hand, the following words point to a less desirable high-fat entrée:

- ✔ Battered
- ✔ Buttered or in butter sauce
- ✔ Creamed or in cream sauce
- ✔ Deep-fried
- ✔ Escalloped
- ✔ Fried
- ✔ Golden brown
- ✔ In a plum sauce
- ✔ In cheese sauce
- ✔ Sautéed
- ✔ Sweet-and-sour
- ✔ With peanuts or cashews

If you think that ordering one kind of sauce rather than another doesn't matter, check out the kilocalorie counts per tablespoon for the following salad dressings. Remember that the energy in food is properly expressed in kilocalories, not calories, which are a thousand times smaller:

- ✔ **Blue cheese:** 82 kilocalories
- ✔ **Creamy Italian dressing:** 52 kilocalories
- ✔ **Low-fat French dressing:** 22 kilocalories
- ✔ **Red-wine vinegar:** 2 kilocalories

Planning at Each Meal and in Specific Kinds of Restaurants

You can make good choices at every meal, whether breakfast, lunch, or dinner. Every kind of food offers you the opportunity to select a low-fat, low-salt alternative. You just need to think ahead and remain aware of the possibilities. Helping you choose healthy meals is the purpose of this section.

When you go to any one of the types of restaurant discussed here, take a look at the waiters and waitresses. Are they overweight or obese? Usually they're not, and yet they eat the food you're about to eat on a regular basis. Therefore, you can order food in this restaurant and know that you have plenty of good healthy options. (Check out Chapter 4 for an introduction to ethnic foods and how to prepare them yourself.)

Breakfast

The good choices at breakfast are fresh foods, which usually contain plenty of fibre. Fresh fruit and juice are good ways to start the meal, followed by low-fat yoghurt or fromage frais. Alternatively, go for hot cereals such as oatmeal, or high-fibre cold cereals such as shredded wheat, or bran cereals. Always add skimmed or semi-skimmed milk instead of whole milk. Enjoy egg whites but not yolks, or ask for an omelette with two whites for every yolk.

Less desirable options are foods such as bacon, fried potatoes, croissants, pastries, and doughnuts.

Appetisers, salads, and soups

Raw and plain food beats items cooked and covered with butter or sour cream, and that rule applies to starters, salads, and soups too. Raw carrots and celery are enjoyable at any time and to almost any extent. Clear soups are always healthier. Tomato and chilli sauces – known as salsa – are a popular accompaniment for crackers and crisps instead of high-fat dips. A delicious green salad is also nutritious and filling.

In contrast, olives, nachos, and avocados contain lots of fat, and nuts, crisps, and cheese before dinner add lots of kilocalories. Fried onion appetisers are currently very popular, and they're often dripping with fat. Watch out for sour cream dips and mayonnaise dips, because they're also full of fat.

Seafood

Most fish are relatively low in fat and a healthy choice. But even the best fish can compromise your nutrition plan when fried. Fish that stand out in the low-fat category are cod, bass, halibut, swordfish, and tuna canned in water. Most of the shellfish varieties are also low fat. Stay away from herring, tuna in oil, and fried anything.

Chinese food

You can eat great Chinese food and not have to worry about upsetting your diet plan. Any of the soups on the menu are delicious and fill you up. Stick to vegetable dishes with small amounts of meat in them. Avoid fried dishes, whether they're meats, tofu, or rice and noodles. Steamed dishes are a much better option. Sweet-and-sour pork really throws off your kilocalorie count and your fat intake, however, so steer clear. And also stay away from the almond biscuits and sticky banana fritters that often follow a Chinese meal.

French food

Although the old style of preparing French food promotes a lot of cream and gravy, a new style, called nouvelle (new) cuisine, emphasises the freshest ingredients, usually cooked in their own sauce. This style has revolutionised French restaurants. Still, some French chefs cling to the old ways, and their food isn't for you, unless you're prepared to share your meal.

Most desserts in French restaurants are high in carbohydrate. Limit yourself to a taste or, better yet, don't tempt yourself – refuse the cake or crème brulée. See if the pastry chef has a fruit dish, such as poached pears, that's both delicious and good for you.

Indian food

Rice, and naan and paratha breads are good carbohydrate choices, but avoid foods made with coconut cream because of the fat content. Meat, fish, and poultry cooked in the tandoori manner (baked in an oven) are fine, but Indian chefs like to fry many foods; keep those to a minimum. Avoid ghee, which is clarified butter. Fried appetisers such as samosas and creamy dishes don't help your blood glucose. Chicken tikka and chapati are fine – they're made with delicious spices (for taste) but little fat.

Italian food

Stick to tomato-based sauces and avoid the creamy, buttery, cheesy sauces. Minestrone soup is a hearty vegetable soup that's low in fat. Pasta in general is fine as long as the sauce isn't fatty. The problem with the pasta, however, is that the quantity is almost always too great. Share it or take half home. Sausage, because of all the added fats, is a poor choice, whether served with pasta or placed on pizza. If you love the taste of basil in pesto sauce, ask for a low-fat version of this classic dish. And ask whether the kitchen staff can make garlic bread with roasted garlic alone, without the butter that often accompanies it. The taste is truly delicious. Avoid Caesar salad and dishes made with a lot of cheese, such as cheese-filled ravioli.

Japanese food

Japanese food is generally fine to eat, particularly sushi, miso soup, and broiled fish. Stay away from the tempura, which is deep-fried. Limit your rice intake to a maximum of 1 to 2 exchanges, which is 70 to 140 grams (2½ to 5 ounces) at a meal.

Mexican food

Mexican food is increasingly popular, but Mexican restaurants offer you many temptations to slip from your healthy eating plan. They often start with crisps, nachos, and cheese. Ask the waiting staff to keep them off the table. Have salsa, not guacamole, as an appetiser. Stay away from anything refried; the word means just what it says. Avoid all dishes laden with cheese, as well as dishes heavy in sausage. Chicken with rice, grilled fish, and grilled chicken are excellent options. Tortillas, burritos, and tostadas are delicious and good for you as long as you avoid the addition of a lot of cheese, sour cream, or guacamole. And keep in mind the importance of moderation. Mexican restaurants are known for large servings, so take some home.

Thai food

Other than the tendency to provide larger-than-needed portions, Thai restaurants do little that isn't healthy. The creative use of spices, emphasis on fish, and use of fresh vegetables make this cuisine a good choice for you. Just watch out for the spices.

Enjoying Your Food

If you're conscientious in planning a delicious restaurant meal ahead of time, you deserve to really enjoy the food. But you need to continue thinking about healthy eating (and drinking) habits even as you sit down to the meal. All the great planning can come undone if you're careless at this point. Think about the following advice as you eat:

✔ After carefully controlling the intake of food on your plate, don't add significant kilocalories by tasting or finishing the food on your companion's plate.

✔ If you have a glass of wine, consider the number of kilocalories.

✔ Remember that the meal is a social occasion. Spend more time talking to your companions and less time concentrating on the food.

✔ Remove the skin if you're eating poultry, and allow the sauce to drip off the morsel of food on your fork if you're eating a dish cooked in sauce.

✔ Try using some behaviour modification to prolong the meal and give your brain a chance to know that you're eating: Eat slowly, chew each bite thoroughly, and put your fork down between each bite.

Finishing with Dessert

For many people, the early courses of a meal are just a prelude to their favourite part, which is dessert. Most people have a sweet tooth, and dessert is often the way to satisfy that need. The Italians don't call the part of the menu that features the desserts the *dulci* (which means 'sweets') without reason. Dessert, in many restaurants, is a showpiece. The pastry chef tries to show how sweet he or she can make the dessert while creating a culinary work of art. The terms *decadent* or 'death by chocolate' are commonly used to describe the richness of these desserts.

Does this mean that you can't have any dessert at all? No. Making a wise choice simply requires a certain amount of awareness on your part. You need to ask yourself the question, 'Is the taste of this dessert worth the potential damage it does to my blood glucose and kilocalorie intake?' If you can answer this question with a 'yes', have the dessert, but check your blood glucose and adjust your medications as needed after eating it. Then return to your nutritional plan without spending a lot of time regretting your lapse. You may even do a little extra exercise to counteract the kilocalories.

On the other hand, if you answer the question with a 'no', ask yourself these questions to help you avoid temptation:

✔ Are you going to remember the dessert ten minutes after you've eaten it?

✔ Can you share the dessert or just taste it?

✔ Do you really need or want the dessert?

✔ Is a fruit dessert available that you can enjoy instead?

To help you avoid that high-kilocalorie dessert even further, think in terms of the number of minutes of active aerobic exercise you need to do to account for the kilocalories you consume in a dessert. If your exercise is walking, double these times. Here are some examples:

- ✔ Brownie: 32 minutes
- ✔ Cheesecake: 40 minutes
- ✔ Chocolate cream pie: 32 minutes
- ✔ Hot fudge sundae: 38 minutes
- ✔ Ice cream cone: 44 minutes
- ✔ Strawberry milkshake: 47 minutes

You may decide that a particular dessert is worth your time, but that's a decision only you can make.

Chapter 18

Packing a Picnic Lunch

· ·

In This Chapter

▶ Getting out and about for fitness

▶ Putting together a perfect picnic

▶ Basking in barbecue bliss

▶ Packing a healthy lunchbox

· ·

So many people now eat away from the home that parks and shopping centres often resemble one giant, mobile, outdoor restaurant. However, eating while doing other things, such as walking, can encourage mindless munching. Far better to sit down and really savour your food, chewing carefully and slowly so that your brain has time to receive, recognise, and act on the hormonal messages from your intestines, which tell you that you've eaten enough. If you eat while concentrating on other things – such as crossing the road without getting run over – your brain is more likely to filter out these messages. The result is that you keep on eating past the point where you feel full, and set off into the realms of excess.

That's what makes the traditional British picnic so great. You walk or cycle to a local beauty spot, carrying your food with you, so that exercise whets your appetite. Then you select your spot under a tree, by a river or lake, on the beach, or just in the middle of a field or park, before laying out your meal. Wherever you sit, you can really savour your food while communing with nature: singing birds, the hum of honey bees, and the lazy swish of a horse's tail.

Walking and Rambling for Health

Without getting too carried away, conjuring up lovely childhood memories of outdoor picnics is easy. Well guess what? You can still enjoy the pleasures of outdoor eating as an adult. Getting into the great outdoors atmosphere can help you develop a healthy lifestyle and get you exercising.

Just select your venue and pack your lunch. Don't take the car unless you promise yourself that you're going to park far enough away to leave a good 20 minutes' walk to get to your final destination.

Don't go venturing into woods or secluded places on your own if you have diabetes and are prone to hypoglycaemic episodes or blackouts. Always take someone with you, tell someone else where you're going, and ensure that someone in your party carries a mobile phone with him or her.

If you plan to go swimming, wait at least an hour after eating before you do so. Don't go swimming alone, especially if you're at risk of hypoglycaemia before lunch.

Perfect picnic bites

Sandwiches, baguettes, and rolls are the mainstay of picnic foods. If you take foods such as chicken, eggs, pâté, and mayonnaise, which spoil rapidly in the heat, always transport them in an insulated chill box with plenty of ice-packs to keep them fridge-fresh. This section gives you some great ideas for picnic sandwiches that don't wilt, even when you do. We don't give strict quantities as picnics are dynamic events, and the quantity of fillings is a very personal thing.

Pecorino, pesto, and sun-dried tomato baguette

Slice a wholemeal baguette down the middle lengthwise, leaving the two halves joined together at the hinge. Spread both sides with some low-fat yoghurt mixed with pesto sauce. Fill with thin slices of pecorino cheese, chopped sun-dried tomatoes, and rocket leaves, and fold over. Wrap in cling-film to transport. Cut into chunky slices when you get to your picnic site.

Hummus, coriander, and carrot baguette

Slice a wholemeal baguette lengthways, leaving the two halves joined together at the hinge. Mix some chopped coriander leaves and grated carrot into some low-fat hummus and spread the mixture over both sides of the roll. Fill the baguette with mixed lettuce leaves and fold over. Wrap in cling-film to transport. Cut into chunky slices at your picnic site.

Rocket, walnut, and gorgonzola rolls

Slice a brown roll in half, lengthways. Mix together some low-fat natural yoghurt and a similar amount of low-fat mayonnaise, and spread onto the cut sides of the roll. Chop the walnuts and mash into some crumbled gorgonzola cheese. Fill the roll with rocket and the cheese and walnut mix. Wrap in cling-film and slice the roll up at the picnic.

Useful items to take on a picnic

When planning your trip, use this checklist of items that often come in useful on a picnic. You may not need them all, but some are sure to come in handy:

- ✔ Black pepper grinder
- ✔ Blanket or rug
- ✔ Bottles of water
- ✔ Corkscrew and bottle opener
- ✔ First aid kit
- ✔ Folding table and chairs
- ✔ Hamper or basket to carry the food
- ✔ Ice or chill box for water and other drinks
- ✔ Insect repellent
- ✔ Knives, forks, and spoons
- ✔ Napkins
- ✔ Plastic bag for rubbish
- ✔ Plastic plates and mugs
- ✔ Spare jumpers in case it turns cold
- ✔ Sprigs of parsley or basil to garnish dishes
- ✔ Sunscreen
- ✔ Tablecloth
- ✔ Thermos of hot water to make fresh coffee or tea
- ✔ Waterproof fold-away hooded jacket in case of rain
- ✔ Wet wipes
- ✔ Wooden cutting board and bread knife

Avocado, cheese, and spinach wrap

Mix the chopped flesh of an avocado with lemon juice to prevent the flesh from browning. Mix together some low-fat natural yoghurt, and a similar amount of low-fat mayonnaise, and spread this dressing over the wrap. Top with thin slices of pecorino cheese, chopped avocado, and baby spinach leaves. Add some torn basil leaves for extra flavour, if you want, before carefully rolling up. Wrap in cling-film to transport, and cut in half when you arrive.

Other picnic options

Picnics don't have to mean sandwiches, rolls, baguettes, or wraps, of course. The best picnic co-author Sarah remembers, prepared by a naval officer used to fine food, included lobster salad, marinated scallops, artichoke hearts, asparagus tips, and home-made chocolate mousse. Chapter 9 shows you how to prepare a variety of salads to make any picnic party proud.

Picnics don't even have to mean cold food. Hot soups and stews survive very well in a wide-mouthed thermos flask, and keep you warm outdoors on a blustery day. Any of the soups from Chapter 8 make great picnic meals. Warm your thermos through with boiling water before adding your soup so it stays as hot as possible until you're ready to slurp the soup down. Or try one of the chilled soups and serve ice-cold on a hot still day.

Healthy energy snacks

If you feel peckish while walking to your chosen picnic site, munch on these healthy snacks rather than a bag of crisps or biscuits. You can also find some delicious and healthy Vegetable Crisps in Chapter 7.

Fruit 'n' nut mix

Make your own trail mix by trying various combinations of nuts and chopped dried fruits, such as almonds, Brazils, cashews, coconut, dates, figs, peanuts, pecans, pumpkin seeds, raisins, sultanas, sunflower seeds, and walnuts.

Peppery balsamic nuts

Sauté some unsalted mixed nuts (for example, cashews, walnuts, or peanuts) in a pan with a tiny amount of olive oil until they start to colour. Add lots of freshly ground black pepper and a dash of balsamic vinegar. Stir well and leave to cool.

Date and walnut mix

Mix together some coarsely chopped Medjool dates with walnut halves for a healthy snack.

Healthy picnic drinks

The main drink to take on a picnic is water, and plenty of it – at least a litre (1¾ pints) per person. You may need more, depending on the heat, how far you have to walk, and how long you intend to stay out. Never skimp, because water is essential to avoid dehydration. And take care with alcohol: Don't drink too much, especially in the heat, because alcohol has a diuretic effect that hastens dehydration. This section provides some great, refreshing drinks that are ideal for a picnic.

Iced lemon tea

Mix left-over brewed tea with cold water, diluting to your preferred strength. Add the juice and zest of two unwaxed lemons and sweeten with a granulated artificial sweetener such as sucralose if you want. Leave to infuse in the fridge until ready to transfer to a thermos flask to keep cold.

Iced mint tea

Mix left-over brewed tea with cold water, diluting to your preferred strength. Add a large handful of chopped, fresh mint, and sweeten to your taste with a granulated artificial sweetener such as sucralose. Leave to infuse in the fridge. Strain and then transfer to a thermos flask to keep cold.

Home-made lemonade

Add the zest and juice of 10 lemons to a litre (1¾ pints) of water. Sweeten to taste with a granulated artificial sweetener such as sucralose. Chill in the fridge. Strain before transferring into your thermos flask.

Cranberry lemonade

Mix cranberry juice with your home-made lemonade to produce an attractively coloured and tasty drink for a hot day.

Picnic desserts

The simplest picnic dessert is undoubtedly lots of fresh fruit. Apples, satsumas, and grapes are ideal, packed in sturdy containers so that they don't bruise.

The classic summer picnic dessert is strawberries and cream. In place of cream, consider serving natural yoghurt or fromage frais flavoured with a little vanilla essence as a healthier alternative. Of course, you don't need cream at all. Strawberries chopped in half and marinated in fresh orange juice are equally delicious. Some people even advise serving them with freshly ground black pepper for a dessert with a difference.

Here are some more interesting picnic desserts.

Raspberry muesli parfait

Mix together some vanilla yoghurt, raspberries, and muesli cereal (see the recipe in Chapter 6). Pile into a plastic container and freeze. Take out of the freezer as you leave the house for your picnic, so that the parfait starts to soften into a refreshing treat ready for your al fresco meal.

Chocolate raspberry bites

Melt some dark chocolate with 70 per cent cocoa solids in a bain marie over a low heat. Mix with an equal quantity of crème fraîche and add a few drops of vanilla essence. Add a handful of fresh, chopped raspberries and spread onto a slice of wholegrain toast. Cut into squares, chill, and serve as petit fours with coffee.

Kiwi fool

Mix some low-fat, natural fromage frais with the mashed flesh of ripe kiwi fruit and chill.

Barbecue Picnics

The smell of food cooking outdoors is unbeatable. Portable barbecues are now widely available, whether fuelled with charcoal or gas. If you fancy barbecuing your picnic meal, here are some tips to help you select healthy options instead of the more usual fatty sausages and burgers. Also check out the great recipe for salmon barbecued on a cedar plank in Chapter 12.

Mighty meats

Select lean cuts of meat such as turkey, chicken, prime steak, and lean lamb. Did you know that grilled rump provides only 168 kilocalories per 100 grams (3½ ounces)? Cubed, lean leg of lamb is also ideal for kebabs and, at 252 kilocalories per 100 grams, is more slimming than using fatty breast of lamb (410 kilocalories per 100 grams).

Take the skin off poultry before eating to reduce the kilocalorie content further – grilled chicken skin provides a massive 501 kilocalories per 100 grams compared with just 148 kilocalories per 100 grams for cooked meat alone. And don't forget more exotic meats – such as buffalo, kangaroo, ostrich, and wild boar – which are also low in fat and high in protein, making them a healthy option.

Oily fish (for example, mackerel, herrings, sardines, and salmon) are rich sources of omega-3 fatty acids, which have a beneficial effect on heart and joint health, and they cook really well on the barbecue thanks to those healthy oils. If foods need additional oil, brush them lightly with olive oil before barbecuing – olive oil is rich in monounsaturated fats, which are good for your heart and circulation.

Plain meats can seem bland. To add flavour, marinate meat and fish with freshly chopped herbs, black pepper, and lemon or lime juice, or even balsamic vinegar. You can also serve grilled meats with salad and hot or cold new boiled potatoes sprinkled with vinaigrette.

Vinegar helps to slow the digestion and absorption of starchy foods such as potatoes, rice, and pasta.

Healthy side dishes

A potato baked in foil in the embers of a barbecue provides only 77 kilocalories per 100 grams compared with 149 kilocalories if roasted – half the kilocalories! This swap may seem enticing, but remember that baked potato is rapidly digested to increase your blood glucose levels, and so eat a small one.

Add antioxidant-rich orange, yellow, red, and dark green Mediterranean-style vegetables to your barbecue. Capsicum peppers, celeriac, cherry tomatoes, chunky sweet potatoes, courgettes, mushrooms, and onions taste great brushed with olive oil and sprinkled with herbs before being chargrilled. Weight for weight, red peppers contain three times as much vitamin C as citrus fruits (green peppers have over twice as much). And tomatoes contain lycopene, a powerful antioxidant that protects against coronary heart disease and cancer. Strangely, barbecuing tomatoes releases more lycopene than eating them raw!

You can liven up salads with freshly-chopped herbs – basil, chives, coriander, mint, oregano, or parsley for extra flavour, vitamins, and minerals. And, while waiting for food to cook, fill up on healthy crudités – capsicum peppers, carrot, cauliflower, celery, cucumber, and radishes with a low-fat dip.

Keeping foods fresh

To avoid food poisoning, remember to keep food for barbecuing properly refrigerated beforehand. A rise in temperature from just 4 to 8°C (40 to 47°F) more than doubles bacterial growth rates. Defrost frozen produce thoroughly, in the fridge, for slow, safe thawing.

Keep your meat and fish in the fridge at a temperature below 5°C (41°F) until just before you leave on your picnic. Store raw meat at the bottom of the fridge, covered, and separate from cooked foods.

If your recipe calls for marinating, always marinate food in the fridge. Don't mix different sorts of raw foods (for example, fish and chicken) – especially in the same marinade; always keep them in separate containers. And, if you intend to use some marinade as a sauce on cooked food, put a portion aside before placing raw food in the remaining marinade. Similarly, never mix raw foods with cooked.

See the next section, 'Sensible food handling', for other important tips, and then transport your food in an insulated chill box along with plenty of ice-packs.

Sensible food handling

Hand in hand with ensuring that you eat fresh food goes the need to make sure that you don't introduce bugs during preparation and cooking. Always carry out the following:

- ✔ Avoid barbecuing any products that are past their use-by date.

- ✔ Cook pork, sausages, burgers, and chicken through to the centre. Although they may look cooked on the outside, you need to pierce the thickest part with the point of a clean, sharp knife to check that the centre isn't still raw. If the juices run clear, the meat is ready for eating; if the juices are pink, continue cooking until they run clear.

- ✔ Cover food to help keep flies at bay.

- ✔ Keep food and chill boxes out of bright sunshine.

- ✔ Keep pets away from food outdoors.

- ✔ Keep separate tools, chopping boards, and plates for raw and cooked foods, and for other produce such as vegetables.

- ✔ Keep your grill clean with a wire brush or a loosely scrunched-up ball of aluminium foil. Wipe with a little vegetable oil to help reduce food sticking.

- ✔ Leave a gap of 2½ centimetres (1 inch) between pieces of food on the barbecue to help them cook evenly.

- ✔ Make sure that barbecued food is cooked thoroughly, and serve piping hot rather than merely warm.

- ✔ Use long-handled tools, such as tongs, for handling and cooking food to help keep hands away from the heat.

- ✔ Use paper towels rather than repeatedly using cloth towels.

- ✔ Wash your hands thoroughly before preparing foods and again before eating.

General barbecue tips

Before we leave the pleasures of eating in the great outdoors, here are some useful additional pointers to make sure that your barbecuing experience is as safe and enjoyable as possible.

- ✔ Avoid windy positions and use a windbreak if necessary. Keep plenty of space around the barbecue so that fences, plants, and garden furniture don't scorch. Having a fire blanket close to hand is also a good idea.

✔ Don't start cooking too soon – let the coals heat up for 45 minutes first – you want heat rather than flame. To improve flavours, try sprinkling coals with fresh herbs, or tie a bunch of herbs to the outside of your barbecue for a pleasant aroma that also helps to deter flies.

✔ Use tongs to turn food, as a fork only pierces it and allows delicious juices to drain away too soon. And try cooking fish loosely wrapped in foil, so that it partly steams and doesn't dry out or fall apart.

✔ When barbecuing during the day, ensure that you have plenty of shade to avoid sunburn and iced water to avoid dehydration. You don't want to end up as red as that lobster you've just lovingly prepared.

Burning citronella candles helps to repel insects. If you don't like the smell of citronella, lavender is a good alternative.

Munching Through a Packed Lunch

Many people pack a lunchbox to take to work. Often you can keep your lunch fresh in the staff fridge, so that fillings such as chicken, fish, pâté, and egg are easier to keep chilled and fresh.

Sandwiches, wraps, and rolls

Choose your bread carefully when making sandwiches. Where possible, select wholemeal, wholegrain, mixed grain, malted, granary, rye, or brown breads. These breads have much less impact on your blood glucose levels than highly processed white bread. Here are some ideas to get your mouth watering.

Poached salmon and spinach

Mash together some cold, poached salmon with low-fat yoghurt and a little horseradish sauce to make the filling. Use two slices of wholegrain bread with a layer of baby spinach leaves in the middle.

Smoked salmon and egg mayonnaise

Mash together a hard-boiled egg with some low-fat natural yoghurt, and season with black pepper. Spread over two slices of wholegrain bread and sandwich together with a layer of smoked salmon in the middle. You can also add salad leaves or mustard and cress if you like.

American pastrami on rye

Pile pastrami, red onion rings, sliced gherkin, sliced tomatoes, and salad leaves between 2 slices of rye bread – or make open sandwiches if you prefer. Moisten with low-fat natural yoghurt mixed with a little wholegrain mustard.

Italian wrap

Mix together some low-fat yoghurt and pesto sauce, and spread over a tortilla. Fill with slices of buffalo mozzarella, torn basil leaves, chopped sundried tomatoes, and mixed leaves before carefully rolling up, for a tasty wrap.

Chicken salad wrap

Mix together some low-fat yoghurt and low-fat mayonnaise, and spread over a wrap. Fill with chopped cooked chicken, rocket leaves, sliced cherry tomatoes, and a few long, thin strips of cucumber (without the peel). Season with black pepper and then wrap.

Spicy prawn roll

Cut a brown roll down the middle lengthwise, leaving the two pieces joined together at the hinge. Mix together equal amounts of low-fat yoghurt and low-fat mayonnaise. Use to bind together a handful of chopped, cooked prawns and season with a little cayenne pepper. Fill the roll with the prawn mayonnaise and some baby spinach leaves.

Tuna and sweetcorn roll

Cut a brown roll down the middle, leaving the two pieces joined together at the hinge. Mash together some low-fat yoghurt and some drained tuna flakes, and mix in some drained sweetcorn kernels. Pile into the roll, together with some lettuce leaves and, if you like, some chopped cherry tomatoes.

Salads in a box

Instead of the usual sandwiches, rolls, and baps, which can get rather samey when you have them every day – even with different, inventive fillings – try something different. Use left-overs to make the following, tasty lunch options as economically as possible. In fact, plan ahead and deliberately cook extra pasta, rice, or boiled potatoes to pack for lunch the next day.

Lunchbox rice salad

Mix together cold left-over rice (brown or white) with a handful of chopped or grated vegetables such as broccoli, carrots, celery, peppers, or sweetcorn. Season with low-sodium soy sauce, lemon or lime juice, or vinaigrette plus chopped mixed herbs to make a simple salad for work or school.

Sprinkling vinaigrette on starchy foods such as rice, potatoes, or pasta helps to reduce blood glucose swings. Vinegar contains acetic acid, which increases the acidity of stomach contents and slows stomach emptying. As a result, digested carbohydrate takes longer to reach the small intestines where it's absorbed, and blood glucose levels rise more slowly.

Lunchbox potato salad

Mix together left-over, cold new potatoes with chopped red pepper, a chopped boiled egg, mustard, and cress, and bind together with a little vinaigrette or low-fat mayonnaise to make a great potato salad.

Where possible, eat new potatoes rather than 'old' ones: The different starch structure that new potatoes contain means that they have less effect on your blood glucose levels. As new potatoes cool, their ability to affect your blood glucose level reduces even more, because the starch they contain becomes more resistant to digestion.

Lunchbox pasta salad

Mix together left-over cold pasta (preferably wholemeal brown pasta) with sweetcorn and chopped mixed vegetables, and a few teaspoons of pesto sauce to make a great healthy lunch.

Peanut butter pasta salad

Mix together cold left-over pasta with a handful of shredded red and green cabbage, a dash of low-sodium soy sauce, a dash of vinegar, and a dollop of pure peanut butter (crunchy or smooth) to make a fantastic Asian salad. You can also add chopped spring onions, diced cucumber, and bean sprouts.

Winter salad

Mix together grated vegetables such as broccoli, carrot, red cabbage, white cabbage, Japanese radish (mooli), red onion, and turnip – whatever needs using up – and moisten with lemon juice and a little low-fat mayonnaise for a deliciously healthy coleslaw. Add a handful of chopped fresh herbs such as chives, coriander, and parsley for even more flavour.

Fruit and nut salad

Chop some pears, apples, celery, and pecan nuts. Mix together with a little lemon juice and low-fat yoghurt for a tasty, healthy side-salad. Mix in some cottage cheese for extra protein.

Enticing Lunchboxes for Kids

Providing balanced nutrition in a school lunchbox for a child with diabetes is essential: You want to provide enough energy to keep him or her going all afternoon. Otherwise, your child's ability to concentrate and retain information is affected, and that's simply unacceptable.

Buying the best box

The first thing to consider is the lunchbox itself. To minimise risks from food spoilage, insert a small ice-pack to help keep food fridge-fresh until lunch time. Some boxes even contain slots to fit an ice-pack in the middle. This ice-pack has the dual purpose of separating drink and yoghurt from crushable sandwiches and fruit. Alternatively, you can add a small ice-pack inside a normal lunchbox – you can usually find room. An ice-pack is especially important when meat is on the menu, and during the hot days of summer. But even in winter, a lunchbox left in a warm room or near a radiator can still cause problems.

And instead of a plain, un-partitioned lunchbox, select one with integral boxes to cut down on packaging such as cling-film and sandwich bags. Some lunchboxes provide a variety of plastic containers to hold grapes, a kiwi, or a hardboiled egg without squishing – and without the need for additional wrapping. This arrangement makes these boxes environmentally friendly, as well as easy to clean when juice cartons and dripping yoghurt tubes are put back in at the end of lunch.

Tips for healthy lunchboxes are available on the Web site www.laptop lunches.co.uk. And to protect fruit, you can get a Banana Guard and a Fruity Face blow-up pouch from www.lakeland.co.uk, which stops apples, peaches, oranges, and so on from getting squished in backpacks.

School lunchbox fillings

This section gives some tips to help you put together a nutritious lunchbox that doesn't have the nutrition police breathing down your neck.

- ✔ Include at least one piece of fruit per day, or a tub of mixed fresh fruit salad kept moist with a little fruit juice. Raisins and dried apricots make a healthy, nutritious snack instead of crisps.

✔ Include at least one salad ingredient in the sandwich filling – for example, cheese and cucumber, chicken and lettuce, ham and avocado, tuna and tomato, or hummus and bean sprouts. You can also grate a little carrot into your sandwich fillings to bulk it up and provide extra vitamins and crunch – bind together with a little yoghurt if you like.

✔ Provide as wide a variety of foods as possible during the week.

✔ Substitute sweetened or fizzy drinks with fresh, unsweetened fruit juice, milk, or even water.

✔ Try cereal bars, gingerbread, carrot cake, flapjacks, or date oatcake rather than sweet cakes, sponge rolls, or biscuits. Digestive biscuits also make a great break-time snack.

✔ Use a carton of yoghurt or fromage frais for dessert as an excellent source of calcium – low-fat varieties contain just as much calcium as whole-fat.

✔ Use brown bread instead of white if your child eats it – or try making a 3-layered club sandwich with brown bread in the middle layer so it's less obvious. Filled wholemeal bread rolls or pitta bread make a tasty change from ready-sliced bread.

✔ Use fresh foods rather than convenience/processed foods wherever possible.

✔ Use raw vegetables (for example, carrot sticks, celery, red pepper strips, or baby tomatoes) to make good finger foods for a healthy snack. You can even provide little pots of dips to dunk them in.

The next sections provide some little healthy novelties that children love to find in their lunchbox as a surprise.

Cucumber chains

Cut a cucumber into 3-centimetre (just over 1-inch) long cylinders and remove the core with a paring knife or apple-corer. Slice the hollow cylinder into 5-millimetre (¼ inch) rings. Make a slit in every other ring and link them together to form a chain.

Cucumber cups

Chop an unpeeled cucumber into chunks and hollow out some of the core. Stuff the cucumber cups with fillings, for example, chopped egg, tuna, cream cheese, or cottage cheese. Add the chopped cucumber flesh to the fillings, or use in an accompanying salad. You can also use the cucumber cups to hold low-fat mayonnaise or other dips for vegetable crudités.

Stuffed tomatoes

Chop the top off medium sized tomatoes and scoop out the seeds. Fill the tomato shells with fillings such as chopped egg, tuna, cream cheese, and so on. Add the chopped tomato flesh to the fillings, or use in an accompanying salad.

Making the most of milk

Milk is almost a perfect food for kids, providing good amounts of vital vitamins and minerals. Milk also acts as an ideal energy source – much better than sweetened drinks and fizzy concoctions swimming in additives such as artificial colourings and sweeteners.

Don't give children cows' milk as their main drink until after they're 1 year old. Semi-skimmed milk is not suitable until after the age of 2 years, providing the child's energy and nutrient intakes are otherwise good. But don't offer skimmed milk until after the age of 5 years (if at all) because young children need the extra energy available from the fat found in milk.

The following facts help to put milk into perspective as a good school lunchbox ingredient – along with an ice-pack to keep it cool and fresh, of course:

- ✔ Milk and milk products (such as yoghurt, fromage frais, and cheese) supply most children with over 30 per cent of their daily calcium requirements – 600 millilitres (1 pint) of milk provides around 720 milligrams of calcium.
- ✔ Milk is the largest dietary source of riboflavin (vitamin B2).
- ✔ Milk supplies around 10 per cent of dietary vitamin A.

Part IV
The Part of Tens

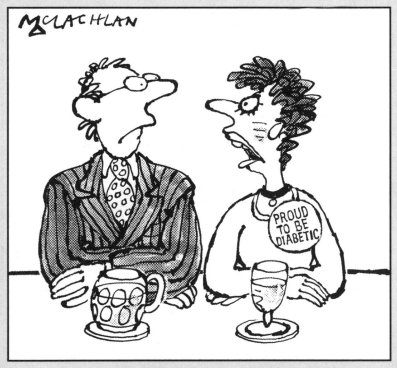

'And _don't_ call me 'sugar'!'

In this part . . .

This part shows you that major improvements can arise from minor changes. It takes you through some basic steps to improve your eating habits, none especially difficult by themselves. You'll realise the tremendous impact that substituting more healthful ingredients can have on your overall nutrition.

You can also find some essential techniques to normalise your blood glucose and thus prevent complications of diabetes. Many of these tips don't relate to diet but approach blood glucose normalisation from a general lifestyle perspective.

This part also offers information on managing the special problems of healthy eating for a child with diabetes. In this situation, you're trying not only to keep the blood glucose normal but also to allow for normal growth and development. This balance requires some special considerations, and we try to offer them.

Chapter 19

Ten (or So) Simple Steps to Change Your Eating Habits

*F*ollowing a nutritional plan can sometimes seem complicated. But really, if you follow a few simple rules, the process becomes much easier. This chapter provides you with ten (or so) simple things that you can do today. None of these things cost anything other than time, but doing them one at a time makes a big difference to your kilocalorie and fat intake. Adding one to another makes the results huge. Your weight, blood pressure, and blood glucose all fall. Who can ask for anything more?

Keeping a Food Diary

Try this little diversion: For the next two days, write down everything you eat and drink – as you eat and drink it. Before you go to bed on the evening of the second day, take a separate piece of paper and try to reconstruct what you've eaten for the past two days without looking at your original list. Then compare the two lists. The differences in the lists are often startling. The point of this exercise is to show you that you're doing a lot of mindless eating, and that trying to follow a nutritional plan from memory usually doesn't work.

As well as showing you what you're eating, a food diary also allows you to select items whose portion size needs reducing (or eliminating altogether). And, when you go to your doctor, the fact that your diary lists lettuce for every meal helps confirm your statement that you eat like a rabbit (not).

Try including something in your diary about how you feel and what you're doing as you eat or drink. This information, besides turning your diary into a more personal statement, allows you to see the associations between your mood and your food. Keeping your exercise record in the diary makes it even more useful, reminding you of when you did (or didn't) exercise.

Finally, your dietitian can easily plug your food intake into a computer program to obtain valuable information such as a kilocalorie breakdown of your diet, amount of salt, levels of saturated fat, and how much cholesterol you tend to eat.

Knowing Why You Eat the Way You Do

You may recognise that you do a lot of your eating for emotional reasons. Try to think back to how you used to eat in your family as a child. What does eating mean to you and your family? Is eating a way of connecting with others in the family, or is it used in some other way? Does eating trigger feelings that you want to have again and that make you feel happy or good in some other way? Or do you associate eating with negative emotions? Do you eat the way you do out of loneliness, boredom, depression, happiness, or anger; as a reward; or as a way to save time? You may come up with several reasons, but you need to understand them and begin to respond to those triggers with other actions besides eating.

After you begin to clarify the emotional aspect of your eating, you can look for ways to have the same emotions without the eating part. What other things can you do to feel happy or connected? For example, if you eat out of boredom, what can you do to keep yourself from feeling bored?

If this activity sounds like psychology, that's because it is psychology! If eating is affecting your life in a negative way, you may want to seek the help of a psychologist to find out exactly what eating means to you. Meanwhile, because that type of counselling is often a long-term process, try doing the other things in this chapter to help gain control of your eating.

All habits, including eating habits, come from repetition. Every time you do something the same way, it encourages you to do it the same way the next time. Breaking this chain helps you to make healthy changes. Here are some things you can do right now until you figure out why you eat:

- ✔ Always leave food on your plate to develop the habit of stopping eating when you're full.

- ✔ Avoid junk food that has kilocalories without nutritional value.

- ✔ Chew your food slowly and pick up all food with utensils, not fingers, after you swallow each bite.

- ✔ Choose non-food rewards, such as new clothes for your new shape.

- ✔ Eat in only one place in your home – your designated eating place – preferably at the table.

- ✔ Eat on smaller plates.

- ✔ Eat three meals and even a couple of healthy snacks every day.

- ✔ Keep food only in the kitchen and out of sight, not on counters.

- ✔ Never eat and do something else at the same time, such as watch TV.

- ✔ Never eat from the bag, the container, or the carton.

- ✔ Select a healthy alternative to eating, such as exercise, a creative hobby, or even conversations with your partner/relatives/friends.

Perform one of these actions at a time. When you successfully make an action part of your behaviour, try a second action. Build up to many changes. The results are delightful.

Eating Every Meal

When you miss meals, you become hungry. If you have type 1 diabetes, you can't safely miss meals, especially if you use insulin. Instead of letting yourself become hungry, eat your meals at regular times so that you don't overcompensate at the next meal (or at a snack shortly after the meal you missed) when you're suffering from low blood glucose. Many people overtreat low blood glucose by eating too many sugar kilocalories, resulting in high blood glucose later on.

Don't miss meals as a weight-loss method, particularly if you take a drug that can lower blood glucose to below normal (hypoglycaemic) levels. For example, a pregnant woman with diabetes especially shouldn't miss meals. She needs to make up for the fact that her baby extracts large amounts of glucose from her blood. Both mother and growing foetus are adversely affected if the mother's body must turn to stored fat for energy.

Eating smaller meals and having snacks in between is probably the best way to eat because doing so raises blood glucose the least, provides a constant source of energy, and allows control of the blood glucose using the least amount of external or internal insulin.

The fact is that following your complete nutritional plan in fewer than three meals is extremely difficult.

Sitting Down for Meals

Eating food with others is one of the pleasures of life. As an added advantage, eating with other people also slows the pace of your eating, which allows your brain to recognise when you're full so that you stop eating at the appropriate time. Sitting down and eating more slowly helps you slow the absorption of carbohydrates, thus slowing the rise in your blood glucose level.

Another advantage of sitting down and eating with others is that they serve as a brake on how much you eat. When people eat alone, they tend to eat more. In the company of others, social controls act as a restraint. And eating while sitting at the table means that you see only the food on the table. When you stand and eat, you can easily walk into the kitchen, where all the rest of the food is waiting (if you're not there already).

You usually limit the food served at the table to what's on your plate, so you aren't exposed to excessive food. You can make sure that the only foods brought to the table are acceptable food options, especially if they're prepared as attractively as possible. A lot of your eating is done because the food looks so good, so make the right foods the best-looking foods.

Drinking Water throughout the Day

Seventy per cent of your body is water, and all your many organs and cells require water to function properly. Most people, especially older people, don't get enough water. Older people often have the additional disadvantage of losing their ability to sense when they're thirsty. The consequences may include weakness and fatigue, not to mention constipation.

Water can replace all the sodas and juice drinks that add unwanted kilocalories to your day. You soon lose your taste for those drinks and discover that you don't need (or miss) the aftertaste of soda and juice that you took for granted. Those drinks also raise your blood glucose very rapidly and are often used to treat low blood glucose.

One person with diabetes admitted to drinking 10 to 12 cans of cola drink daily. His high blood glucose level returned to normal after he broke his cola habit.

Make drinking water a part of your daily routine. Drink some when you brush your teeth. Drink more with meals and snacks. Many people don't want to drink loads of water close to bedtime – in order to avoid the need to get up during the night to visit the bathroom – which is all the more reason to make sure that you get your water ration earlier in the day. Aim to drink at least eight glasses of water per day, each glass being 200 to 300 millilitres (7 to 10 fluid ounces).

Consuming Vegetables throughout the Day

What makes you think that broccoli is only a side dish to accompany your dinner meat or fish? How can you possibly get in your daily three to five servings of vegetables when you think so narrowly? What happens if you drink vegetable juice for breakfast? Suppose you added vegetables to an omelette? How about a salad at lunch instead of that large sandwich containing way too much carbohydrate?

You can find many different kinds of vegetables in the supermarket, and yet most people limit themselves to very few of them. Your whole meal can consist of vegetables with a small amount of protein thrown in just as a garnish. Try a vegetarian restaurant to see for yourself how delicious freshly prepared vegetables can be.

We're not talking about the starchy vegetables, such as beans, peas, and lentils, which really belong in the starch list of food exchanges, but vegetables that contain much less carbohydrate. These vegetables include asparagus, cabbage, carrots, cauliflower, chard, green beans, kale, onions, pak choi, summer squash, turnips, and water chestnuts.

Use these vegetables in meals and for snacks. They fill you up but add very few kilocalories. Some are just as good when frozen and defrosted as they are when fresh, because they're flash-frozen immediately after picking. Especially good snack vegetables include baby carrots, cucumbers, and pieces of sweet red pepper.

Reducing Added Fat

Recipes that are handed down within families often contain much unnecessary added fat. The same is also true for recipes created by chefs who aren't conscious of the harmful effects of high fat intake. The recipes in this book are carefully selected to minimise added fat: Try to do the same when you cook at home.

Cooking food doesn't generally require the extra fat. Although olive oil is better for you than animal fats such as lard and butter, it still has plenty of kilocalories – in fact, just as many as animal fats. A gram of fat contains 9 kilocalories, no matter what the source.

Try halving the amount of fat suggested in a recipe to see what happens. See whether the taste suffers or if preparing the food is more difficult.

How much difference does reducing the fat make in terms of kilocalories? Each gram of oil supplies 9 kilocalories, and so adding 240 millilitres (9 fluid ounces) of oil to a recipe adds over 2,000 kilocalories (assuming for a moment that 1 millilitre of fat weighs around 1 gram). You get rid of 1,000 kilocalories if you simply cut the fat in half. If your recipe serves four people, each person is getting 250 kilocalories less fat. Is that a worthwhile reduction? You bet!

Chapter 20 contains great ideas on making smart food choices, including some food substitutions.

Removing the Attached Fat

Many foods, such as sausage and luncheon meats, contain so much fat that lowering their fat content isn't possible. Avoid these foods as much as possible. But other protein sources, such as chicken, steak, roast beef, and pork, often have large amounts of visible fat attached to them, so you can remove this fat before you prepare the food. In the case of poultry, removing the skin removes most of the fat. Selecting white meat rather than dark further reduces the fat in poultry.

As fat cooks on a grill, it often flames, which causes the meat to burn. Removing the fat before you cook it makes the cooking process safer (because the burning fat doesn't spray around), and the resulting meat is much lower in kilocalories.

Leaving Out the Salt

Many people add a lot of salt to their food, with the result that they taste mostly salt and not much of the food. Try getting rid of the salt in your recipes, as is already the case for most recipes in this book. You can always add salt later if you miss its flavour. At first, you may find that the food tastes bland because it takes around six weeks for your taste buds to adapt to tasting lower salt levels. Then you begin to discover the subtle tastes that are in the food but were overpowered with salt.

Why do you need to cut back on your salt intake? Because salt raises blood pressure. Recent studies, particularly the United Kingdom Prospective Diabetes Study (1998), show that you can slow or prevent diabetes complications if you reduce blood pressure.

 You can try the approach of slowly removing salt from your recipes: For example, if a recipe calls for a teaspoon of salt, add only ¾ teaspoon. You aren't going to notice the difference. Next time, try ½ teaspoon. And so on. The recipes in this book use very little, if any, salt.

Adding Taste with Condiments, Herbs, and Spices

This section explores a case of getting something for almost nothing. If you like a lot of distinctive flavours in your food, try using various condiments, herbs, and spices to replace the flavours of fat and salt. Experimenting with these flavours can bring entirely new tastes to old favourite recipes. Try breaking free from old habits of eating – ones that aren't so good for you – and replacing them with new tastes.

Foods that you associate with a bland taste, such as some fish, come alive when you add the right herbs and spices. Not only do they taste different, but they also smell wonderful and exotic. And they have the additional advantage of improving your nutritional balance.

Examples of condiments that add great taste and few kilocalories are salsa, hot sauce, mustard, and horseradish. Herbs that add flavour include rosemary, thyme, and basil. Herbs are best added toward the end of cooking to preserve their flavour if fresh, or at the beginning of cooking to bring out their flavour if dried.

Using Healthy Cooking Methods

The best methods of cooking are those that don't add fat and which, instead, allow the fat naturally present in a food to drain away. Such methods include grilling, dry roasting, boiling, steaming, and barbecuing. Grilling a beefburger, for example, often eliminates as much fat from a moderate-fat burger as buying a reduced-fat burger to begin with. Frying, sautéing, and other methods that depend on butter or fat add exactly the things that you want to remove – unless you use only the merest hint of oil spray.

If you must use fat, use a cooking spray that reduces the amount of added fat.

Chapter 20

Ten Easy Substitutions in Your Eating Plan

In This Chapter

▶ Making better choices with fish, beans, meats, and sweets

▶ Replacing 'bad' fats with 'good' fats

▶ Switching from larger to smaller portions

*O*ne of your major weapons in the lifelong battle against complications of diabetes is your ability to choose. You can choose to exercise every day. You can choose to take your medications. Perhaps your most effective resource is your skill in making the right food choices. The consequences of choosing the right foods are immediate and enormous:

✔ In the short term, you feel better in general. Your body, like any complicated machine, prefers the correct fuel.

✔ In the medium term, you notice more normal values when you test your blood glucose levels. As a consequence of these more normal levels, you sleep better, you don't have to go to the bathroom as often, and your sexual activity benefits too. If you're a woman, you're less likely to develop vaginal thrush, whereas if you're a man you're less likely to develop erectile dysfunction. And both sexes can benefit from an improved libido.

✔ In the long run, you also reduce your risk of developing the complications of diabetes, such as eye, kidney, and nervous system diseases.

If you have type 2 diabetes (check out Chapter 1 for the different types of diabetes), you can achieve all these benefits by making the correct food choices. With type 1 diabetes, you do have other considerations, but good food choices are just as important. Take a look at the suggestions in this chapter. None of them is especially difficult to follow. With these suggestions, you generally save money and usually lose weight. Do you need any further incentives?

Catching Fresh Fish

You've had a long day, and you want to pick up something to make for dinner. You stop in front of the frozen foods and find a breaded frozen fish fillet. The instructions to prepare it are simple, and so you're tempted to put the box in your basket. Don't! Put the package back neatly on its shelf and head over to the fresh fish department.

You can buy a nice 110-gram (4-ounce) piece of swordfish, tuna, salmon, herring, or mackerel, grill it with herbs for ten minutes or less, and end up with the right amount of protein and far less fat and carbohydrate kilocalories. The breaded frozen fish is often too large for a single meal and has excess kilocalories that you simply don't need.

Your grilled fish tastes better too. Frozen fish just can't duplicate the taste of ultra fresh fish, and so make friends with your fishmonger or local fishermen to get the best produce available.

Spilling the Beans

You know that your muscles are made of protein, and so naturally when you think of protein, you think of meat. Protein, however, comes from many sources. Vegetables have proteins too, and they don't have the fat that meats provide.

People often think that you can't survive on vegetable protein alone because sources of vegetable protein lack some of the building blocks required for muscle growth. As any vegetarian knows, this simply isn't true. Soybeans, for example, contain all the different building blocks that you need to build your own muscle protein.

Even without soybeans, you can get all the building blocks you need if you eat several different vegetable protein sources together, such as rice and beans or yoghurt with chopped nuts.

The best non-meat sources of protein are legumes such as dried beans and peas. Other protein sources include nuts and seeds, but they contain quite a bit of fat, which means that the kilocalorie count swells, although the fat is mostly healthy monounsaturated fat. The following vegetable protein sources provide the equivalent of 30 grams (1 ounce) of animal protein:

- 35 grams (1.3 ounces) of sunflower seeds
- 65 grams (2.3 ounces) of cooked soybeans
- 90 grams (3.2 ounces) of pecan nuts
- 160 grams (5.7 ounces) of silken tofu (soft)
- 165 grams (5.9 ounces) of baked beans

Choosing the Least Fatty Meats

You're sick of beans, and your spouse spends more time finding new air fresheners for the house than showering you with affection. You need real meat. At this point, you can make some good choices that save plenty of fat and kilocalories.

If the cut of meat's name contains the words 'loin', you're choosing a lower fat selection. Cuts from the leg also tend to have lower fat content. Examples include tenderloin, sirloin, and leg of lamb. For help in selecting low-fat meats, ask your butcher. And remember to trim off any visible fat both before and on your plate.

The difference between lean cuts and fatty cuts is sometimes as much as 70 kilocalories per 30 grams (1 ounce). If you eat the higher fat meat, you get an extra 200 kilocalories or more, almost all in the form of saturated fat – to work this amount off takes 40 minutes of brisk walking!

Poultry and wild game, such as pheasant, goose, and duck, are also low-fat meat alternatives, *if you remove the skin.* The way you cook meat also makes a big difference in the fat count; grilling, barbecuing, and braising are always preferred to frying and sautéing.

Choosing Fruits to Replace Sweet Desserts

Replacing sweet desserts with fruit may seem difficult if you frequently eat in restaurants, but can be less tricky than you think. Chapter 16 contains several delicious recipes that are excellent examples of lower-kilocalorie, lower-fat options for dessert. These recipes usually include unique ways to prepare fruits or mix fruits together for delicious new tastes. Look for similar offerings on the menus of the restaurants you visit, and try the recipes from this book at home.

At home, of course, you're in charge. The tradition of offering a bowl of fresh fruit at the end of a meal seems to have disappeared in the United Kingdom, but you can revive it for your family and guests. Fresh fruit is available 12 months a year, although the options are generally fewer in the winter months compared to the summer. You don't have to limit fruit to the role of replacing dessert at the end of a meal. Starting a meal with grapefruit or melon is a delicious substitute for a plate of pasta, risotto, or some other higher-kilocalorie appetiser. Ending the meal with a delicious peach or some grapes or plums is just as satisfying as that sugary, fatty pie, cake, or ice cream.

How do you benefit from this change? If you end your meal with a typical piece of carrot cake, you take in 339 kilocalories, consisting of 11 grams of fat and 56 grams of carbohydrate. Desserts you sometimes find in restaurants called something like Death by Chocolate, or Chocolate Decadence, typically contain 340 kilocalories with 15 grams of fat and 51 grams of carbohydrate. Choose a sweet peach instead, and you get only 60 kilocalories, consisting of 15 grams of carbohydrate and no fat.

You don't have to put dessert chefs out of business. They're some of the most creative people in the culinary arts. But just as the chefs who create entrées now veer towards more nutritious main dishes, dessert chefs also need to embrace the abundance of available fresh fruits to prepare wonderful desserts.

Adding Fibre to Your Diet

Choosing fruits as described in the preceding section has another benefit: Fruits contain fibre, which is especially desirable for someone with diabetes. Although fibre is a carbohydrate, you can't break it down into nutrients that add kilocalories. Fibre has many benefits, but the most important are the following:

- Insoluble fibre stays in the intestine to reach the large bowel, where it helps to prevent constipation and – probably – cancer of the colon.
- Soluble fibre dissolves in water and slows absorption of carbohydrate in the small intestines to help avoid rapid rises in blood glucose and fat levels.

The next question is how do you get more fibre? Breakfast is the easiest place to make a change:

- Eat low-fat muffins made with fruit and whole grains.
- Eat unrefined cereals like oats in place of processed cereal.
- Eat wholegrain bread in place of refined white bread.

You can add more fibre at other meals if you choose pasta instead of pota-toes and higher fibre rice like basmati instead of white rice. Among fruits, those from temperate climates, such as apples and plums, generally provide more fibre than hot-climate fruits like bananas.

Making the Right Fat Selections

Vegetable sources of fat are often more healthy than animal fats. However, even among the vegetable fats, some are better and some are worse. The better ones (such as olive oil and rapeseed oil) don't raise cholesterol, whereas the worse ones (such as corn oil, cottonseed oil, palm oil, and margarine) lower the good cholesterol. You don't want to lower the good cholesterol.

Animal fats belong to a group called *saturated* fats, some of which raise cho-lesterol levels, and that's not desirable. Some animal fats are quite high in cholesterol, such as the fat in an egg yolk. You can overcome this by selecting omega-3 enriched eggs from hens fed a diet rich in these healthy fats.

And don't forget the *trans fats,* those evil man-made fats that often hide in food labels under the term 'partially hydrogenated corn or vegetable oils or fats'. You find these in chips and many store-bought biscuits and ready-meals. Always read food labels! (See Chapter 5 to find out how to decipher food labels.)

Whether you eat animal fat or vegetable fat, all fats contain an enormous 9 kilocalories of energy per gram. Although fat is an efficient way for your body to store excess energy, you want to limit your daily fat intake to 30 per cent or less of your total kilocalories.

Finding a Cow That Makes Low-Fat Milk

You may think that if scientists can clone sheep and send a man to the moon they can produce a cow that makes low-fat milk. Unfortunately, getting cows to produce low-fat milk isn't yet possible, because newborn calves depend on this extra energy. In any case, extracting the fat after milking is easy, in order to provide a more healthy lower-fat option. If you currently drink regular whole milk, start weaning yourself from the fat by changing to semi-skimmed milk for a while, and then consider moving on to skimmed milk.

Many people believe that they can never adapt to drinking skimmed milk. But your taste buds quickly become used to it, and after a while, you find that regular milk tastes too creamy!

Does drinking skimmed milk rather than whole milk really make a difference? Do bees like nectar? If you switch your milk from whole milk to semi-skimmed you go from 66 kilocalories down to 46 kilocalories per 100 millilitres (approximately 3½ fluid ounces). Moving down to skimmed milk takes you down even lower to 32 kilocalories per 100 millilitres (3½ fluid ounces) – less than half the kilocalories of whole milk. If you drink a 300-millilitre (10½-fluid ounce) glass of milk, that's just 96 kilocalories for skimmed, compared with 198 kilocalories for whole milk: A significant saving on a daily basis.

When ordering your morning café latte, specify low-fat milk (skinny or lite versions); if you don't ask, the server automatically uses full-fat milk.

Other dairy products that are available in low-fat form include hard cheeses like cheddar, as well as softer versions like cream cheese. Yoghurt is another popular food that you can purchase in low-fat varieties.

Low fat doesn't necessarily mean low kilocalorie. Ingenious food manufacturers have found ways to entice you to buy their low-fat foods by adding lots of carbohydrate (sweetener), meaning that the kilocalorie count is often still pretty high. Read the label!

Snacking on Low-Fat Foods

Eating regular snacks during the day smooths out your glucose control and stops you approaching a meal in an already-hungry state. Your choice of snacks can add a lot of kilocalories, especially fat kilocalories, or they can satisfy you without damaging your nutritional plan.

Instead of high-fat potato crisps, choose air-popped popcorn. Instead of a glass of full-cream milk, choose semi-skimmed or even skimmed. Other satisfying snacks that don't mess up your plan include three breadsticks, one matzo, or three rice cakes. (Check out Chapter 15 for some great snack ideas.)

Use your microwave oven to warm or cook your snack, and in the process improve your level of snack satisfaction. For example, an apple in the microwave becomes a baked apple – somehow more delicious than a raw apple but no more kilocalorific. Just make sure that you don't also have a baked worm.

Finding Free Foods

When dietitians talk about 'free foods', they aren't referring to foods you can tuck into your shopping basket and not pay for when you leave the supermarket (likely to attract the attention of the local constabulary). They mean foods that have so few kilocalories that you can eat them and not have to list them in the food diary (see Chapter 19 for more on keeping a food diary).

A long list of free foods exists, including the following:

- ✓ Black coffee, tea, club soda, and sugar-free drinks
- ✓ Cabbage, celery, cucumber, spring onions, and mushrooms
- ✓ Cranberries and rhubarb
- ✓ Salad greens
- ✓ Seasonings and condiments (see Chapter 19)
- ✓ Sugar-free varieties of sweets, gum, and jam rather than regular sweets, gum, and jam, which are full of sugar

Enjoy these foods and drinks with meals, as snacks, or any way you want.

These free foods have so few kilocalories that they're useless as a treatment for low blood glucose.

Playing with Portions

Many restaurants offer the same food items as appetisers and main dishes. The fact is that the quantity served as an appetiser is generally the right amount of food for your nutritional plan, whereas the main dish is often twice as much or more. In addition, the main dish can cost at least three times as much as the appetiser. Therefore, we heartily recommend that you order the appetiser for your main dish.

Some restaurants have a children's menu containing the same food as the main menu but in smaller portions. No law exists to prohibit an adult from ordering off the children's menu. Just ignore the annoyed facial expression of your server, who rapidly calculates the loss in tip.

If you've ever ordered a tasting menu in a restaurant, you know that you get a large number of different foods but very little of any of them. The chefs know that you don't need enormous quantities, but you do want the feeling that you're getting a lot. Your appetiser–main dish comes on a small plate and psychologically satisfies you.

Unless you're in a restaurant that you know gives appropriate portions, use Dr Rubin's 'half portion plan' to save yourself a lot of kilocalories. The plan works as follows: As soon as your food arrives, cut the food into two portions. Push one portion to the side. You can take the amount home in a doggy-bag, or leave it. Eat the other portion, knowing that you're tasting the delicious food without ruining your nutrition programme. Don't cheat! If you try to decrease your portion by eating until you've finished about half without cutting in advance, you end up eating too much or eating the whole thing.

Debbie, who has diabetes, eats in a restaurant known for its large portions. Wisely, she shares the meal with her spouse. Unwisely, she orders a dessert because she feels that she's eaten so little of her main dish. She orders a piece of apple pie that's served, for some reason, on a large plate. Although the piece is enormous, psychologically she feels that she's received only a small portion and goes ahead and eats it all. Needless to say, her blood glucose suffers.

Chapter 21

Ten Strategies to Normalise Your Blood Glucose

In This Chapter

▶ Knowing your blood glucose level

▶ Exercising and taking medications to stay in control

▶ Reacting immediately to foot and dental problems

▶ Keeping a positive attitude while planning for unexpected situations

▶ Staying aware of new developments and using expert help

▶ Avoiding methods that don't work

In *Diabetes For Dummies*, 2nd Edition (Wiley), Dr Sarah Jarvis and Dr Alan Rubin describe the management of diabetes in detail. This chapter gives you the highlights of that extensive discussion. Although this book is about eating, controlling your blood glucose requires much more from you than a nutritional plan to help normalise your glucose control.

Doctors consider your blood glucose level to be normal when it measures less than 5.6 mmol/l (millimoles per litre) – that's 100 mg/dl (milligrams/decilitre) – if you've eaten nothing for 8 to 12 hours. If you have eaten, your blood glucose is normal if it measures less than 7.8 mmol/l (140 mg/dl) two hours after eating. If you never see a blood glucose level higher than 7.8 mmol/l (140 mg/dl), you're doing very well indeed. See Chapter 1 for a full explanation of mmol/l and mg/dl.

Knowing Your Blood Glucose

No excuse is adequate for you not having a good idea of your blood glucose level at all times, although people make some pretty far-out excuses for not doing so – close to 'The dog ate my glucose meter'. The ability to measure blood glucose accurately and rapidly is the greatest advance in diabetes care since the discovery of insulin. Yet many people don't track their blood glucose.

How can you know what to do about your blood glucose if you don't know what it measures in the first place? Sure, pricking your finger hurts, but the needles are now so fine that you barely feel them, and new glucose monitoring devices are launched on a regular basis. Join organisations such as the Diabetes Research and Wellness Foundation (www.drwf.org.uk Tel: 02392 637808) and Diabetes UK (www.diabetes.org.uk Tel: 0207 424 1000) to keep up-to-date with developments.

The number of glucose meters now available is vast, and they're all good. However, they do vary in things such as overall size, method of calibration, size of display, range of blood glucose over which they supply an accurate reading, time taken to deliver a reading, and whether or not you can download data to your computer or obtain an average reading over a week or fortnight. Meters are available at most chemists, and you can ask your diabetes nurse to supply you with one on loan from the NHS.

If you have very stable blood glucose levels, test once a day – some days in the morning before breakfast, other days in the evening before supper. Varying the time of day that you test your blood glucose gives you and your doctor a clearer picture of your control under different circumstances. If your diabetes requires insulin, or is unstable, you need to test at least before meals and at bedtime in order to select your insulin dose.

Painless devices for measuring blood glucose are right around the corner. The closeness of this great advance is a particularly good reason to keep aware of new developments (see 'Staying Abreast of New Developments', later in this chapter, about tracking advancements).

Using Exercise to Control Your Glucose

When people are asked how much exercise they do, about a third admit that they do none at all. If you're a person with diabetes and consider yourself to be a part of the group that doesn't exercise, you aren't taking advantage of a major health tool – not just for controlling your blood glucose but also for improving your physical and mental state in general. In one recent study, a large group of people without diabetes, but who had a high chance of developing the condition (because both parents had diabetes), took part in a regular exercise programme. An amazing 80 per cent who stayed on the programme didn't develop diabetes.

Don't think that exercise means hours of exhaustion followed with a period of recovery. We're talking about a brisk walk, lasting no more than 60 minutes, every day and not necessarily all at once. If you want to do more, that's fine, but just about anyone can do this much. People who can't walk for some reason can still get their exercise by moving their arms. To lose weight as a result of exercise, you need to do 90 minutes a day, every day.

Exercise can provide the following benefits to your overall health:

- Helps with weight loss
- Lowers bad cholesterol and triglyceride fats and raises good cholesterol
- Lowers blood glucose levels because the glucose is used for energy
- Lowers blood pressure
- Reduces stress levels
- Reduces the need for drugs and insulin injections

When we see a new person with diabetes, we give him or her a bottle of pills. These pills aren't taken by mouth; they're spilled on the floor and picked up every day. This method is our way of making sure that each new patient gets at least a little exercise every day.

Taking Your Medications

Over the last ten years, a number of new drugs became available for treating diabetes, helping you to maintain good glucose control to avoid the complications of diabetes. Now, with the right combination of medications (and using some of the other tools in this chapter), just about anyone can achieve excellent diabetes control. But no medication works if you don't take it.

The word *compliance* applies here. Compliance refers to the willingness of people to follow instructions – specifically, taking their medications. People tend to start off very compliant at the beginning of treatment, but as their condition improves, compliance falls off. And therefore diabetes control falls off as well.

The fact is that, as you get older, the forces contributing to a worsening of your blood glucose tend to get stronger. You want to do all you can to reverse that tendency. Taking your medications is an essential part of your overall programme.

If you find all the medications you take confusing, get yourself a medication box that holds each day's medications in separate compartments. You can then make sure that the compartment for each day is empty by the next day. These useful devices are widely available in chemists as well as in healthfood stores (because people use them to store all those vitamin tablets).

Seeking Immediate Help for Foot Problems

The failure to seek immediate help for any foot problems leads to a lot of grief in diabetes. Your doctor may see you and examine your feet only once every two or three months. You need to look at your feet every day. At the first sign of any skin breakdown or other abnormality (such as discoloration), see your doctor straight away. In diabetes, foot problems can go from minor to major in a very brief time. Don't take risks in this area, because seeing your doctor is so important – major problems may mean amputation of toes or more. (See Chapter 1 for more information about foot problems as they relate to diabetes.)

You can reverse most foot problems, if you catch and treat them early. You may require a different shoe or need to keep weight off the foot for a time – minor inconveniences compared to an amputation.

Besides inspecting your feet daily, here are some other actions you can take:

- Ensuring that nothing is inside your shoe before you put it on
- Testing bath water with your hands to check its temperature, because numb feet can't sense if the water is scalding hot
- Wearing new shoes for only a short time before checking for damage

Taking immediate action goes for any other type of infection you develop too. Infections quickly raise your blood glucose level while you're ill. Try to avoid taking oral steroids for anything if you possibly can – talk to your doctor about alternatives. Steroids really make your glucose shoot up.

Brushing Off Dental Problems

Keeping your teeth in excellent condition is important, but especially if you have diabetes. 'Excellent condition' means brushing them twice a day and using dental floss at the end of the day to reach where the toothbrush can't go, as well as regular visits to the dentist for cleaning and examination.

Many people with diabetes have dental problems as a result of poor dental hygiene. As a side effect, controlling your blood glucose is much harder (strange but true, probably as a result of inflammation). After receiving appropriate dental treatment, these people often require much less medication.

People with diabetes don't have more cavities than people without diabetes, but they do have more gum disease if their glucose isn't under control. Gum disease results from the high glucose that bathes the mouth – a perfect medium for bacteria. Keeping your glucose under control helps you avoid losing teeth as a result of gum disease, as well as the further deterioration in glucose control.

Maintaining a Positive Attitude

Your mental approach to diabetes plays a major role in determining your success in controlling the disease. Think of diabetes as a challenge – like algebra, or asking someone out. As you overcome challenges in one area of your life, the skills you master help you in other areas. Looking at something as a challenge allows you to use all your creativity.

When you approach something with pessimism and negativity, you tend not to see all the possible ways in which you can succeed. You may take the attitude that 'It doesn't matter what I do'. That attitude leads to failure to take medications, failure to eat properly, failure to exercise, and so forth.

Simply understanding the workings of your body, which comes with treating your diabetes, probably makes you healthier than the couch potato who understands little more than the latest sitcom.

Some people do get depressed when they find out that they have diabetes. If you're depressed and your depression isn't improving after several weeks, consider seeking professional help.

Planning for the Unexpected

Life is full of surprises – like when you're first told that you have diabetes. You probably weren't ready to hear that news. But you can make yourself ready to deal with surprises that may damage your glucose control.

Most of those surprises have to do with food. Someone may offer you the wrong kind of food or too much or too little food; or the timing of food may not correspond to the requirements of your medication. You need to have plans for all these situations before they occur.

You can always reduce your portions when the food is the wrong kind or excessive, and you can carry portable kilocalories (like glucose tablets) when food is insufficient or delayed.

Other surprises have to do with your medication, such as leaving it in your luggage – which is heading to Warsaw while you're flying to Hawaii. Keep your important medications with you in your carry-on luggage, not in checked luggage. Again, your ability to think ahead can prevent you from getting separated from your medication.

Not everything is going to go right all the time. However, you can minimise the damage if you plan ahead.

Staying Abreast of New Developments

The pace of new discoveries in diabetes is so rapid that keeping on top of the field is difficult even for the experts. So, keeping up-to-date is even more difficult for you. You don't have access to all the publications, the drug company representatives, and the medical journals that experts see every day.

However, you can keep current in a number of ways. The following tips can help you to stay up-to-date on all the advances:

- Join a diabetes organisation, such as Diabetes UK (www.diabetes.org.uk) or the Diabetes Research and Wellness Foundation (www.drwf.org.uk). You start to receive the association's excellent newsletters, which often contain the cutting edge of diabetes research as well as available treatments.

- Obtain a copy of *Diabetes For Dummies,* 2nd Edition (Wiley), which explains every aspect of diabetes for the non-professional.

- Sign up for a diabetes awareness course. Such courses give you a basis for a future understanding of advances in diabetes. Diabetes UK and the Diabetes Research Awareness Foundation often run day or residential courses.

- Use the Internet to search for Web sites providing information about diabetes in the United Kingdom and worldwide.

Don't hesitate to question your doctor or ask to see a diabetes specialist if your doctor's answers don't satisfy you.

The cure for your diabetes problem is possibly in next week's newspaper. Give yourself every opportunity to find and understand that cure.

Using the Experts

The available knowledge about diabetes is huge and growing rapidly. Fortunately, you can turn to a multitude of people for help. Take advantage of these people at one time or another, including the following:

- Chiropodist to trim your toenails and advise on foot problems
- Diabetes hospital specialist, who is aware of the latest and greatest in diabetes treatment
- Diabetes nurse to give you a basic understanding of this disease
- Dietitian to help you plan your nutritional programme
- Eye doctor (ophthalmologist) to examine your eyes regularly
- General practitioner, who takes care of your diabetes as well as all your other medical concerns
- Mental health worker, if you run into adjustment problems
- Pharmacist, who can help you understand your medications

Take advantage of any or all these people when you need them. Most are available on the National Health Service, and you can pay to see some privately as well, if you want.

Avoiding What Doesn't Work

Not wasting your time and money on worthless treatments is important. When you consider that, worldwide, over 230 million people are living with diabetes, they provide a huge potential market for people with 'the latest wonder cure'. Before you waste your money, check out any claims with your diabetes experts.

You can find plenty of treatments for diabetes on the Internet. One way you can ensure that the claims are based on science is to look for verification from the Health on the Net Foundation, which you can find at www.hon.ch. The site's stamp of approval means that it adheres to principles with which every legitimate scientist agrees.

Don't make any substantial changes in your diabetes management without first discussing them with your doctor.

Chapter 22

Ten Healthy Eating Habits for Children with Diabetes

*A*n epidemic of excessive weight and obesity is taking hold among children: More youngsters now have type 2 diabetes than ever before. Several factors are responsible for this epidemic, including:

- Excessive intakes of high-kilocalorie fruit drinks and other kilocalorific beverages
- More time spent in front of the television and the computer rather than exercising
- Over-consumption of high-fat foods

Children pay a high price for their overweight condition in the form of low self-esteem and less acceptance from their peers, not to mention the risk of developing type 2 diabetes.

For overweight children, the old joke about looking too short for your weight really is true. Children often grow out of their overweight condition. As a parent, your job is to help them maintain their weight until they grow older and taller, not necessarily to help them lose weight.

This chapter describes how you can help your diabetic child to achieve healthy eating habits. You're an enormous force in your child's life, and you can do a great deal, as he or she grows up, to create a person with a life of quality as well as quantity.

Setting an Example

Children resemble their parents not just in physical appearance but also because they tend to pick up their parents' mannerisms. Your children are constantly studying you. They follow the example you set with your eating. If they observe you overeating and dieting, they assume that's the appropriate way to behave.

You set a positive dietary example when you eat the same foods that you want your child to eat, keep the quantities of food that you eat moderate, and select food that's low in fat and salt and high in fibre. You also set a good example when your child observes that exercise is a part of your daily routine.

If your child needs to lose weight, the chances are that you do as well. Try to do the following to set a good example:

✔ Avoid fatty snacks, such as biscuits and cakes

✔ Keep dairy products low-fat

✔ Reduce your use of butter and margarine

✔ Serve seafood and skinless poultry instead of meat

✔ Substitute low-sugar jam, salsa, or mustard for butter

✔ Use meat for taste instead of as a main dish

Engaging Children in Shopping

Taking your child to the supermarket is a great opportunity to explain good food-buying habits. Let your child read the nutrition labels (see Chapter 5 for a full explanation of nutrition labels) and explain the meaning of each type of nutrient to him or her. When reading the labels, do the following:

✔ Point out that you're looking for foods low in total fat, saturated fat, cholesterol, and salt.

✔ Look for words like 'partially hydrogenated oil'. These words refer to *trans fats,* which not only raise bad cholesterol, but also lower good cholesterol at the same time.

✔ Have your child compare the carbohydrate and protein content of foods as well as the other substances named on the label, especially fibre, but also calcium, iron, vitamin A, and vitamin C. Explain how each of these substances plays a part in good nutrition. (See Chapter 2 of *Diabetes For Dummies,* 2nd Edition, by Dr Sarah Jarvis and Dr Alan Rubin (Wiley) for an explanation of the purpose of these nutrients.)

✔ Let your child look at labels side by side, such as those on a bottle of fruit drink compared with a container of low-fat milk. Or compare regular and semi-skimmed milk.

If you purchase foods without labels (such as fresh fruits and vegetables), you can still explain the contents of those foods. Create a food basket that mirrors healthy eating guidelines (see Chapter 2 on healthy eating) so that your child can see the amounts of each food group that need to make up a diet.

Tell your child how advertising and food displays entice you to buy high-kilocalorie, low-nutrition food, especially at the checkout where you don't have time to change your mind and put it back. (Look in Chapter 5 for more information on this topic.)

Involving Children in Food Preparation

When you ask children to describe their earliest memories, they often talk happily about helping their grandmother or mother make some kind of food.

Preparing food together is a great bonding experience between you and your child, and also provides you with the opportunity to explain good nutrition. If you follow a recipe and tell your child to measure half the fat listed in the recipe, or leave out the salt altogether, that lesson stays with the child for life.

Have your child create his or her own nutrition plan for a day and discuss every part of it, pointing out what's carbohydrate, protein, fat, the balance among those foods, and how they affect his or her diabetes. Use healthy eating guidelines (see Chapter 2 for details) or advice from your child's dietitian to help you make your plans.

Never prepare one meal for your child with diabetes and another for the rest of the family. Everyone can benefit from the better choices you make with your child's nutritious food. The child also realises that eating isn't punishment for a person with diabetes because the whole family eats the same way. Really, no such thing as a 'diabetic' diet exists – a healthy eating diet is for everyone.

Keeping Problem Foods Out of Sight and Good Foods in Easy View

If crisps or creamy biscuits sit on the kitchen counter, can you blame your child (or yourself) for grabbing a handful every time he or she sees them? Don't buy these foods in the first place. If you do, keep them out of sight. After all, think about what happens when you walk up to a buffet table. You can more easily avoid what you don't see.

On the other hand, keep fruits and vegetables in plain sight, along with other acceptable snacks, such as air-popped popcorn. Having a special device for drinking water is also a good idea, because it makes water into something special and, therefore, more desirable. Even having a pitcher of water in the refrigerator beats going to the sink, where the association is with washing hands and dishes rather than nutrition.

Again, your child follows your example. If you raid the freezer for ice cream, don't be surprised to see your child doing the same thing. And don't forget the great benefit to you when you set an example for your child: You get excellent nutrition as well.

Explaining the Meaning of Portions

Your child has no more of an idea of the meaning of portions than you did before you started reading this book. In Chapter 1, we show you how to recognise a portion of various kinds of foods. Explain this information to your child so that he or she can readily select the amount of food that corresponds with a portion. Thinking in terms of a tennis ball representing a medium fruit, or a domino representing 28 grams (1 ounce) of cheese is much easier for a child than thinking in terms of measurements. These terms also introduce a certain amount of fun into the process of selecting how much to eat.

Missing No Meals

Your child must know that missing meals isn't appropriate for the following reasons:

✔ If he or she has type 1 diabetes, a missed meal is a fairly certain prelude to a *hypoglycaemic* (low blood glucose) reaction. Breakfast is especially important because he or she is going from the fasting (sleeping) state, when energy needs are minimal, to the state of activity, when kilocalories are essential. A school-age child has trouble with morning classes when no food energy is available.

✔ If he or she misses a meal, the resulting extreme feeling of hunger leads to over-compensating during the next meal. Overeating at that meal can make your child go from low to very high blood glucose very rapidly.

✔ If he or she misses a meal, your child may come to think that irregular eating is acceptable. The best way to encourage weight control is to encourage the regular eating of smaller meals and snacks, which is a programme that anyone can follow for life as a fairly certain way of getting good, balanced nutrition. After the initial weight loss, people rarely continue to succeed when their weight loss programme calls for missing meals.

Try to standardise your child's eating as much as possible:

✔ Encourage three moderate-sized meals and two low-sugar snacks daily.

✔ Offer water or semi-skimmed milk for a beverage, not fizzy drinks or other beverages with a lot of sugar. Diet drinks that emphasise sweetness just make a child believe that sweetness is essential in a liquid.

✔ Offer food about the same time each day and in the same quantities.

Ensuring Good Restaurant Eating

A high-kilocalorie, high-fat diet isn't good for you no matter where you eat it. Certain places, such as fast-food restaurants, promote these types of diets most of the time. If your child is permitted to choose, he or she makes choices that promote unhealthy weight gain. A film producer who ate only McDonald's food for one month developed serious abnormalities of his liver, a very high cholesterol level, and other unhealthy changes (see the film *Super Size Me*). He developed these health problems mainly because he made the poor choices of eating the large portions of burgers, soft drinks, and fries.

If you eat at fast-food places with your kids, review Chapter 17 so that you're prepared to point out the best menu selections. If the foods for the restaurant you frequent aren't in the chapter, find out where you can get nutritional information. For example, visit the fast-food company's Web site or write to the company if you can get the address. Alternatively, publications exist that list the foods in these restaurants with their nutrient content.

If you go to restaurants other than fast-food places, encourage your child to find out what's in the food that he or she orders. Considering what you pay for the food; you're entitled to know what you're getting. Point out the fact that portions, even children's portions, are usually too large. Set an example in the restaurant and order two starters rather than a starter and a main course dish – or take home half of your food in a 'doggy-bag'.

Don't tell your child how long to take eating. Better to let children decide what's best because they know when they're full. If your child leaves food on the plate, don't point out that starving people in some remote country would love to get their hands on the leftovers. Don't try to regulate your child's food intake and tell him or her to stop eating or keep eating. Instead, set an example and stop when you know you've had enough. If your child has type 1 diabetes, discuss the need for enough carbohydrate at each meal.

In addition, avoid buffets. You and your child are bound to overeat when the food is unlimited. You want to get your 'money's worth', and you probably end up with large portions and no idea what's in them.

Monitoring TV Food Ads with Your Child

Like it or not, your child spends a certain amount of time in front of the television every day. The ads that he or she views are most likely for high-kilocalorie, high-sugar, high-fat snack foods. Sitting with your child for some of the viewing time and discussing the nutritional content of the food in the adverts is important and valuable. Even if you keep that kind of food out of your shopping trolley and your house, your child's eventually going to visit a friend's home and find that food.

If you discuss the food in advance, your child is in a position to turn it down or at least to know how eating it affects his or her nutrition plan. Don't expect your child to act perfectly with food all the time, whether at home or away. Do you? We confess that we sometimes stray from perfect eating ourselves.

Your child needs to see how poor food choices affect his or her blood glucose. Such an observation is often enough to prevent your child from making that particular choice again. On the other hand, you never want to nag your child about eating off their nutritional plan. Instead, accept the mistake and suggest that your child moves back to appropriate eating with the next meal.

Making Friends with the Dietitian

The dietary needs of growing children are complicated enough, but when you factor in diabetes as well, the situation is beyond the knowledge of most parents. When a child is first diagnosed with diabetes, a dietitian is involved with drawing up the child's nutritional plan from the very beginning. If your child is old enough, involve him or her in the plan's details; any child of ten or older benefits from involvement with his or her food choices. A nutritional plan for diabetes isn't something that you impose upon your child, but something you work out together.

You and the dietitian need to take your child's food preferences into consideration. Otherwise, your child doesn't want to follow any plan that you devise. Work out a diet with the dietitian that's about 50 to 60 per cent carbohydrate, 20 per cent protein, and 30 per cent fat with less than 10 per cent saturated fat.

Ask the dietitian to show you and your child how to count the carbohydrates in a meal. Knowing the carbohydrate count is the easiest way to determine how much insulin to take.

Using the Experts

You can make use of expert advice to help with your child's nutrition. Diabetes UK (www.diabetes.org.uk) offers plenty of good advice, as do many other organisations.

A useful resource is the diabetes portal at www.diabetes.co.uk, which includes lots of information and links to useful sites, plus daily global news and an archive of diabetes-friendly recipes.

Part V
Appendixes

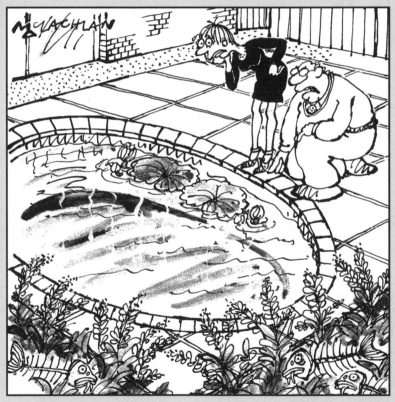

'The koi carp have gone again – that's the <u>very</u> last time you bring your Dieting and Nutrition Club round for afternoon tea!'

In this part . . .

Did you think that you were finished with this book? Not so fast! We couldn't leave you without adding a few helpful appendixes chock-full of extra information on diabetes.

In Appendix A, you can read about dietary supplements which can help you with your health in general, and your diabetes in particular. Appendix B shows you how to use diabetic exchanges to work out a proper diabetic diet. The exchanges help you know what and how much food should be eaten to maintain normal weight and normal blood glucose levels, the key to prevention of diabetes complications.

Appendix C is a cooking glossary that defines terms that you find in this book. Appendix D offers a handy list of weights and measures so you can convert any quantity in a recipe to another system of measurement.

Appendix E shows you where you can find more great recipes for a person with diabetes, both in books and on the Web.

Appendix A

Investing in Food Supplements for Optimum Health

⋅⋅⋅

*Y*our body needs a wide range of vitamins, minerals, and trace elements to process glucose properly. Although diet should always come first, many people do not obtain enough of these vital nutrients from their food alone. This is partly because of poor diet choices, partly because of modern farming and processing techniques, and partly because some soils are deficient in trace elements such as selenium. In addition, many crops are picked unripe, flown around the world, chilled, and stored before use, which reduces their nutrient content even further.

In 2002, the *Journal of the American Medical Association* published a scientific review of over 150 clinical trials involving vitamin and mineral supplements. This showed that lack of many micronutrients is a risk factor for heart disease, stroke, some cancers, osteoporosis, and other major health problems. And, in an accompanying paper, the authors even state that, 'Pending strong evidence of effectiveness from randomised trials, it appears prudent for all adults to take vitamin supplements.' This is especially true for people with diabetes, whose need for vitamins and minerals is increased as a result of their changed metabolism and by the increased amount of minerals and water-soluble vitamins that are lost in their urine. In fact, a systematic review of evidence for the effectiveness and safety of herbal, vitamin, and mineral therapies for people with diabetes was published in *Diabetes Care* in 2003. Across nearly 60 controlled clinical trials, 3 out of 4 had a positive effect on glucose control. In this Appendix we look at the most important supplements, with the best evidence to support their use.

What to Look for in Supplements

A number of supplement formulations are available, such as tablets, capsules, powders, pastilles, oils, syrups, teas, infusions, effervescent formulations, tinctures, and even gels. Deciding what supplements to buy is often confusing. Checking labels can help you make your selection, because the list of ingredients, including non-active ingredients such as sugar, colourings, and fillers, is listed in descending order by weight. Some supplements may contain sugar or other carbohydrate as a sweetener, and you need to take this into account as part of your daily intake.

The separate nutrition information panel lists the amount of each active ingredient, and its percentage of the *recommended daily amount* (RDA) where appropriate.

When reading labels, check

✔ Whether the supplement provides a complete range of nutrients or whether it is a more specific formulation, providing, for example, just the B group vitamins.

✔ Whether the range of ingredients provided suits your particular needs.

✔ The doses of each nutrient – in the case of vitamins and minerals, how does the dose compare with the RDA?

✔ The form in which the supplement is delivered. For example, good supplements supply vitamin E in its natural form, such as *d-alpha tocopherol,* rather than the less active, synthetic form, *dl-alpha tocopherol.*

✔ That the product suits your particular dietary requirements. For example, is it suitable for vegetarians? Is it gluten, yeast, lactose, or dairy free? Does this matter to you?

Confusingly, food supplements are not allowed to have overt health claims on their labels by law. This makes it difficult to know what some supplements are designed to do. They may, however, use general, agreed statements such as *May help to maintain a healthy heart,* or *May help to replenish the vitamin C lost during colds,* to help you select the right product for your needs.

How to Take Supplements

Take your vitamin and mineral supplements immediately after food – just four bites of food or a glass of juice will do. Don't take them on an empty stomach, as some can make you feel sick or cause indigestion. Wash them down with water or orange juice rather than with coffee or tea, which can interfere with their absorption.

Where taking two or more capsules of the same preparation a day, spread these out over the day, if possible, to maximise absorption and obtain more even blood levels.

Let your doctor know which supplements you are thinking about taking, and check for any potential interactions with your prescribed drugs beforehand. And monitor your blood glucose levels closely, especially over the first few days of starting a new supplement, to see if it affects your glucose control. Ask your doctor how to adjust your dose of medication as your blood glucose control starts to improve. This will help you to avoid *hypoglycaemia* (low blood glucose levels).

If you are pregnant or planning a pregnancy, or if you are breastfeeding, do not take any supplements unless they are specifically designed for use during pregnancy. Always check with a doctor or pharmacist if you are unsure.

Do not exceed the manufacturers' recommended doses.

Reducing Diabetes Complications with Supplements

Persistently raised glucose levels damage your cells, and can produce a variety of complications affecting your eyes, kidneys, nervous system, and peripheral circulation. Several supplements, especially the antioxidants, seem to provide some protection against diabetes complications.

Diabetic eye problems

Raised glucose levels damage tiny capillaries that can bleed into the retina, leading to a slowly progressive loss of vision (diabetic retinopathy).

Vitamin C helps to protect against the blood vessel damage linked with eye damage and may protect against eye complications, including cataracts. One study shows that taking 300 micrograms of vitamin C daily decreases the risk of cataracts by 70 per cent.

People with the highest intakes of vitamin E, another important antioxidant in the body, are 50 per cent less likely to need cataract surgery than those with the lowest intakes.

Antioxidants found in extracts from the bark of the French maritime pine (known commercially as Pycnogenol® – see the section 'French maritime pine bark' later in this appendix) bind to blood vessel wall proteins in the eye to repair areas of weakness and seal leaking blood vessels in the retina. Pycnogenol can reduce the progression of diabetic retinopathy and preserve vision. Taking 50 milligrams three times a day for two months can significantly improve visual sharpness.

The risk of age-related *macular degeneration* increases in people with diabetes. Macular degeneration reduces the fine vision needed for reading and recognising faces. People with macular degeneration have around 70 per cent less of the carotenoids, lutein, and zeaxanthin in the macula than those with healthy vision. Taking lutein supplements ranging from 10 milligrams to 30 milligrams per day can significantly increase lutein concentrations within the macula and protect eyesight.

Herbal remedies derived from Ginkgo biloba and bilberries can also improve eye health.

Diabetic kidney problems

Antioxidants also provide some protection against diabetic kidney problems (nephropathy). Several studies suggest that taking a vitamin-like substance called *alpha-lipoic acid* (ALA – see the section on it later in this appendix) can reduce the leakage of protein through the kidneys into the urine. In a trial involving 84 people with diabetes, protein leakage increased over 18 months in those not taking ALA, while it did not worsen in those taking 600 milligrams of ALA per day, suggesting that ALA helps to preserve kidney function.

Diabetic nerve problems

People with diabetic nerve problems (neuropathy) appear to have lower vitamin B6 levels than those with diabetes who do not develop neuropathy. Taking 50 milligrams of vitamin B6 three times daily for four months can significantly improve symptoms in two-thirds of those affected.

Foot ulcers

Low magnesium levels can increase the risk of developing diabetic foot ulcers threefold. Doctors don't yet know whether or not magnesium supplements can improve pre-existing foot ulcers, however.

Improving Glucose Control with Supplements

A variety of vitamins and minerals are involved in processing glucose in the body. Chromium and magnesium are particularly helpful for glucose control.

Chromium

Chromium is an essential trace element which, together with vitamin B3, forms part of a complex called *glucose tolerance factor* (GTF). GTF increases the number of insulin receptors present on muscle and fat cell membranes, improving insulin sensitivity and allowing more glucose to enter these cells. Chromium is found in brewer's yeast, egg yolk, red meat, cheese, fruit, whole grains, vegetables, and black pepper. Chromium deficiency is common, however, and an estimated nine out of ten adults do not get enough from their diet. People with diabetes appear to have particularly low chromium levels compared to people without diabetes, probably because they lose twice as much chromium through their urine.

Research suggests that in people with Type 2 diabetes chromium supplements can improve blood glucose levels and help to deliver better long-term glucose control. Taking 200 micrograms of chromium per day can lower the amount of hypoglycaemic medication needed. It is only useful in people who have low chromium levels, however, so does not benefit everyone.

Look for supplements that provide chromium already incorporated into GTF from chromium-enriched yeast cultures for the best effect.

Magnesium

Magnesium is an essential mineral needed for the action of most enzymes in the body. It is naturally found in seafood, meat, eggs, dairy products, whole grains, pulses, nuts, and green leafy vegetables. Food processing removes significant amounts so that an estimated 80 per cent of people do not obtain the recommended 300 milligrams per day from their diet.

People with diabetes are three times more likely to have low magnesium levels than people without diabetes. A diet rich in magnesium may even help to prevent the onset of Type 2 diabetes, especially in people who are overweight. When over 127,000 adults without diabetes were monitored for 12 to 18 years, those with the highest magnesium intake were a third less likely to develop diabetes than those with the lowest intake, even when taking other factors such as age, weight, exercise, family history of diabetes, smoking, and alcohol consumption into account.

Taking magnesium supplements totalling around 300 milligrams daily can improve glucose levels and lower insulin requirements in people with diabetes.

Magnesium citrate is the most readily absorbed form, while magnesium gluconate is less likely to cause intestinal side effects such as diarrhoea.

Selenium

Selenium is a *trace element* – an element found in extremely small quantities – that is essential for the body's main antioxidant enzymes to work properly, especially those known as *glutathione peroxidases*. These enzymes help to protect the body from some of the damage linked with premature aging and diabetes complications.

Selenium levels in the population are low; intakes have halved over the last 50 years due to soil deficiencies, and because we now import wheat from selenium-deficient regions in Europe rather than from America. Selenium levels are lower than normal in people with diabetes.

Selenium has an insulin-like action that stimulates uptake of glucose and improves glucose control. It is thought to activate proteins that tell the cells when insulin is present.

The standard dose for selenium in a supplement is 50–200 micrograms daily, but be aware that excess selenium is toxic, so don't take more than 300 micrograms daily long-term.

Vanadium

Vanadium is a trace element that is found in some foods such as parsley, black pepper, seafood (especially lobster and oysters), radishes, lettuce, whole grains, sunflower seeds, soybeans, buckwheat, carrots, and garlic. It appears to improve glucose control in people in diabetes, although how it works is not fully understood. In people with type 2 diabetes, vanadium supplements can lower glucose concentrations by 20 per cent. Its use is controversial, however, as long-term safety is not known.

Zinc

Zinc is an essential trace element found especially in red meat, seafood (especially oysters), offal, brewer's yeast, whole grains, pulses, eggs, and cheese. It is involved in the production of insulin and some people with type 2 diabetes may have an inherited inability to transport enough zinc into the pancreatic cells that need it to make insulin. Zinc supplements of 15 milligrams per day may help to lower glucose levels in some people with type 1 diabetes.

Maintaining Good Health with Vital Vitamins

Some vitamins are particularly important for people with diabetes, especially vitamins that are also antioxidants, such as vitamins C and E.

Vitamin C

Vitamin C is structurally similar to glucose and plays a role in glucose tolerance. Food sources include berries – especially blackcurrants – kiwi fruit, citrus fruit, green sprouting vegetables, guavas, mangoes, and capsicum peppers.

Vitamin C protects proteins in the circulation from damage by raised glucose levels. This damage, known as *glycosylation,* also affects the blood pigment, *haemoglobin*. Taking supplements supplying 1 gram of vitamin C per day can reduce levels of glycosylated haemoglobin by 18 per cent within 12 weeks.

Vitamin C is acidic. If you are prone to indigestion, take the non-acidic form known as Ester-C.

Vitamin C can interfere with some laboratory tests used to assess blood and glucose levels in urine, so if taking vitamin C, let your doctor know.

Vitamin E

Vitamin E consists of eight different substances, of which the most active is *d-alpha-tocopherol*. Vitamin E is an antioxidant that protects body fats from oxidation and strengthens capillaries and muscle fibres. Food sources include wheatgerm oil, avocado, butter or margarine, oily fish, nuts, and seeds.

Usual doses range from 100 milligrams to 727 milligrams. It is best taken together with vitamin C and/or ALA (see the section on ALA later in this appendix) as these help to regenerate vitamin E after it has performed its antioxidant actions.

Folic acid

Folic acid is a B vitamin needed to process a harmful amino acid called homo-cysteine. Folate is the natural form of this vitamin, and is found in green leafy vegetables. Folate is less active in the body than the synthetic form, folic acid, which is used to fortify foods such as breakfast cereals.

When your folic acid intake is low, your homocysteine levels rise, and this hastens hardening and furring up of the arteries, especially in people with diabetes. For every 400 micrograms per day increase in dietary intake of folic acid/folate intake, the risk of developing peripheral artery disease decreases by over one-fifth.

People with type 2 diabetes tend to have lower levels of folic acid compared with similar people without diabetes, and are more likely to have raised levels of homocysteine as a result. Taking supplements of 600 micrograms per day can improve homocysteine levels.

Metformin, a drug used to treat insulin resistance, can lower folic acid levels enough to produce a 4 per cent increase in homocysteine levels after just four months' treatment. This effect is counteracted by taking folic acid supplements which, at a relatively low dose of 250 micrograms per day, can lower total homocysteine by 14 per cent after 4 weeks and by almost 22 per cent after 12 weeks.

Absolutely Fabulous Antioxidants

Antioxidants such as vitamin C and E neutralise harmful substances called free radicals to prevent oxidising reactions in the body. In people with diabetes, production of free radicals is particularly high, and this contributes to the complications that develop when long-term glucose control is poor. Although diet should always come first, fruit and vegetables alone cannot supply the optimum quantities of antioxidants needed when you have diabetes. The most important antioxidants for people with diabetes are vitamin C, vitamin E, selenium, alpha-lipoic acid, carotenoids, co-enzyme Q10, and pycnogenol.

Alpha-lipoic acid (ALA)

Known as ALA for short, this vitamin-like substance speeds energy production in cells, and regenerates vitamins C and E to enhance their effectiveness. People with diabetes who take alpha-lipoic acid supplements have significantly lower levels of harmful oxidation reactions than those not taking ALA, even when glucose control is poor. The usual dose is 50 to 100 milligrams daily when taken as a general antioxidant, but higher doses of 600 milligrams are sometimes taken under the supervision of a nutritional therapist when diabetes complications are present.

Monitor blood glucose levels carefully as ALA stimulates glucose uptake into muscle cells to lower raised glucose levels.

Carotenoids

Carotenoids are antioxidant plant pigments found in dark green, leafy vegetables (spinach, for example) and yellow, orange, or red fruits and vegetables, including carrots, yams, apricots, mangoes, and tomatoes. Some research suggests that people at high risk of developing type 2 diabetes who have a high carotenoid intake from fruit and vegetables (especially carrots and pumpkins) are half as likely to develop poor glucose tolerance as those with low intakes. Supplements are also available at doses of 6– 15 milligrams of mixed carotenoids daily.

Excess carotenoids tinge the skin yellow-orange. The discolouration is harmless but looks like cheap fake tan. Not a good look. It resolves when you reduce your intake.

Co-enzyme Q10

Co-enzyme Q10 (CoQ10) acts together with vitamin E to provide a powerful antioxidant defence. It is also needed to process oxygen in cells, and to generate energy-rich molecules. CoQ10 appears to improve glucose control in people with type 2 diabetes by increasing energy levels within beta-cells so they can make insulin more effectively. Lack of CoQ10 is linked with coronary heart disease and congestive heart failure.

CoQ10 supplements are important for people taking statin drugs to lower cholesterol levels, as statins block production of CoQ10 in the body.

The usual does of CoQ10 is 30 milligrams to 100 milligrams daily. Higher amounts of up to 600 milligrams should only be used under medical supervision.

French maritime pine bark

The bark of the French maritime pine (Pycnogenol®) contains a rich blend of antioxidants that can reduce hardening and furring up of the arteries and abnormal blood clots, and lower your risk of coronary heart disease and stroke. Doses of 125 milligrams of Pycnogenol® per day are as effective as 500 milligrams of aspirin at reducing abnormal blood clotting, even in smokers. But, unlike aspirin, Pycnogenol® does not produce intestinal side effects such as peptic ulceration, and does not increase bleeding time.

Pycnogenol® also improves fasting blood glucose levels in a dose-dependent fashion up to a dose of 200 milligrams per day, but how it does this is not fully understood.

Absorbing Essential Fatty Acids

Omega-3 fish oils and conjugated linoleic acid are useful supplements for people with diabetes. Although diet should always come first, it is now difficult to eat enough oily fish to provide optimum levels of omega-3s, as levels of pollutants in the sea mean we are advised to limit our consumption to no more than four portions per week. Women and girls who are pregnant, or trying for a child, are advised to eat no more than two portions weekly.

Omega-3 fish oils

Omega-3 fish oils have a beneficial effect on insulin sensitivity and glucose tolerance. People who eat the most fish are 60 per cent less likely to develop glucose intolerance or diabetes over a four-year follow-up period than those who eat no fish, even when taking age, weight, and carbohydrate intake into account. And giving infants cod liver oil during the first year of life can lower the risk of a child developing type 1 diabetes by over a quarter. There is also some evidence that a good intake of omega-3s may reduce the risk of developing type 2 diabetes, but this is not yet certain.

Always monitor glucose levels carefully when taking any supplement, including omega-3 fish oils, so you can adjust your medication depending on how it affects your blood glucose levels.

Conjugated linoleic acid (CLA)

Conjugated linoleic acid (CLA) is found in beef, lamb, and dairy products. It is made by bacteria in the stomach of ruminant animals (cows, for example) and we cannot produce it ourselves. CLA helps to reduce *central obesity*, in which the main deposits of fat are located around the abdomen, and improve insulin sensitivity as it transports fatty acids away from fatty tissues to muscle cells where they are burned for fuel.

Trials show CLA can reduce the size of visceral fat cells (around the waist) while increasing lean body mass – building muscle at the expense of fat. Twenty-five middle-aged men with metabolic syndrome and abdominal obesity who took 4.2 grams of CLA per day showed a significant decrease in waist size, compared with the placebo, after just four weeks. And in a study involving 22 people with type 2 diabetes, three-quarters showed improvements in insulin levels after eight weeks, with a moderately reduced blood fasting glucose level.

You can take 3 grams to 6 grams of CLA daily, divided into two separate doses.

Appendix B

Exchange Lists

· ·

*T*his appendix includes food exchange lists that are the basis of a popular meal-planning approach to help people with diabetes eat the right number of calories from the correct energy sources. Dietitians recommend certain foods, but the patient has the choice to use whatever foods he or she wants. For more information on how to use the exchange method of balancing your diet, see Chapter 2.

Listing the Foods

Thousands of different foods are available, and each one is grouped on the basis of the energy source (carbohydrate, protein, or fat) that is most prevalent in the food. Fortunately, the food content of one type of fish – salmon, for example – is just about the same as another type of fish, such as halibut. Therefore, a diet that calls for one meat exchange can use any one of a number of choices or exchanges. You can exchange one for the other, so your diet is never boring.

Listing all food sources in this space isn't possible, but you can get more information from a dietitian, in books, or on the Internet.

Starch

Tables B-1 and B-2 list starch exchanges. Each exchange contains 15 grams of carbohydrate plus 3 grams of protein and 0 to 1 grams of fat, which amounts to 80 kilocalories per exchange. Foods containing whole grains also provide around 2 grams of fibre.

Table B-1	Starch Exchanges	
Cereals, Grains, Pasta	*Bread*	*Dried Beans, Peas, Lentils (Higher in Fibre)*
Bran cereals, 10g	Bagel, ½	Baked beans, 65g
Cooked cereals, 115g (cooked), 55g	Beefburger roll, ½	Beans and peas
Muesli, 3 tablespoons	Breadsticks, 2	Broad beans, 90g
Oatmeal (cooked), 110g	Hot dog roll, ½	Peas, green, 70g
Pasta (cooked), 70g	Muffin, ½	Lentils (cooked), 65g
Puffed cereal, 20g	Pitta bread, 15cm across, ½	
Rice (cooked), 65g	Raisin bread, 1 slice	
Shredded wheat, 20g	Tortilla, 15cm across, 1 piece	
	White bread, 1 slice	
	Wholemeal bread, 1 slice	

Table B-2	More Starch Exchanges	
Crackers/Snacks	*Starchy Vegetables*	*Starchy Foods with Fats*
Matzo, 20g	Corn on the cob, 1	Chow mein noodles, 25g
Melba toast, 5 slices	Potato (baked), 85g	Chips, 10 (85g)
Popcorn (no fat), unsweetened, 35g	Potato (mashed), 100g	Sweet muffin, 1
Pretzels, 25g	Squash (winter), 110g	Pancakes, 10cm, 2
Wholemeal crackers, 4	Sweetcorn kernels, 80g	Waffle, 11cm, 1
	Yam (sweet potato), cooked, 40g	

Meat and meat substitutes

Meats are divided into very lean, lean, medium-fat, and high-fat lists based on the fat they contain. They all contain no carbohydrate and 7 grams of protein. The fat content changes the kilocalorie count for each exchange as follows:

	Fat (grams)	*Kilocalories*
Very lean	0–1	35
Lean	3	55
Medium-fat	5	75
High-fat	8	100

Very lean meat and substitutes:

- ✔ Poultry: Chicken or turkey (white meat, no skin), 30g
- ✔ Fish: Fresh or frozen cod, flounder, haddock, halibut, trout, fresh tuna, or tuna canned in water, 30g
- ✔ Shellfish: Clams, crab, lobster, scallops, shrimp, or crab sticks, 30g
- ✔ Game: Venison, buffalo, or ostrich, 30g
- ✔ Cheese with 1 gram of fat or less per 30g; non-fat or low fat cottage cheese, 55g; fat-free cheese, 30g
- ✔ Other:
  - Egg whites, 2
  - Hot dogs with 1 gram or less fat per 30g, 30g
  - Kidney, 30g
  - Processed sandwich meats with 1 gram or less fat per 30g, 30g
  - Sausage with 1 gram or less fat per 30g, 30g

One very lean meat plus one starch exchange:

- ✔ Beans, peas, or lentils, 100g

Lean meat and substitutes:

- ✔ Beef: Choice grades of lean beef trimmed of fat, such as round sirloin and flank steak, tenderloin, roast (rib, chuck, rump), steak (T-bone, porterhouse, cubed), or minced, 30g

✔ Pork: Lean pork; canned, cured, or boiled ham; Canadian bacon; tenderloin or centre loin chop, 30g

✔ Lamb: Roast, chop, or leg, 30g

✔ Veal: Lean chop or roast, 30g

✔ Poultry: Chicken, turkey (dark meat, no skin), chicken white meat (with skin), domestic duck or goose (well-drained of fat), no skin, 30g

✔ Fish:

  • Herring, 30g

  • Oysters, 6 medium

  • Salmon (fresh or canned), 30g

  • Sardines (canned), 2 medium

  • Tuna (canned in oil, drained), 30g

✔ Game: Wild goose (no skin) or rabbit, 30g

✔ Cheese:

  • 4.5 per cent-fat cottage cheese, 55g

  • Grated Parmesan, 2 tablespoons

  • Cheeses with 3 grams or less fat per 30g, 30g

Medium-fat meat and substitutes list:

✔ Beef: minced, roast, or steak, 30g

✔ Pork: loin, chops, escalope, or cutlet, 30g

✔ Lamb: chops, leg, roast, or minced, 30g

✔ Veal: Cutlet or escalope, 30g

✔ Poultry: Chicken (dark meat with skin), ground turkey or ground chicken, or fried chicken (with skin), 30g

✔ Fish: Any fried fish, 30g

✔ Cheese: With 5 grams or less fat per 30g

  • Feta or mozzarella, 30g

  • Ricotta, 60g

✔ Other:

  • Egg, 1

  • Sausage with 5 grams or less fat per 30g, 30g

- Soy milk, 240ml
- Tempeh, 40g
- Tofu, 115g

High-fat meat and substitutes list:

✔ Pork: Spare ribs, minced pork, or pork sausage, 30g

✔ Cheese: All regular such as Emmenthal, cheddar, and Edam, 30g

✔ Other: Processed cured meats such as bologna, salami, or frankfurter, 30g

✔ Bacon, 3 slices

High-fat meat plus one fat exchange:

✔ Hot dog (beef, pork, or combination), 1

High-fat meat plus two fat exchanges:

✔ Peanut butter, 2 tablespoons

Fruit list

Each exchange in Table B-3 contains 15 grams of carbohydrate (60 kilocalories) but no protein or fat. The list includes fresh, frozen, canned, and dried fruit and juice.

Table B-3	Fruit Exchanges	
Fruit	*Dried Fruit*	*Fruit Juice*
Apple, 115g	Apple, 4 rings	Apple, 125ml
Apple sauce, 130g	Apricots, 8 halves	Cranberry, 75ml
Apricots, 4	Dates, 2½	Grape, 75ml
Apricots (canned), 130g	Figs, 1½	Grapefruit, 125ml
Banana (23cm), ½	Prunes, 3	Orange, 75ml
Blackberries, 110g	Raisins, 2 tablespoons	Pineapple, 125ml
Blueberries, 110g		Prune, 75ml

(continued)

Table B-3 *(continued)*

Fruit	Dried Fruit	Fruit Juice
Cantaloupe melon (12.5cm diameter), ⅓		
Cherries, 12		
Cherries (canned), 125g		
Figs, 2		
Fruit cocktail, 125g		
Grapes, 15		
Grapefruit, ½		
Honeydew melon, ⅛		
Kiwi, 1		
Mango, ½		
Nectarine, 1		
Orange, 1		
Papaya, 210g		
Peach, 1		
Peaches (canned), 130g		
Pear, 1 small		
Pears (canned), 130g		
Persimmons, 2		
Pineapple, 150g		
Pineapple (canned), 80g		
Plums, 2		
Raspberries, 125g		
Strawberries, 185g		
Tangerines, 2		
Watermelon, 385g		

Milk list

Each exchange has 12 grams of carbohydrate and 8 grams of protein. Each exchange may have 0 to 8 grams of fat, so the kilocalorie count is 90 to 150.

Skimmed and very low fat milk list: Add 0 kilocalories for fat content.

- Skimmed milk, 240ml
- Non-fat or low fat buttermilk, 240ml
- Evaporated skimmed milk, 120ml
- Dry non-fat milk, 80ml
- Plain, non-fat yogurt, 180ml
- Non-fat or low fat fruit-flavoured yogurt sweetened with alternative sweetener, 240ml

Reduced-fat milk list: Add 45 kilocalories for fat content.

- Semi-skimmed milk, 240ml
- Plain low fat yogurt, 180ml

Whole milk list: Add 72 kilocalories for fat content.

- Whole milk, 240ml
- Evaporated whole milk, 120ml
- Goats' milk, 240ml

Vegetable list

Each exchange has 5 grams of carbohydrate and 2 grams of protein, which equals 25 kilocalories. Vegetables have 2 to 3 grams of fibre. Remember that starchy vegetables such as lentils, sweetcorn, and potatoes are on the starches list, earlier in this chapter. The serving size for all is 90g of cooked vegetables or 100g of raw vegetables.

- Artichoke (½ medium)
- Asparagus
- Aubergine
- Beans (fresh green)

- Bean sprouts
- Cabbage
- Carrots
- Cauliflower
- Courgettes
- Greens (chard, kale)
- Kohlrabi
- Mangetout
- Okra
- Onions
- Peppers (green)
- Sauerkraut
- Summer squash
- Swede
- Turnips
- Water chestnuts

Fats

These foods have 5 grams of fat and little or no protein or carbohydrate per portion. The calorie count is, therefore, 45 kilocalories. The important thing in this category is to identify the foods that are high in cholesterol and saturated fats and avoid them. See Table B-4.

Table B-4	Fat Exchanges
Unsaturated Fats	*Saturated Fats*
Almonds, 6	Butter, 1 teaspoon
Avocado, 30g	Coconut, 2 tablespoons
Cashews, 1 tablespoon	Cream, single, 2 tablespoons
Margarine, 1 teaspoon	Cream cheese, 1 tablespoon
Margarine (diet), 1 tablespoon	Cream, double, 1 tablespoon

Unsaturated Fats	Saturated Fats
Mayonnaise, 1 teaspoon	Cream, sour, 2 tablespoons
Oil (corn, olive, soybean, sunflower, peanut), 1 teaspoon	
Olives, 10 small	
Peanuts, 10 large	
Pecans, 2 whole	
Salad dressing, 1 tablespoon	
Salad dressing (low fat), 2 tablespoons	
Seeds (pine nuts, sunflower), 1 tablespoon	
Seeds (pumpkin), 2 teaspoons	
Walnuts, 2 whole	

Other carbohydrates

This list contains cakes, pies, puddings, and other foods with lots of carbohydrate (and often fat). They have 15 grams of carbohydrate. Because the protein and fat content is so variable, the total number of kilocalories in each item varies as well. Examples are too numerous to list but include, for example:

- ✔ Ice cream, 65g
- ✔ Brownie, 5cm square
- ✔ Ginger nuts, 3

Free foods

These foods contain less than 20 calories per serving, so you can eat as much of them as you want without worrying about overeating and without worrying about serving size.

- ✔ **Condiments:** Horseradish, ketchup (1 tablespoon), mustard, pickles (unsweetened), low-calorie salad dressing, taco sauce, and vinegar
- ✔ **Drinks:** Bouillon, sugar-free drinks, sparkling water, coffee, and tea

✔ **Fruit:** Cranberries, unsweetened, and rhubarb

✔ **Non-stick pan spray**

✔ **Salad greens:** Endive, any type of lettuce, and spinach

✔ **Seasonings:** Basil, celery seeds, chilli powder, chives, cinnamon, curry, dill, flavouring extracts (vanilla, for example), garlic, garlic powder, herbs, lemon juice, lemon, lime, mint, onion powder, oregano, paprika, pepper, pimento, soy sauce, spices, wine (used in cooking), and Worcestershire sauce

✔ **Sweet substitutes:** Sugar-free candy, sugar-free gum, sugar-free jam or jelly, and sugar substitutes such as saccharin, sucralose, and aspartame

✔ **Vegetables:** Cabbage, celery, cucumbers, spring onions, hot peppers, mushrooms, and radishes

Using Exchanges to Create a Diet

Foods in exchange lists make it easy to create a diet with great variation. The menus in this section are adjusted to reflect the lower carbohydrate and higher protein that is generally recommended for people with diabetes. Table B-5 shows exchange amounts for diets of 1,500 kilocalories. Table B-6 offers a sample menu.

This diet provides 150 grams of carbohydrate, 125 grams of protein, and 45 grams of fat, keeping it in line with the 40 per cent carbohydrate, 30 per cent protein, and 30 per cent fat programme.

You can have the total menu in Table B-6 on one day.

Table B-5	1,500 Kilocalories
Breakfast	*Lunch*
1 fruit exchange	3 lean-meat exchanges
1 starch exchange	1 vegetable exchange
1 medium-fat meat exchange	2 fat exchanges
1 fat exchange	1 starch exchange
1 low fat milk exchange	2 fruit exchanges

Dinner	Snack
4 lean-meat exchanges	1 starch exchange
2 starch exchanges	½ low fat milk exchange
2 vegetable exchanges	1 lean-meat exchange
1 fruit exchange	
2 fat exchanges	
½ low fat milk exchange	

Table B-6	A Sample Menu at 1,500 Kilocalories
Breakfast	**Lunch**
125ml apple juice	85g skinless chicken
1 piece of toast	90g cooked green beans
1 teaspoon margarine	4 walnuts
1 egg	1 slice bread
240ml skimmed milk	
Dinner	**Snack**
115g lean beef	55g cottage cheese
1 piece of bread	½ muffin
90g peas	120ml skimmed milk
90g broccoli	
⅓ cantaloupe melon	
2 tablespoons salad dressing	
Salad of free foods	
115g low fat yogurt	

Table B-7 shows the exchange amounts for a 1,800-kilocalorie diet. This diet provides 180 grams of carbohydrate, 135 grams of protein, and 60 grams of fat, which maintains the appropriate 40:30:30 division of calories.

Table B-7	1,800 Kilocalories
Breakfast	**Lunch**
1 fruit exchange	3 lean-meat exchanges
1 starch exchange	1 vegetable exchange
1 medium-fat meat exchange	2 fat exchanges
2 fat exchanges	2 starch exchanges
1 low fat milk exchange	2 fruit exchanges
	½ low fat milk exchange
Dinner	**Snack**
4 lean-meat exchanges	2 starch exchanges
2 starch exchanges	2 lean-meat exchanges
2 vegetable exchanges	½ low fat milk exchange
1 fruit exchange	
3 fat exchanges	

Using the example of the 1,500-kilocalorie diet, you can easily make up a 1,800-kilocalorie diet.

Appendix C

A Glossary of Key Cooking Terms

al dente: Cook to slightly underdone with a chewy texture, usually applied to pasta.

bake: Cook with hot, dry air.

barbecue: Cook on a grill, using charcoal, wood, or gas.

baste: Spoon melted butter, fat, or other liquid over food.

beat: Mix solid or liquid food thoroughly with a spoon, fork, whisk, or electric beater.

bind: Add an ingredient to hold the other ingredients together.

blanch: Plunge food into boiling water until it softens, to bring out the colour and loosen the skin.

blend: Mix foods together less vigorously than beating, usually with a fork, spoon, or spatula.

boil: Heat liquid until it rolls and bubbles.

bone: Remove the bone from meat, fish, or poultry.

braise: Brown foods in fat and then cook slowly in a covered casserole dish.

bread: Coat with breadcrumbs.

brown: Cook quickly to darken the outside of the food and seal in the juices.

caramelise: Dissolve sugar and water slowly and then heat until the food turns brown.

ceviche: Raw seafood placed in an acid, such as fruit juice, to 'cook'.

chop: Cut food into small to large pieces.

curdle: Cause separation by heating egg- or cream-based liquids too quickly.

deglaze: Pour liquid into a pan of meat – after roasting or sautéing and after removal of fat – to capture the cooking juices.

degrease: Remove fat from the surface of hot liquids.

de-vein: Remove the dark brownish-black vein that runs down the back of a prawn or lobster.

dice: Cut into cubes the size of dice.

dilute: Add water to make a liquid, such as a sauce, less strong.

drain: Remove liquid by dripping through a strainer.

drippings: The juice left after meat is removed from a pan.

dry steaming: Cooking foods such as vegetables in their own natural juices rather than adding additional moisture.

dust: Sprinkle lightly with sugar or flour.

emulsify: Bind hard-to-combine ingredients, such as water and oil.

fillet: Cut meat, chicken, or fish away from the bone.

fold: Mix together without breaking.

fry: Cook in hot fat over high heat until brown.

fumet: A heavily concentrated stock.

garnish: Decorate food.

grate: Shred food in a grater or food processor.

grease: Lightly cover a pan with fat to prevent food from sticking.

grill: Cook on a rack under a source of heat such as a grill.

hors d'oeuvres: Bite-sized foods served before dinner.

infusion: Extract flavour from a food into a hot liquid.

julienne: Cut vegetables and other foods into matchstick-sized strips.

knead: Work dough to make it smooth and elastic.

leaven: Cause to rise before and during baking.

marinate: Place in a seasoned liquid (a marinade) to tenderise and enhance flavour.

meringue: Egg whites beaten with sugar and baked in low heat.

mince: Chop food very fine.

pan-roast: A two-step process that first sears and seals a thicker piece of meat or chicken in a pan on the hob and then finishes that piece in the oven, in the same pan you started with.

parboil: Partially cook food in boiling water.

pare: Remove skin from a fruit or vegetable.

phyllo: A tissue-thin layer of dough.

pickle: Preserve food by submerging in a salty brine or vinegar.

pilaf: A rice dish seasoned with herbs and spices, combined with nuts, dried fruits, poultry, and vegetables.

pinch: The amount of food you can take between two fingers.

poach: Submerge food in a liquid that is barely boiling.

proof: Test yeast – to find out whether it's active – by mixing with warm water and sugar.

purée: Break food into small particles to create a smooth consistency (examples are apple sauce and mashed potatoes).

reduce: Boil down a liquid to concentrate the taste of its contents.

roast: Cook in dry heat.

sauté: Brown food in very hot fat.

sear: Subject foods such as meat to extremely high heat for a short period of time to seal in juices.

shred: Tear or cut into very small, thin pieces.

simmer: Cook over low heat, never boiling.

soufflé: A baked food made light by folding in whipped egg whites.

steam: Cook food over a small amount of boiling water.

stock: A liquid in which solid ingredients (like chicken meat and bones, vegetables, and spices) are cooked and then usually strained out.

steep: Place dry ingredients in hot liquid to flavour the liquid (tea is an example).

stew: Slowly cook meat and vegetables in liquid in a covered pan.

stir-fry: Quickly cook meat or vegetables in a wok with a little oil.

sweat: Cook over low heat in a small amount of fat (usually butter) to draw out juices to remove rawness and develop flavour.

toast: Brown by baking.

vinaigrette: A dressing of oil, vinegar, salt, pepper, and various herbs and spices.

whip: Beat rapidly to add air and lighten.

zest: The outermost coloured peel of an orange or other citrus fruit.

Appendix D

Conversions of Weights, Measures, and Sugar Substitutes

· ·

Do you know how many teaspoons are in a tablespoon? Or how many grams are in a pound? And how do you choose between all those sugar substitutes on the market? What if you need to convert an oven temperature from Fahrenheit to Celsius? This appendix offers some information to help you answer those questions.

Conversions

The following list provides some common measurement conversions.

1 teaspoon = 5 millilitres (ml)

1 tablespoon (tbsp) = 15ml

1 teaspoon (tsp) = ⅓ tablespoon

1 tablespoon = 3 teaspoons

2 tablespoons = 30ml (1 fluid ounce)

4 tablespoons = 60ml (2 fluid ounces)

1 pound = 16 ounces = 450 grams (g)

1 fluid ounce = 2 tbsp

10ml = 1 centilitre (cl)

10cl = 1 decilitre (dl)

10dl = 1 litre (l)

1 litre = 1,000ml

1 pint = 600ml

½ pint = 300ml

Table D-1 explains how to convert specific measurements. For example, if you have 3 *ounces* of mushrooms, how many *grams* of mushrooms do you have? To find out, multiply 3 by 28.35 (you have 85.05 grams).

Table D-1	Conversion Methods	
To Convert	*Multiply*	*By*
Ounces to grams	Ounces	28.35
Grams to ounces (dry)	Grams	0.035
Fluid ounces (liquid) to millilitres	Ounces	30.00
Pounds to grams	Pounds	453.59
Pounds to kilograms	Pounds	0.45
Inches to centimetres	Inches	2.54
Centimetres to inches	Centimetres	0.39

Temperatures

To convert degrees Fahrenheit (°F) to degrees Celsius (°C) is slightly more complicated. It involves subtracting 32 from the Fahrenheit number and then dividing by 1.8. To convert degrees Celsius to degrees Fahrenheit, you need to multiply by 1.8 and then add 32. It's much easier to look it up in a table such as Table D-2!

Table D-2 shows you the equivalent Fahrenheit and Celsius temperatures (with a few tweaks here and there to get round figures). Most ovens in the UK are calibrated according to the Celsius scale.

Table D-2	Temperature (Degrees)
Fahrenheit	*Celsius*
32	0
212	100
250	120
275	140
300	150

Fahrenheit	Celsius
325	160
350	180
375	190
400	200
425	220
450	230
475	240
500	260

Sugar Substitutes

The new approach to nutrition for people with diabetes doesn't emphasise the elimination of sugar from your diet entirely as long as you count the kilo-calories that you consume, although it's a good idea to keep your sugar intake to a minimum. When a recipe calls for only a few teaspoons of sugar, you may want to use table sugar (also known as *sucrose*). When the recipe calls for 4 tablespoons (50 grams) of sugar or more, then substitution with a non-caloric or low calorie sweetener of your choice definitely saves you kilo-calories and is kinder to your blood glucose levels. There are also sweeteners other than table sugar that do contain kilocalories but offer other advantages, such as not raising your blood glucose as fast. (Chapter 2 tells you more about sweetness options in more detail.)

The following natural sweeteners contain kilocalories that are added into the total kilocalorie count. They're absorbed and metabolised differently to glucose, so they affect your blood glucose differently.

- Fructose, found in fruits and berries
- Sorbitol and mannitol, sugar alcohols occurring in plants
- Xylitol, found in strawberries and raspberries

Artificial sweeteners are often much sweeter than table sugar. Therefore, much less of this type of sweetener is required to achieve the same level of sweetness as sugar. The current artificial sweeteners (from oldest to newest) include the following:

- Acesulfame-K
- Aspartame
- Saccharin
- Sucralose

If you plan to substitute another sweetener for sugar, check the manufacturer's instructions on the label to find the measurements needed to achieve equal sweetness. Table D-3 is a handy guide.

The best sugar alternative to use is sucralose, sold as Splenda. Unlike most other sweeteners, Splenda is heat stable so you can use it in cooking and baking, and it works best from a technical point of view as an ingredient. It is more like sugar than most other artificial sweeteners, and volume for volume has the same sweetness.

1 teaspoon of Splenda provides ½ gram of carbohydrate and 2 kilocalories of energy.

Table D-3	Sucralose Equivalents
Sugar	*Sucralose (Splenda Granulated)*
1 teaspoon	1 teaspoon
1 tablespoon	1 tablespoon
28g (1 oz)	2 tablespoons
57g (2 oz)	4 tablespoons
85g (3 oz)	6 tablespoons
100g (4 oz)	8 tablespoons

Appendix E

Other Recipe Sources for People with Diabetes

• •

So many cookbook recipes are available for people with diabetes that you can make a different healthy recipe every day and never eat the same one twice. You can find a number of excellent books and even more recipes on Web sites. You can generally count on the recipes in books to contain the nutrients they list, but Web recipes are not always as reliable; you need to evaluate the site before accepting the recipes. You can trust the sites that we list here.

Cookbooks for People with Diabetes

The books listed in this section offer recipes for home-cooked meals, and contain plenty of great recipes and ideas.

Claydon, Anne, Markham, Diana, and Toms, Graham: *The Diabetes Guide: Lifestyle Tips and Over 80 Recipes,* edited by Adam Daykin, Virgin Books, 2006

Diabetes UK: *Healthy Cookbook: Diabetes,* Dorling Kindersley, 2000

Perham, Molly: *Real Food for Diabetics,* Foulsham, 2001

Worrall Thompson, Antony: *Healthy Eating for Diabetes,* Kyle Cathie, 2003

Worrall Thompson, Antony: *Antony Worrall Thompson's GI Diet,* Kyle Cathie 2005

Worrall Thompson, Antony: *The Diabetes Weight Loss Diet,* Kyle Cathie 2007

Food and Recipe Web Sites for People with Diabetes

In this section, we list the best of the currently available Web sites for people with diabetes.

- The nutrition section of the Diabetes UK Web site at `www.diabetes.org.uk` contains a ton of useful information about nutrition as well as loads of recipes.

- The diabetes portal site at `www.diabetes.co.uk` provides further information about diabetes, as well as lots of links to delicious recipes.

- The food section of the BBC website has information aimed at people with diabetes, including several recipes. You can find these at: `http://www.bbc.co.uk/food/recipes/mostof_diabetes.shtml`

- The Vegetarian Society has some good vegetarian recipes, some of which are especially useful for people with diabetes. These are available at `http://www.vegsoc.org/cordonvert/recipes2/diabetic.html`

Index

• *D* •

• Z •

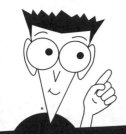

FOR DUMMIES®

Do Anything. Just Add Dummies

PROPERTY

UK editions

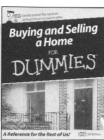

978-0-7645-7027-8

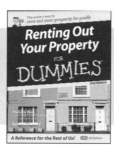

978-0-470-02921-3

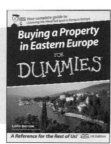

978-0-7645-7047-6

PERSONAL FINANCE

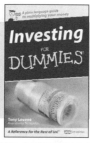

978-0-7645-7023-0

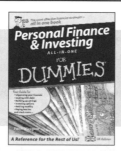

978-0-470-51510-5

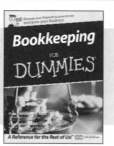

978-0-470-05815-2

BUSINESS

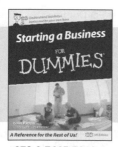

978-0-7645-7018-6

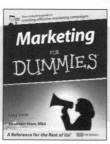

978-0-7645-7056-8

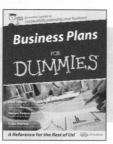

978-0-7645-7026-1

Answering Tough Interview
Questions For Dummies
(978-0-470-01903-0)

Arthritis For Dummies
(978-0-470-02582-6)

Being the Best Man
For Dummies
(978-0-470-02657-1)

British History
For Dummies
(978-0-470-03536-8)

Building Self-Confidence
For Dummies
(978-0-470-01669-5)

Buying a Home on a Budget
For Dummies
(978-0-7645-7035-3)

Children's Health
For Dummies
(978-0-470-02735-6)

Cognitive Behavioural Therapy
For Dummies
(978-0-470-01838-5)

Cricket For Dummies
(978-0-470-03454-5)

CVs For Dummies
(978-0-7645-7017-9)

Detox For Dummies
(978-0-470-01908-5)

Diabetes For Dummies
(978-0-470-05810-7)

Divorce For Dummies
(978-0-7645-7030-8)

DJing For Dummies
(978-0-470-03275-6)

eBay.co.uk For Dummies
(978-0-7645-7059-9)

English Grammar For Dummies
(978-0-470-05752-0)

Gardening For Dummies
(978-0-470-01843-9)

Genealogy Online
For Dummies
(978-0-7645-7061-2)

Green Living For Dummies
(978-0-470-06038-4)

Hypnotherapy For Dummies
(978-0-470-01930-6)

Life Coaching For Dummies
(978-0-470-03135-3)

Neuro-linguistic Programming
For Dummies
(978-0-7645-7028-5)

Nutrition For Dummies
(978-0-7645-7058-2)

Parenting For Dummies
(978-0-470-02714-1)

Pregnancy For Dummies
(978-0-7645-7042-1)

Rugby Union For Dummies
(978-0-470-03537-5)

Self Build and Renovation For
Dummies
(978-0-470-02586-4)

Starting a Business on
eBay.co.uk For Dummies
(978-0-470-02666-3)

Starting and Running an Online
Business For Dummies
(978-0-470-05768-1)

The GL Diet For Dummies
(978-0-470-02753-0)

The Romans For Dummies
(978-0-470-03077-6)

Thyroid For Dummies
(978-0-470-03172-8)

UK Law and Your Rights
For Dummies
(978-0-470-02796-7)

Writing a Novel and Getting
Published For Dummies
(978-0-470-05910-4)

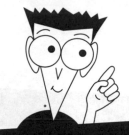

FOR DUMMIES®

Do Anything. Just Add Dummies

HOBBIES

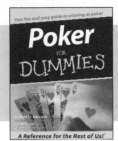

978-0-7645-5232-8

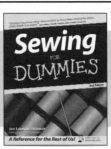

978-0-7645-6847-3

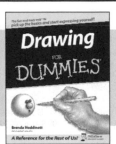

978-0-7645-5476-6

Also available:

Art For Dummies
(978-0-7645-5104-8)

Aromatherapy For Dummies
(978-0-7645-5171-0)

Bridge For Dummies
(978-0-471-92426-5)

Card Games For Dummies
(978-0-7645-9910-1)

Chess For Dummies
(978-0-7645-8404-6)

Improving Your Memory
For Dummies
(978-0-7645-5435-3)

Massage For Dummies
(978-0-7645-5172-7)

Meditation For Dummies
(978-0-471-77774-8)

Photography For Dummies
(978-0-7645-4116-2)

Quilting For Dummies
(978-0-7645-9799-2)

EDUCATION

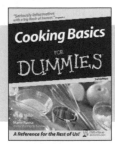

978-0-7645-7206-7

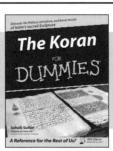

978-0-7645-5581-7

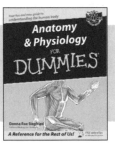

978-0-7645-5422-3

Also available:

Algebra For Dummies
(978-0-7645-5325-7)

Algebra II For Dummies
(978-0-471-77581-2)

Astronomy For Dummies
(978-0-7645-8465-7)

Buddhism For Dummies
(978-0-7645-5359-2)

Calculus For Dummies
(978-0-7645-2498-1)

Forensics For Dummies
(978-0-7645-5580-0)

Islam For Dummies
(978-0-7645-5503-9)

Philosophy For Dummies
(978-0-7645-5153-6)

Religion For Dummies
(978-0-7645-5264-9)

Trigonometry For Dummies
(978-0-7645-6903-6)

PETS

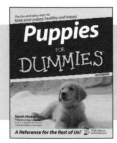

978-0-470-03717-1

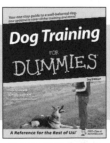

978-0-7645-8418-3

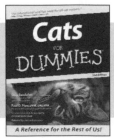

978-0-7645-5275-5

Also available:

Aquariums For Dummies
(978-0-7645-5156-7)

Birds For Dummies
(978-0-7645-5139-0)

Dogs For Dummies
(978-0-7645-5274-8)

Ferrets For Dummies
(978-0-7645-5259-5)

Golden Retrievers
For Dummies
(978-0-7645-5267-0)

Horses For Dummies
(978-0-7645-9797-8)

Jack Russell Terriers
For Dummies
(978-0-7645-5268-7)

Labrador Retrievers
For Dummies
(978-0-7645-5281-6)

Puppies Raising & Training
Diary For Dummies
(978-0-7645-0876-9)

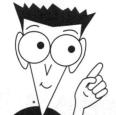

FOR DUMMIES®

The easy way to get more done and have more fun

LANGUAGES

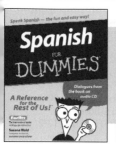
Spanish
978-0-7645-5193-2

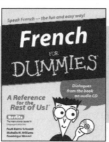
French
978-0-7645-5193-2

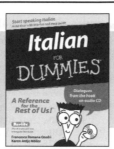
Italian
978-0-7645-5196-3

Also available:

Chinese For Dummies
(978-0-471-78897-3)

Chinese Phrases
For Dummies
(978-0-7645-8477-0)

French Phrases For Dummies
(978-0-7645-7202-9)

German For Dummies
(978-0-7645-5195-6)

Hebrew For Dummies
(978-0-7645-5489-6)

Italian Phrases For Dummies
(978-0-7645-7203-6)

Japanese For Dummies
(978-0-7645-5429-2)

Latin For Dummies
(978-0-7645-5431-5)

Spanish Phrases
For Dummies
(978-0-7645-7204-3)

Spanish Verbs For Dummies
(978-0-471-76872-2)

MUSIC AND FILM

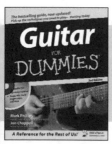
Guitar
978-0-7645-9904-0

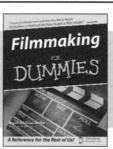
Filmmaking
978-0-7645-2476-9

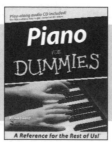
Piano
978-0-7645-5105-5

Also available:

Bass Guitar For Dummies
(978-0-7645-2487-5)

Blues For Dummies
(978-0-7645-5080-5)

Classical Music For Dummies
(978-0-7645-5009-6)

Drums For Dummies
(978-0-471-79411-0)

Jazz For Dummies
(978-0-471-76844-9)

Opera For Dummies
(978-0-7645-5010-2)

Rock Guitar For Dummies
(978-0-7645-5356-1)

Screenwriting For Dummies
(978-0-7645-5486-5)

Singing For Dummies
(978-0-7645-2475-2)

Songwriting For Dummies
(978-0-7645-5404-9)

HEALTH, SPORTS & FITNESS

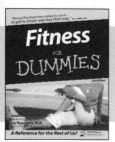
Fitness
978-0-7645-7851-9

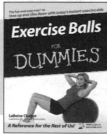
Exercise Balls
978-0-7645-5623-4

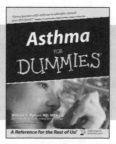
Asthma
978-0-7645-4233-6

Also available:

Controlling Cholesterol
For Dummies
(978-0-7645-5440-7)

Dieting For Dummies
(978-0-7645-4149-0)

High Blood Pressure
For Dummies
(978-0-7645-5424-7)

Martial Arts For Dummies
(978-0-7645-5358-5)

Pilates For Dummies
(978-0-7645-5397-4)

Power Yoga For Dummies
(978-0-7645-5342-4)

Weight Training
For Dummies
(978-0-471-76845-6)

Yoga For Dummies
(978-0-7645-5117-8)

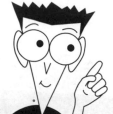

FOR DUMMIES®

Helping you expand your horizons and achieve your potential

INTERNET

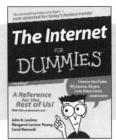

978-0-470-12174-0

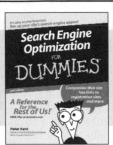

978-0-471-97998-2

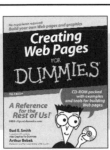

978-0-470-08030-6

Also available:

Building a Web Site For Dummies, 2nd Edition (978-0-7645-7144-2)

Blogging For Dummies (978-0-471-77084-8)

Creating Web Pages All-in-One Desk Reference For Dummies, 3rd Edition (978-0-470-09629-1)

eBay.co.uk For Dummies (978-0-7645-7059-9)

Web Analysis For Dummies (978-0-470-09824-0)

Web Design For Dummies, 2nd Edition (978-0-471-78117-2)

DIGITAL MEDIA

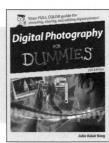

978-0-7645-9802-9

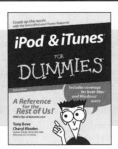

978-0-470-04894-8

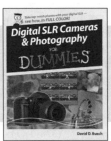

978-0-7645-9803-6

Also available:

BlackBerry For Dummies (978-0-471-75741-2)

Digital Photo Projects For Dummies (978-0-470-12101-6)

Digital Photography All-In-One Desk Reference For Dummies (978-0-470-03743-0)

Photoshop CS3 For Dummies (978-0-470-11193-2)

Podcasting For Dummies (978-0-471-74898-4)

Zune For Dummies (978-0-470-12045-3)

COMPUTER BASICS

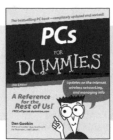

978-0-7645-8958-4

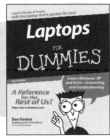

978-0-470-05432-1

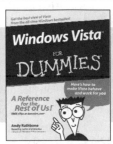

978-0-471-75421-3

Also available:

Macs For Dummies, 9th Edition (978-0-470-04849-8)

Office 2007 All-in-One Desk Reference For Dummies (978-0-471-78279-7)

PCs All-in-One Desk Reference For Dummies, 3rd Edition (978-0-471-77082-4)

Upgrading & Fixing PCs For Dummies, 7th Edition (978-0-470-12102-3)

Windows Vista All-in-One Desk Reference For Dummies (978-0-471-74941-7)

Windows XP For Dummies, 2nd Edition (978-0-7645-7326-2)

Available wherever books are sold. For more information or to order direct go to www.wiley.com or call 0800 243407 (Non UK call +44 1243 843296)